Nursing Care of Older People

Nursing Care of Older People

Edited by

Andrew Hindle

Strategic Health Lead for Older People and Long Term Conditions, Dudley Primary Care Trust

and

Alison Coates

Lead for Teaching and Learning (Nursing), Birmingham University

With Consultant Editor **Paul Kingston**

Professor of Health and Social Care, Director Centre for Ageing and Mental Health, Staffordshire University

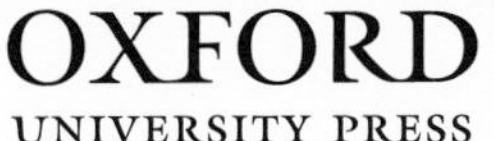

OXFORD
UNIVERSITY PRESS
Great Clarendon Street, Oxford OX2 6DP

Oxford University Press is a department of the University of Oxford.
It furthers the University's objective of excellence in research, scholarship,
and education by publishing worldwide in

Oxford New York

Auckland Cape Town Dar es Salaam Hong Kong Karachi
Kuala Lumpur Madrid Melbourne Mexico City Nairobi
New Delhi Shanghai Taipei Toronto

With offices in

Argentina Austria Brazil Chile Czech Republic France Greece
Guatemala Hungary Italy Japan Poland Portugal Singapore
South Korea Switzerland Thailand Turkey Ukraine Vietnam

Oxford is a registered trade mark of Oxford University Press
in the UK and in certain other countries

Published in the United States
by Oxford University Press Inc., New York

British Library Cataloguing-in-Publication Data
Data available

Library of Congress Cataloging in Publication Data
Data available

Typeset by Glyph International, Bangalore, India
Printed in Italy
on acid-free paper by
L.E.G.O.S.p.A—Lavis TN

ISBN 978-0-19-9563111

1 3 5 7 9 10 8 6 4 2

This book is dedicated to those health and social care professionals who go the extra mile to improve care, dignity, and make a positive difference to the quality of lives of older people.

Preface

'The greatest virtues are those which are most useful to other people'.

Aristotle

With an increasing ageing population, the nature of nursing older people is constantly changing—particularly across a wide range of care environments. However, the fundamentals of care do not change and this book materialized via a programme that set out to ensure and embed high-quality standards, and to improve care for older people, with dignity at the core of practice. Nursing older people is not only about treating illness; it is also undeniably about caring with dignity, and delivering personalized and responsive holistic care. *Nursing Care of Older People* has thus been written with the aforementioned remit for pre-registration nurses, qualified nurses, and other healthcare professionals who deliver care to older people. The book is relevant to those who work with older people who have physical, mental, and learning disability health needs throughout the UK and beyond. We have endeavoured to discuss skills that nurses require, irrespective of where they practise.

Nursing Care of Older People has been written by a wide range of specialist and experienced nurses, healthcare professionals, and academics. The book also gives prominence to the importance of carers of older people, including a specific chapter on this subject. In addition, there is an Online Resource Centre that students can use alongside the text.

The front cover of this book was chosen as portraying a positive image of older people, while being realistic that age is taking its toll. We hope that the reader will take from it the message that nursing older people can be very rewarding—particularly when time is taken to listen and to acknowledge that older people are no different from younger people, except that their lives have been enhanced by a wealth of experiences.

Andrew Hindle and
Alison Coates

Acknowledgements

We are grateful to Professor Paul Kingston at Stafford University for his counsel and guidance as consultant editor.

Alison and Andrew express their profound gratitude to Geraldine Jeffers at OUP for her motivation, patience, and unstinting professional guidance and support to two people embarking on their first experience of editing.

We also thank Holly Edmundson at OUP for her assistance in collating various elements of the book.

Our grateful thanks are also extended to all those who reviewed drafts of this book.

Andrew also thanks his wife Linda for her encouragement, continued support, and patience over the length of this project.

Andrew Hindle and Alison Coates

Contents

About the authors xiii
How to use this book xvi
Online Resource Centre xviii

Part 1: Communication and dignity 1

Chapter 1 Introduction 3
Chapter 2 Dignity, values, attitudes, and person-centred care 9
Chapter 3 Hearing and sight loss 23
Chapter 4 The law and the older person 43
Chapter 5 Carers, families, and single householders in the community 55

Part 2: Patient safety 67

Chapter 6 Mobility and falls 69
Chapter 7 Medicines management 83

Part 3: Care settings 95

Chapter 8 Primary and community care 97
Chapter 9 Hospital care 109

Part 4: Changes in the ageing process 121

Chapter 10 Key medical disorders of older adults 123
Chapter 11 Dementia, mental health, and the older adult 141
Chapter 12 Learning disabilities and the older adult 154
Chapter 13 Nutrition and fluids 168
Chapter 14 Elimination and continence and the older adult 185
Chapter 15 Hygiene, infection control, and the older adult 201
Chapter 16 Pain and its pharmacological management in older adults 213
Chapter 17 Sleep in older people 234
Chapter 18 End-of-life care 245

Index 261

Detailed contents

About the authors xiii
How to use this book xvi
Online Resource Centre xviii

Part 1
Communication and dignity **1**

Chapter 1 Introduction **3**
Andrew Hindle and Alison Coates
Why this book? 3
Nursing older people is a dominant aspect of nursing practice 4
How this book will help you deliver care to older people 4
Part 1: Communication and dignity 4
Part 2: Patient safety 5
Part 3: Care settings 5
Part 4: Changes in the ageing process 5
Conclusion 7
References 7

Chapter 2 Dignity, values, attitudes, and person-centred care **9**
Jo Galloway
Introduction 9
Ageism 9
Additional care needs 10
Health and social care policy 11
Dignity 11
Adult protection and elder abuse 13
Person-centred care 16
Conclusion 20
Questions and self-assessment 20
References 21
Statutes 22
For further reading and information 22

Chapter 3 Hearing and sight loss **23**
Andrew Hindle, Debbie Lynch, and Darren McHale
Introduction to hearing and sight loss 23
Section one: Hearing loss 24
Introduction to hearing loss 24
Definitions 24
Acoustics 24
Anatomy and physiology 24
Common ear conditions 26
Experiences of deaf and hard-of-hearing people 27
What is it like to have a hearing loss as a result of the ageing process? 29
How to communicate effectively with people who have hearing loss 29
Aids to communication 30
Additional aids to communication 30
Perspectives of people with hearing loss 31
Conclusion to hearing loss 32
Questions and self-assessment 32
Section two: Sight loss 33
Introduction to sight loss 33
Common causes of sight loss 33
Visual disturbance 35
Supporting people with sight loss 35
Questions and self-assessment 41
References 41
For further reading and information 42

Chapter 4 The law and the older person **43**
Herman Wheeler
Introduction 43
Ageism, age discrimination, and abuse 44
Legal assertions and their implications 45
Ethics, sources of law, and the older person's right to care 45
Confidentiality 48
Informed consent 48
The law and end-of-life issues for the older adult 50
Conclusion 53
Questions and self-assessment 53
References 53
Statutes 54
Cases 54

Chapter 5 Carers, families, and single householders in the community 55
Andrew Hindle
Introduction 55
Single householders 55
Older people and loneliness 56
Families 57
Who is a carer? 57
Support for carers 61
Ethnicity 63
Conclusion 64
Questions and self-assessment 64
For further reading and information 64
References 64
Statutes 65

Part 2
Patient safety 67

Chapter 6 Mobility and falls 69
Andrew Hindle
Introduction 69
Definition of a fall 69
Facts about falls 69
National Service Framework for Older People Standard 6: Falls 70
Multifactorial falls risk assessment 70
Home environment and community: Falls prevention and strategies, and falls health promotion 75
Medicines and falls 76
Osteoporosis 76
Other consequences of falls (negative connotations) 77
Further nursing aspects of falls and falling, and home environment prevention and advice 78
Physical activity and exercise programmes 78
The perspective of an occupational therapist 80
Conclusion 80
Questions and self-assessment 81
References 81
For further reading and information 82

Chapter 7 Medicines management 83
Maggi Banning
Introduction 83
What is medicines management? 84
Why older people? 84
The nursing role 85
Older people and concordance/adherence to medication 85
Medication errors 87
Conclusion 91
Questions and self-assessment 91
References 92
For further reading and information 93

Part 3
Care settings 95

Chapter 8 Primary and community care 97
Kay Norman
Introduction 97
Self-care 98
Personalized care plans 101
Nursing in the older person's home 101
Intermediate care 105
Long-term care 105
Conclusion 107
Questions and self-assessment 107
References 107
Statutes 108
For further reading and information 108

Chapter 9 Hospital care 109
Professor Wilf McSherry and Judith Bennion
Introduction 109
Experience of older people within acute care 111
Care organization and delivery 112
A systematic approach to care delivery 114
Patient comfort rounds 115
Key responsibilities/skills of the nurse 115
Importance of communication 117
Discharge planning 118
Conclusion 119
Questions and self-assessment 119
References 119

Part 4
Changes in the ageing process 121

Chapter 10 Key medical disorders of older adults 123
Dr Jen Benbow and Professor Susan Mary Benbow
Introduction 123

Physiological changes of ageing 124
Psychosocial aspects of chronic illness 124
Key endocrine conditions 126
Key neurological conditions 128
Key cardiovascular conditions 131
Key respiratory conditions 135
Key musculoskeletal conditions 136
Conclusion 137
Questions and self-assessment 138
References 138
For further reading and information 140

Chapter 11 Dementia, mental health, and the older adult 141
Alison Coates

Introduction 141
Dementia 142
Delirium (acute confusional state) 145
Depression 146
Anxiety disorders 148
Bipolar affective disorder 149
Schizophrenia 149
Alcohol 150
Conclusion 151
Questions and self-assessment 151
References 151

Chapter 12 Learning disability and the older adult 154
Kim Scarborough

Introduction 154
Terminology 155
Rights and principles 155
Communication strategies and people with learning disabilities 156
Causes of learning disability, and effect on health and ageing 159
Dementia and people with learning disabilities 160
Pain management 163
Health initiatives and meeting the needs of people with learning disabilities 163
Challenges in services for older people with learning disabilities 163
Specialist services for people with learning disabilities 164
Conclusion 165
Questions and self-assessment 165
References 165

Chapter 13 Nutrition and fluids 168
June Copeman

Introduction 168
Nutrition consequences of normal ageing 168
Hydration and fluid consequences of normal ageing 169
Nutritional status of older people 170
Nutritional requirements and nutritional guidelines 170
Promote healthy active life 172
Nutrition screening and nutrition assessment 174
Food selection, choice, and consumption 176
Strategies to improve the nutrition intake in individuals 178
Why eating can be difficult for older people 179
Organizational initiatives to improve nutrition 181
Conclusion 182
Questions and self-assessment 182
References 183
For further reading and information 184

Chapter 14 Elimination and continence and the older adult 185
Alison Coates and Gill Davey

Introduction 185
Normal urinary elimination and the ageing process 185
Common causes and types of urinary incontinence 186
Investigations to determine the cause of urinary incontinence 187
Other assessments 188
Treatment for stress incontinence 188
Treatment for urgency incontinence 189
Skin care and incontinence 191
Assessment process 191
Faecal incontinence 193
Skin care 196
Nursing care 196
Conclusion 198
Questions and self-assessment 199
References 199
For further reading and information 200

Chapter 15 Hygiene, infection control, and the older adult **201**
Debbie Weston

Introduction 201
The problem of healthcare-associated infections 202
The chain of infection 203
The principles of infection control 205
Conclusion 209
Questions and self-assessment 210
References 210

Chapter 16 Pain and its pharmacological management in older adults **213**
Amelia Williamson-Swift

Introduction 213
Pain physiology and ageing 213
Introduction to acute pain and persistent pain 216
Assessment of pain in the older adult 220
Pharmacological management of pain in the older adult 223
Conclusion 229
Questions and self-assessment 231
References 231
Statutes 233
For further reading and information 233

Chapter 17 Sleep in older people **234**
Lesley Hayes

Introduction 234
Normal sleep patterns 235
Addressing underlying health issues that affect sleep quality 238
Assessment 239
Locus of intervention 240
Conclusion 241
Questions and self-assessment 241
References 242
For further reading and information 244

Chapter 18 End-of-life care **245**
Lisa Beeston

Introduction 245
What is meant by 'end of life?' 245
The evidence base for best practice and care 246
Service user and carer review 247
Conceptualizing end-of-life care for our own practice 247
Issues of loss 253
Illness trajectories and symptoms 254
Liverpool Care Pathway 255
Care after death 255
Conclusion 257
Questions and self-assessment 257
References 257
Statutes 259
For further reading and information 259

Index 261

About the authors

Editors

Andrew Hindle is the Strategic Commissioning Lead for Older People and Long-term Conditions at Dudley NHS, England. A registered and district nurse, Andrew has worked in strategy and commissioning since 2004, including within the regional Champions for Older People Programme, to ensure quality care for this client group.

Alison Coates is Lead for Teaching and Learning (Nursing) at the University of Birmingham. She has extensive experience of nursing older people with both physical and mental health needs, and of teaching on this area of care.

Contributors

Maggi Banning, Senior lecturer in advanced clinical practice. EdD, M.Sc., PGDE, B.Sc. (hons), SCM, SRN Brunel University, School of Health and Social care.

Lisa Beeston (MSc Prof Ed; BSc Hons; RGN; Oncology Cert; Counselling Cert; FETC). Senior Lecturer, Faculty of Health, Staffordshire University.

Jen Benbow, MB, BS, MRCP, is an Advanced Trainee in Geriatric Medicine, Liverpool Hospital, Sydney, Australia.

Susan Mary Benbow, MB, ChB, MSc, FRCPsych, is Professor of Mental Health & Ageing, Staffordshire University, Stafford, UK & Director, Older Mind Matters Ltd.

Judith Bennion BSc (Hons), SRN, Matron for General Medicine, Shrewsbury and Telford Hospital NHS Trust.

Alison Coates MA, BA (hons), Dip Ad Ed, RGN, RMN, is the Lead for Teaching and Learning (Nursing) at the University of Birmingham in the College of Medical and Dental Sciences, School for Health and Populations Sciences.

June Copeman MEd, MSc, BSc, RD, is Subject Group Lead, Nutrition and Dietetic, Faculty of Health and Social Science, Leeds Metropolitan University.

Gill Davey MSc, RN, is Continence Service Manager/Clinical Nurse Specialist, Dudley Primary Care Trust.

Jo Galloway, Deputy Director of Nursing, Quality and Safety, NHS Warwickshire. Registered Nurse, BA (Hons) Health and Social Policy, MSc Health Studies, PGCert learning and Teaching in Higher Education. Or RN, BA(Hons), MSc, PGCert.

Lesley Hayes MA, BA (Hons), Dip HE, RN, PGCHPE is a Lecturer in Nursing at Staffordshire University.

Andrew Hindle MA (Gerontology), DN, BSc (hons), RGN, is Strategic Commissioning Lead: Older people and Long Term Conditions, Dudley NHS.

Debbie Lynch, BA (hons), Principal Safeguarding and Quality Manager, Royal National Institute of blind people, Qualifications.

Mr Darren McHale BSc (Hons) MSc (Audiological Science), Consultant Clinical Scientist, Head of Audiology Services, The Shrewsbury and Telford Hospital NHS Trust.

Wilfred McSherry, PhD, MPhil, BSc (Hons), PGCE (FE), PGCRM, RGN, NT, ILTM Professor in Dignity of Care for Older People, Centre for Practice and Service Improvement, Faculty of health, Staffordshire University. Professor Harald Deaconess, University College Bergen, Norway.

Kay Norman MSc, PGDHE, BSc (Hons), RGN, Principal Lecturer in Community Based Care Faculty of Health, Staffordshire University.

Kim Scarborough MSc, BSc(Hons), PGC(HE), PGCM, RNT, RNLD, is Senior Lecturer in Learning Disabilities, University of the West of England and a National Teaching Fellow.

Debbie Weston RGN, BSc (Infection Control) Deputy Lead Nurse Infection Prevention and Control, East Kent Hospitals University NHS Foundation Trust.

Herman Wheeler, PhD, MA Law, LLB, PGD (Law), MEd (Psychology), BEd (Hons), DN (Lon), RMN, RGN, RNT, is a Chartered Psychologist and Lecturer at the University of Birmingham in the College of Medical and Dental Science, School of Health and Population Sciences.

Amelia Williamson Swift, MSc, PGCE (HE), RGN is a Lecturer in Nursing at the University of Birmingham in the College of Medical and Dental Science, School for Health and Populations Sciences.

How to use this book

Nursing Care of Older People is an evidence-based and practical guide to meeting the holistic health needs of older patients. This brief tour shows you how to get the most out of this textbook package.

NURSING PRACTICE INSIGHTS

Nursing practice insights outline specific skills, practical tools and tips for delivering the highest standard of care.

NURSING PRACTICE INSIGHT: EFFECTIVE ASSESSMENT

- Be aware of changes and risks within the home.
- Take time to talk to the person whom you are visiting.
- Listen to their story and ask what they see as their problems/concerns.
- Ask how you can help.
- Suggest services available that may be appropriate to help with concerns (for example, voluntary services

ing
ocial
ome
mily
vhat
tred

Case study

Clare is a 62-year-old lady with Down's syndrome. Clare has come to accident and emergency (A&E) after a fall. The care staff where she lives have reported that she has started wandering around, appears more confused, and that her behaviour has changed. Clare seems upset and uncooperative.

- What might be causing Clare to be upset and uncooperative?

CASE STUDIES

Case studies link theory, evidence and models to nursing practice through the use of short patient scenarios.

ILLUSTRATIONS

Illustrations of underlying physiology, processes, concepts and assessment tools reinforce learning.

DOLOPLUS-2 SCALE BEHAVIOU

NAME : Christian Name :

Behavioural Records

SOMATIC REACTIONS

1• Somatic complaints
- No complaints ....
- Complaints expressed upon inquiry only ....
- Occasionnal involuntary complaints ....
- Continuous involontary complaints ....

STUDENT ACTIVITY

Student activity boxes ask you to explore specific topics on your own or with your mentor in order to develop appropriate nursing skills and knowledge.

Student activity

- Discuss with your mentor the types of assessment used within your area.
- Look at the types of documentation that are currently used for assessment for varying types of care. Are they easy to complete and understand?
- How have the patients been involved with this process?

achieve a safe discharge.

tal

he

se

si-

Reflection point

At this point, it might be useful to reflect upon the study relating to Charles' admission and identify v safeguards would need to be put in place to facilitat safe discharge home.

REFLECTION POINTS

Reflection points allow you to reflect on key issues and think more critically about the subject. At the end of each chapter readers are asked how the chapter will inform their practice, a helpful activity for portfolios of learning.

REFERENCES

Assignments are supported by directions to online resources, further reading material as well as references to evidence-based guidelines and research literature.

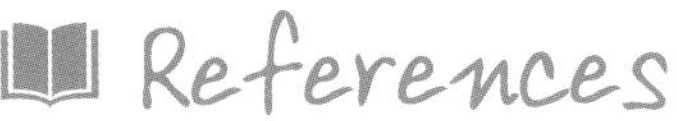

Alexopoulos, G. (2002) *The Cornell Scale for Depression in Dementia*, available online at http://www.afmc.us/Documents/quality_improve/depression/CornellScaleGuidelines.pdf [accessed 15 February 2010]

How to use the Online Resource Centre

Nursing students need to put theory into practice on placement and this book has a dedicated website to help you get started. Just bookmark the address and go there when instructed to in the book: www.oxfordtextbooks.co.uk/orc/hindle/

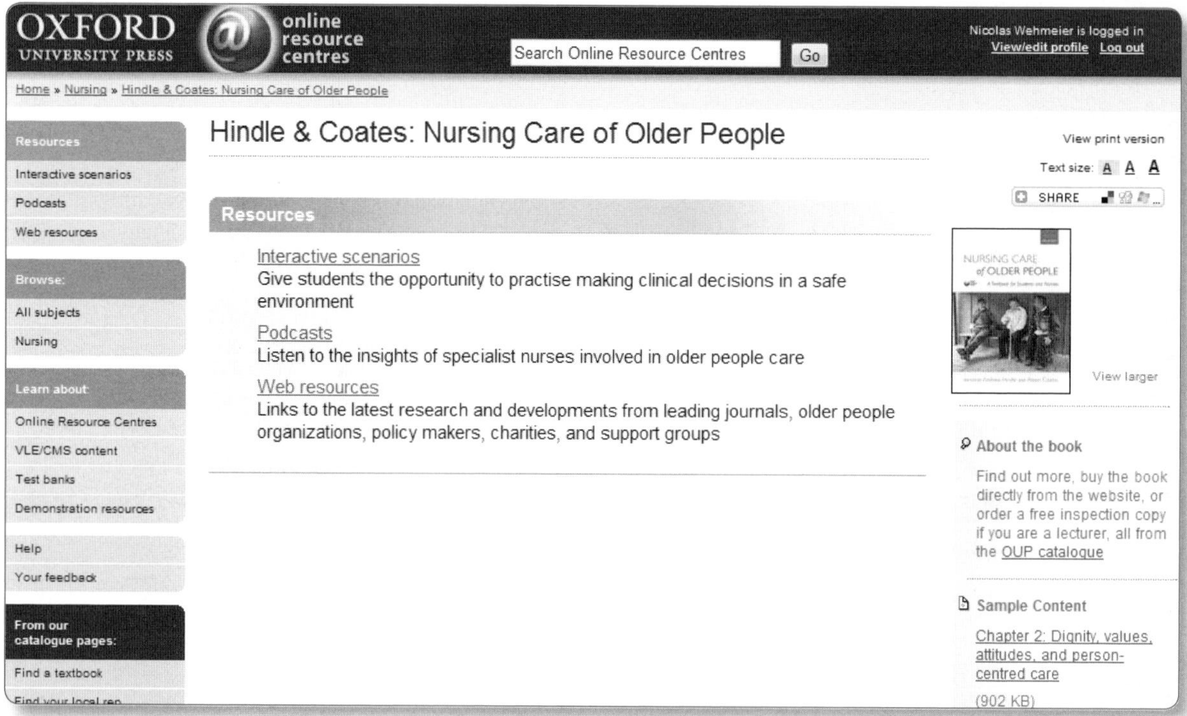

Students can:

- Find bonus material for chapters such as extra artwork—wherever you see this symbol you'll be directed to go online and find additional learning tools
- Practise making clinical decisions using our interactive scenarios—the authors outline best nursing practice
- Listen to the insights of specialist nurses involved in older people care
- Get ahead with 'insider' sources of further information and guidelines

Lecturers and mentors:

can use all of the above in their teaching materials.

Part 1

Communication and dignity

Introduction

Andrew Hindle and Alison Coates

Working with older people is likely to be a significant part of many nurses' practice. Two-thirds of in-patients in acute hospital beds are over the age of 65 and much of community nursing is concerned with caring for older adults. The ageing population in the UK has brought a sharp rise in the number of people living longer. In 2006, 15 per cent of the population were over 65 years of age. By 2016, that proportion will rise to 18.2 per cent, and by 2026, to 20.3 per cent. The fastest population increase has been in the number of people aged 85 and over—often referred to as the 'oldest old'—who accounted for 1.3 million of the UK's population in 2008 (ONS, 2009).

Whilst many older people enjoy an active life, and others maintain their health with the help of regular nursing advice and care, there are also mounting numbers of frail, vulnerable older people who require more comprehensive, holistic, and person-centred care. Sadly, their needs have often not been met, and there have been a number of incidences and reports of poor quality practice—notably in hospitals and care homes, where a lack of appropriate leadership has resulted in poor assessment and adherence to care plans, inadequate discharge arrangements, and inappropriate use of medication. The UK charity Age UK (previously Age Concern and Help the Aged) has highlighted such issues and concerns regarding the care of older people in a number of published reports, such as *Hungry to be Heard* (2006), which identifies the scandal of malnourishment of older people in hospital, and campaigns such as *Down But Not Out* (2008), in which the problem of older people not being diagnosed with and treated for depression is highlighted.

Meeting older people's health needs through high-quality assessment, care, and standards enables them to maintain and optimize their independence, which in turn provides quality to their lives.

Why this book?

It is the experience of the editors that many students come into nursing wanting to provide high-quality care, but that sometimes, unfortunately, they can witness older people receiving care that is not in keeping with the professional standards that we all aim to provide. Nevertheless, the nursing community wants to ensure that older people receive the best nursing care possible, and we believe that one way to achieve this is by ensuring that nurses of the future are fully equipped and prepared to take on this challenging and rewarding role. The Nursing and Midwifery Council (NMC) captures our aims perfectly in its *Guidance for the Care of Older People* (2009):

The essence of nursing care for older people is about getting to know and value people as individuals through effective assessment, finding out how they want to be cared for from their perspective, and providing care which ensures that respect, dignity and fairness are maintained.

NMC (2009)

The inspiration for this book stemmed from an initiative called The Champions for Older People Programme, which aimed to address and improve dignity and care for older people. The Champions Programme developed from the *National Service Framework for Older People* (DH, 2001a), in which it was identified that care environments—and in particular hospitals—did not provide education and training programmes for staff aimed at caring for older adults. The Champions Programme identified nurses from across every hospital in the West Midlands and these nurses attended workshops led by expert speakers who focused on improving care for older people. The topics addressed by these expert speakers form the basis of this book.

Nursing older people is a dominant aspect of nursing practice

Currently, the content of preregistration nursing curricula relating to older people varies greatly across universities depending on the curriculum philosophy. Some universities integrate aspects of older people's care into large nursing modules; others have specific modules on care of older people in each of the adult, mental health, and learning disabilities branches.

The NMC has reviewed preregistration nursing programmes and is considering the requirements on the future workforce of nurses, which are due to be published in September 2010. These include meeting the needs of an increasingly older population. Teaching and learning about older people's health needs, including assessment and care planning, whilst maintaining respect and dignity, will be fundamental for all nursing courses.

The modern National Health Service (NHS) has a focus on patient choice and developing a quality-driven service, so nurses that care for older people require a wide range of skills to deliver these priorities. They need to be prepared for different patterns of care, including working with patients' families and carers, meeting mental health needs, supporting self-care, rehabilitation, and ensuring that high standards of care are met across all care environments including the hospital, community, intermediate care and care home. There is no doubt that caring for older people can be a very rewarding career for nurses and there are increasing opportunities for career development (DH, 2006a; Scottish Executive, 2006).

How this book will help you deliver care to older people

This book includes the fundamental areas of care provided to older people who may have physical, mental, or learning disability health needs, whether the setting and care environment is in a hospital or the community. It covers all aspects of daily living and the key elements of a holistic assessment. Each chapter includes learning outcomes, case studies, and nursing practice insights, as well as informs the reader on where he or she can access further specialist knowledge. The book is divided into four parts focusing on:

- communication and dignity;
- patient safety;
- care settings; and
- changes in the ageing process.

Part 1: Communication and dignity

Dignity, values, attitudes, and person-centred care

It is relevant to begin this book with a chapter identifying the importance of maintaining dignity, because this is at the core of nursing care. Dignity has been high on the national agenda following its emphasis in the review under the National Service Framework for Older People, *A New Ambition for Old Age* (2006b), which led to a national dignity-in-care campaign. Dignity, of course, should be applied whatever the age group, but an examination on dignity and older people is needed because of the ageism that pervades our society and the specific care needs of older people—particularly where they are vulnerable and communication or functional abilities are diminished.

A person-centred assessment is included, because it enables the nurse to identify the person's individual needs and preferences in order to inform a plan of care.

Incorporated into this chapter is an overview of *adult protection and elder abuse*. This includes the main forms of abuse and the possible signs of abuse that can occur. The legislation for the recognition and prevention of abuse of vulnerable adults is also explored.

Hearing and sight loss

This chapter is particularly significant because many older people have sight and hearing impairments that can have a major impact on their quality of life. Nurses who care for older people will be confronted with sight and hearing loss on a daily basis. The chapter therefore provides an introduction to the anatomy and physiology of the eye and ear, and age-related changes, along with an overview of conditions that can arise and the management of these. There is also an insight into the difficulties and challenges that older people with sensory loss face, coupled with communication strategies and practical tips to ensure that nurses have a heightened awareness and provide high-quality care.

Law and ethics

This chapter addresses the subject of the law as it relates to health care. Whilst the author identifies that there is no single area of the law that deals uniquely with older people, this chapter highlights areas of the law that have particular relevance to the care of older people and nursing practice. The reader will develop an understanding of the ethical and legal frameworks in which they, as nurses, should make decisions and deliver care.

Carers, families, and single householders in the community

The ageing population has major implications on the organization of support and care for older people. This chapter will focus on some of these implications relating to the impact on single householders', families', and carers' support.

The important role that carers have in supporting older people in the community is covered, as is identifying and addressing the needs of carers themselves. The chapter also discusses social isolation and loneliness, and the interventions for prevention and managing loneliness.

Part 2: Patient safety

Mobility and falls

Falls in older adults can have serious consequences, and can result in hospital admission and a loss of independence. Ensuring safe mobility, with assessment of risk and appropriate interventions, is an important component in sustaining older people's independence, and helping to maintain confidence and self-esteem. The chapter covers the impact that a fall can have on an older person, the causes of falls (both intrinsic and extrinsic), osteoporosis, risk assessment and care management, falls prevention, and strategies including exercise intervention programmes.

Medication management

In the UK, older people comprise more than 18 per cent of the population and receive 59.7 per cent of prescriptions dispensed by community pharmacists and dispensing doctors (ICHSC, 2008). This statement alone explains why medicine management is so relevant to older people. This chapter will enable the reader to develop an understanding of the issues related to medication management and why it is particularly important for older people, including the implications of poly-pharmacy, adverse side effects, the importance of medication reviews, and key nursing roles and responsibilities, including supporting older people to take their medication in a safe and effective way.

Part 3: Care settings

Primary/community care

Most people access health care in the UK through primary and community services (DH, 2004). Indeed, for many, it is the only setting in which they will receive healthcare advice and treatment, so it is important for all nurses to have an understanding of how primary and community health care can support older people—with a particular emphasis on maintaining their independence. This chapter explains the role of the multidisciplinary team, and its importance in assessing and meeting the needs of the older person. It also addresses the importance of self-care, self-management programmes, hospital admission avoidance, tele-care and tele-health, personalized care plans, and single assessment processes. There are also sections on the different care environments, including the patient's own home, intermediate care, and care homes.

Hospital care

Older people are the primary users of hospital care and the National Audit Office (2007) identified that 60 per cent of acute hospital beds are occupied by older people. Caring for older people in hospital is complex and often undervalued. This chapter considers older people's experiences, how care and services can be organized in hospital, models for delivering care, key nurse responsibilities, and what factors should be considered when the older person is discharged. The author highlights that underpinning all care should be a commitment to maintaining the dignity and independence of older adults.

Part 4: Changes in the ageing process

Key medical conditions

As people age, they are more likely to develop health problems and long-term conditions. This chapter identifies the key physiological changes that occur as we age and the psychosocial impact of long-term illness, and summarizes some of the major health conditions affecting older people and the nursing management of each condition, including:

- diabetes;
- Parkinson's disease;
- stroke;
- ischaemic heart disease;
- chronic heart failure;
- atrial fibrillation;
- leg ulcers;
- chronic obstructive pulmonary disease;
- community-acquired pneumonia; and
- arthritis.

The multiple roles that nurses can play in the holistic assessment and management of patients with both acute and chronic medical problems is explored.

Dementia and mental health

Mental health problems can affect up to 50 per cent of older people in general hospitals, 60 per cent of those in care homes, and 40 per cent of those that consult their general practitioner (GP) (DH, 2007). Given this statistic, nurses are likely to care for older people with mental health problems in all clinical settings. It is important therefore that they have knowledge of how mental health problems can affect older adults.

This chapter provides an overview of a large and complex subject area, and draws on different approaches to mental health in order for the nurse to develop an understanding of the issues, and to begin developing the nursing care and core skills needed when working with older people who have dementia, depression, and other mental health problems.

Learning disability

With improvements in medicine and living conditions, people with a learning disability are living longer. Older people with a learning disability have greater health needs than the general population because they have a higher incidence of epilepsy, physical disability, mental illness, and sensory loss (DH, 2001b). However, many older people with a learning disability have mental and physical health needs that are often not diagnosed. This chapter covers the causes of learning disabilities, health risks, and life experiences. It aims to identify the barriers to health care that people with a learning disability might encounter, communication strategies and aids to promote effective communication, and specialist support services, and identifies how, as a nurse, you can develop and adapt skills to ensure that you meet the needs of this patient group.

Nutrition and fluids

Nutrition and hydration are central to care. This chapter identifies why older people are at risk from a poor diet and how their nutritional needs should be addressed. The chapter covers the nutrition and hydration consequences of normal ageing, nutritional and fluid requirements and guidelines, the implications of obesity and malnutrition, nutrition screening and nutrition assessment, how environment can impact on intake, dysphagia, the impact of cognitive impairment, and strategies and interventions that nurses can implement to improve intake.

Elimination and continence

This chapter identifies that both urinary and faecal incontinence are symptoms and not a diagnosis. The author takes the reader through the causes and types of incontinence, and highlights that these should not be considered an inevitable consequence of ageing. The chapter covers the investigations to determine the causes, and an overview of assessment and treatment options for both urinary and faecal incontinence.

Hygiene and infection control

Older people are one of the most vulnerable 'at risk' groups with regard to healthcare-associated infections (HCAIs) and are particularly at risk from potentially life-threatening infections. This is because of their increased susceptibility to infections as a result of underlying illness and disease, and the body's ability to fight infection naturally declining with age. The chapter includes the implications of HCAIs, specific risk factors for the development of HCAIs in older people, the various components that facilitate the spread of infection and the importance of hand decontamination, and the correct use of gloves, aprons, and isolation in preventing and breaking the links in the chain of infection.

Pain management

For older people, suffering from pain can have a great impact on their quality of life, so this chapter focuses on the importance of effective, individualized care based on sound knowledge of the underlying physiological, psychological, and pharmacological principles that can promote recovery or restore quality of life. The chapter also differentiates between acute pain and persistent pain, and how to undertake an assessment of pain in the older adult.

Sleep and rest

Sleep can be affected by a wide range of factors, which can be internal, such as chronic illness, and external, such as a change of routine or residence. This chapter focuses on how sleep can impact the lives of some older people and how good-quality sleep can be promoted. The chapter also explores the 'normal' process of the sleep cycle, along with key changes that occur with age, the concept of sleep hygiene, medication and non-medication approaches to sleep, assessment, and the role of the nurse in helping to facilitate good-quality sleep.

End-of-life care

Most deaths in European countries occur in people aged over 65 (WHO, 2004). This has implications for the nursing profession in providing good-quality palliative and end-of-life care for older people. This chapter covers best practice and care, choice of care environment, therapeutic interventions, dignity, issues of loss, illness trajectories and symptoms, care pathways, and care after death. The author raises many questions for the reader to consider and concludes by stating that much of our care focuses on the 'where', 'when', 'what', and 'how' (that is, the environment, behaviours, capabilities, and strategies) of care, but that we need to consider how the 'why', 'who', and 'for whom' (that is, the beliefs, values, spirituality, identity, and purpose) fits in with the care that we provide.

Conclusion

This book is not intended to be an exhaustive account of nursing care for older people; rather, our aim has been to provide an accessible, engaging resource that will help you to improve your skills, deliver safe, effective, quality care, and develop a positive attitude towards older people. At the end of each chapter, you will find references and further reading, and websites through which you can explore the issues highlighted further. You will also be directed to the Online Resource Centre that accompanies this book. The interactive resources that you will find there have been written to support blended learning, and ultimately to help nurses to develop the knowledge and skills required for nursing older people.

It is hoped that this book will be a useful resource throughout the preregistration programme, as well as for qualified staff who wish to update their knowledge and share this resource with colleagues who also care for older people. We hope that this text will help you realize the skills and rewarding career of caring for older people.

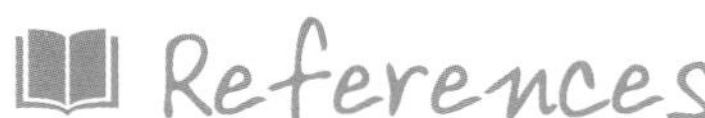

Age UK (2006) *Hungry to be Heard*, available online at http://www.scie.org.uk/publications/guides/guide15/files/hungrytobeheard.pdf.

Age UK (2008) *Down But Not Out*, available online at http://www.ageuk.org.uk/get-involved/campaign/depression-in-later-life-down-but-not-out/.

Department of Health (2001a) *National Service Framework for Older People*, London: DH, available online at http://www.dh.gov.uk/prod_consum_dh/groups/dh_digitalassets/@dh/@en/documents/digitalasset/dh_4071283.pdf.

Department of Health (2001b) *Valuing People: A New Strategy for Learning Disability for the 21st Century*, London: HMSO.

Department of Health (2004) *NHS Improvement Plan: Putting People at the Heart of Public Services*, available online at http://www.dh.gov.uk/en/Publicationsandstatistics/Publications/PublicationsPolicyAndGuidance/DH_4084516.

Department of Health (2006a) *Modernizing Nursing Careers: Setting the Direction*, London: DH.

Department of Health (2006b) *A New Ambition for Old Age: The Next Five Years*, available online at http://www.dh.gov.uk/en/Publicationsandstatistics/Publications/PublicationsPolicyAndGuidance/DH_4133941.

Department of Health (2007) *Health Survey for England 2005: Health of Older People*, London: DH, available online at http://www.dh.gov.uk/en/Publicationsandstatistics/PublishedSurvey/HealthSurveyForEngland/Healthsurveyresults/DH_635.

Information Centre for Health and Social Care, The (2008) *Prescriptions Dispensed in the Community 1997–2007*, London: ONS, available online at http://www.ic.nhs.uk/webfiles/publications/PCA%20publication/Final%20version%20210708.pdf.

National Audit Office (2007) *Improving Services and Support for People with Dementia*, available online at http://www.nao.org.uk/publications/0607/support_for_people_with_dement.aspx.

Nursing and Midwifery Council (2009) *Guidance for the Care of Older People*, available online at http://www.nmc-uk.org/General-public/Older-people-and-their-carers/Care-and-respect-every-time-new-guidance-for-the-care-of-older-people/.

Office for National Statistics (2009) *Ageing: Fastest Increase in the Old*, a available online at http://www.statistics.gov.uk/cci/nugget.asp?id=949.

Scottish Executive (2006) *Modernizing Nursing Careers: Setting the Direction*, Edinburgh: Scottish Executive.

World Health Organization Europe (2004) *Better Palliative Care for Older People*, available online at http://www.euro.who.int/__data/assets/pdf_file/0009/98235/E82933.pdf.

Dignity, values, attitudes, and person-centred care

Jo Galloway

Learning outcomes

By the end of this chapter, you will be able to:

- define 'positive ageing' and the contribution that older people make to society;
- discuss ageism, and the stereotypes and labels that are associated with ageing and old age;
- demonstrate an understanding of the importance of dignity and respect for many older patients;
- recognize the possible signs of abuse or neglect, so that concerns can be raised to ensure the safety and empowerment of vulnerable adults;
- identify best practice and opportunities to achieve person-centred care in both community and hospital settings; and
- reflect on your own practice and the standards of care provided within your practice setting, and establish actions that you can take to ensure that patients are treated with dignity and respect, and receive care that is person-centred.

Introduction

Everyone is an individual with their own unique values, attitudes, beliefs, and preferences. To achieve care that is person-centred, the nurse needs to recognize individuality and diversity, whilst consulting with and involving the individual at all stages of their patient journey. When caring for older people, it is important to have an understanding of ageism—that is, stereotypes and labels associated with older people—together with the impact that this can have on their experience and patient outcomes.

This chapter examines values and attitudes relating to the care of older people, and explores best practice regarding the promotion of person-centred care. The principles discussed within the chapter are applicable to both health and social care, and within community or other settings.

Ageism

Ageism is also referred to as 'age discrimination' and relates to discrimination or prejudice against a person, or persons, on the basis of their age. Ageism in health care can relate to receiving a lower standard of service or even to being denied access to a service—for example, being told that symptoms experienced are directly related to old age, not receiving a general practitioner (GP) referral to a consultant on the grounds of age, or not being involved in decision-making about transfer of care arrangements when being discharged from acute hospital care.

A New Ambition for Old Age (DH, 2006a) was informed by older people and argued that age discrimination is now uncommon in English health services; nonetheless, '*deep-rooted negative attitudes and behaviours*' still exist towards older people. The new ambition outlined in this document was that, by 2011, older people and their families will have confidence that older people will be treated with respect for their dignity and their human rights in all care settings.

See also Chapter 18 on ageism on a personal, cultural, and structural level in relation to end-of-life care

Stereotypes and labels

There are a number of stereotypes and labels associated with old age.

- A **stereotype** relates to a standard or convention shared by members of a social group. Stereotypes might include, for example, the perception of older people being incontinent, experiencing confusion, or making no contribution to society.
- A **label** relates to a descriptive phrase or term ascribed to an individual. Labels associated with old age can be similarly derogatory and include a plethora of terms such as 'geriatric' and 'coffin dodgers'.

Values, attitudes, and beliefs

Each person is unique, with their own personal values and beliefs shaped by a number of factors that include culture, religion, and personal experiences.

- **Values** relate to our personal principles, morals, and ideals—that is, what we consider to be important.
- **Attitudes** relate to a person's views, which may be evidenced in the way they behave.
- **Beliefs** relate to those things in which an individual has faith—'religious beliefs', for example—which may not necessarily be founded on fact.

Societal norms change over time, and the healthcare practitioner needs to take account of generational influences and culture to help them in providing care that is patient-centred. In addition to establishing and respecting the values, attitudes, and beliefs of older people, the healthcare practitioner also needs to be aware of their own personal values, attitudes, and beliefs, and needs to ensure that he or she provides non-judgemental, personalized care to their patients.

Spirituality and religion

Religion and spirituality are often perceived as being one and the same thing. Gender (2002) defines 'spirituality' as focusing on answering questions related to the meaning and purpose of life, and 'religion' as relating to the personal or institutional system of organized beliefs, practices, rituals, and/or forms of worship, and states that religion is a means to achieving spirituality. In providing person-centred care, it is important to address spirituality and religious beliefs. Hindu and Muslim women, for example, may prefer to be treated or cared for by a healthcare practitioner of the same gender.

See also Chapter 18 on spirituality in relation to end-of-life care.

Sexuality

'Sexuality' can be defined as:

an individual's self-concept, shaped by their personality, and expressed as sexual feelings, attitudes, beliefs and behaviour, expressed through a heterosexual, homosexual, bisexual or transsexual orientation.

(RCN, 2000)

Sexuality can be expressed through personal thoughts, feelings, behaviours, presentation, intimacy, and roles in life.

Many older people have a number of gender-specific roles, such as wife/husband, partner, civil partner, mother/father, and grandmother/grandfather, and their roles and responsibilities relating to these roles need to be acknowledged—for example, caring responsibilities. Other issues can include the loss of a long-term partner, and the grief and loss that is associated with this. Healthcare practitioners should not take a person's social networks for granted and should ensure that stereotypes of families or social relationships reflect diversity.

Achieving culturally competent care

'Cultural competence' relates to an individual's ability to treat every person with dignity, respect, and fairness, in a way that is sensitively responsive to differences and similarities, and thereby contributes to creating a genuinely inclusive culture. In order to achieve this, nurses need to examine their own values, beliefs, and cultural identity, and understand discrimination and racism in all of its forms. They also need to be able to recognize and continuously develop the skills, roles, and functions needed to perform cultural assessments, to plan, implement, and evaluate culturally sensitive care, and to challenge discrimination and prejudice.

Additional care needs

It is imperative that healthcare practitioners treat all patients as individuals regardless of age, religion, belief, gender, or sexual orientation. A holistic patient assessment is essential to identify patient needs, which may require specific interventions in order to ensure that dignity is maintained and person-centred care is achieved. It is important, for example, to establish whether the patient experiences any sensory impairment, such as hearing or sight loss. If this is the case, the patient's care or treatment plan should reflect care-delivery interventions that are necessary to support effective communication—for example, the use of a portable hearing loop or patient information leaflets that are printed in a specific font and in a larger font size.

See also chapter 3

Health and social care policy

In *High-quality Care for All: NHS Next-stage Review Final Report* (DH, 2008a), the Department of Health sets out the vision for the National Health Service (NHS) as *'an NHS that gives patients and the public more information and choice, works in partnership and has quality of care at its heart'*. The report highlights how achieving the vision will be dependent upon addressing variations in the quality of care and empowering patients. The report sets out the development of the NHS Constitution to empower both patients and staff (ibid.).

Respect and dignity comprise one of six NHS values, which were informed by staff, patients, and the public, and are outlined within the NHS Constitution (DH, 2009). It states:

[W]e value each person as an individual, respect their aspirations and commitments in life, and seek to understand their priorities, needs, abilities and limits. We take what others have to say seriously. We are honest about our point of view and what we can and cannot do.

(DH, 2009)

Other NHS values include commitment to quality of care, compassion, improving lives, working together for patients, and the idea that everyone counts.

Dignity

'Dignity' is a difficult concept to define and has a strong association with respect. 'Privacy' has been defined as *'freedom from intrusion'* and 'dignity' as *'being worthy of respect'* (DH, 2003). A Europe-wide study of dignity and older people identified that it is often easier to describe and provide examples of *indignity*—that is, the opposite of dignity (Doe Consortium, 2005).

Within this study, four types of dignity were identified, as follows.

- **Merit**—This relates to dignity or social status that is ascribed to people because of their role or position in society, or because of what they have achieved. For example, a nurse, or a doctor, or a therapist has status that is recognized by other people. When older people retire, they may be excluded from wider involvement in society and may experience associated loss of their dignity.
- **Moral status**—This is emphasized by the person's moral autonomy or integrity. If an older person is able to live according to their own moral principles, then that person will experience a sense of dignity.
- **Personal identity**—This was found to be the most relevant in the context of older people: *'It relates to self-respect, and reflects an individual's identity as a person. This can be violated by physical interference as well as by emotional or psychological insults such as humiliation'*.
- **Menschenwurde**—This type of dignity *'refers to the inalienable value of human beings'*. It was identified as being grounded in *'what it is to be human'*. Three themes were identified within this type:
  - **(a)** a control of physical functions;
  - **(b)** that human beings are storytelling animals, a core of which is the capacity to build and shape one's identity and understanding of oneself through the development of meaningful stories about our lives; and
  - **(c)** that, as social creatures, human beings require self-respect that comes from them being recognized by others as worthy of respect.

An evaluation on the impact of the *National Service Framework for Older People* (NSFOP) (DH, 2001a) on the experiences and expectations of older people found that there were perceptions of improvements in systems, but that there were also negative personal experiences of using services and ageist attitudes that altered quality of life and standards of care (Manthorpe et al., 2007).

The report into the NSFOP highlighted where dignity is not maintained, including:

- **Being cared for in mixed sex bays and wards that accommodate both men and women**
- **Feeling neglected or ignored whilst receiving care**
- **Being made to feel worthless or a nuisance**
- **Being treated more as an object than a person**
- **Generally being rushed and not being listened to**
- **A disrespectful attitude from staff or being addressed in ways they find disrespectful, e.g. when they have not been asked about their preferences about the preferred form of address to be used**
- **Being provided with bibs intended for babies rather than a napkin whilst being helped to eat**
- **Having to eat with their fingers rather than being helped to eat with a knife and fork**

(DH, 2006a)

More recently, the *Robert Francis Inquiry Report into the Mid-Staffordshire NHS Foundation Trust* (the Francis Report) exposed serious issues relating to patient experience and dignity (DH, 2010a). Included in the report's recommendations is a review of the systems and processes, values, and behaviours that make up a system for the early detection and prevention of serious failures in the NHS. It emphasizes that everyone has a role to play in safeguarding quality of care to patients (DH, 2010a).

Improving dignity

The Royal College of Nursing (2008) gathered the perspectives of nurses, healthcare assistants, and nursing students regarding the maintenance and promotion of dignity in everyday practice. This revealed '*a high level of dignity and sensitivity to dignity issues amongst nursing staff, combined with a strong commitment to dignified care and concern in relation to dignity violations*'.

The findings of this research mirror those of other studies in the identification of three main factors that maintain or adversely affect dignity in care:

1. **The physical environment and the culture of the organisation (Place)**
2. **The nature and conduct of care activities (Processes)**
3. **The attitudes and behaviour of staff and others (People)**

(RCN, 2008)

The government's 'Dignity in Care' campaign was launched in 2006 with the aim of eliminating tolerance of indignity in health and social care services through raising awareness and inspiring people to take action. The Campaign incorporates the 'Dignity in Care Challenge', which comprises ten dimensions for the delivery of high-quality care services that respect people's dignity:

1. **Have zero tolerance of all forms of abuse**
2. **Support people with the same respect you would want for yourself or a member of your family**
3. **Treat each person as an individual by offering a personalized service**
4. **Enable people to maintain the maximum level of independence, choice and control.**
5. **Listen and support people to express their needs and wants**
6. **Respect people's right to privacy**
7. **Ensure people feel able to complain without fear of retribution**
8. **Engage with family members and carers as care partners**
9. **Assist people to maintain confidence and self-esteem**
10. **Act to alleviate people's loneliness and isolation**

(DH, 2006b)

In addition to, and in support of, the Department of Health's Dignity campaign, a number of other national campaigns and best practice guides have been launched by public-sector, professional, and voluntary organizations to raise the profile of dignity and to promote privacy, dignity, and respect in health and social care environments. These include the RCN Dignity Campaign (2008), the Social Care Institute for Excellence (2006) *Adult Services Practice Guide: Dignity in Care*, and the Age UK campaign for demanding quality care for old people (Age UK, 2010).

The Healthcare Commission focused on dignity as a key theme in its annual health check for 2006–07 and carried out a targeted inspection programme to assess the extent to which NHS trusts were meeting the government's core standards relating to dignity in care for hospital in-patients. Based on the scrutiny against standards and the issues identified by other evidence, a number of key themes emerged as the essential elements for ensuring that older people were being provided care in a way that was dignified and that matched their personal needs while in hospital. The themes identified were:

- involving older people in their care;
- delivering personal care in a way that ensures dignity for the patient;
- having a workforce that is equipped to deliver good-quality care;
- strong leadership at all levels; and
- a supportive ward environment.

See chapter 9

The Healthcare Commission (2007: 9) states that '*Dignity (including nutrition and privacy) is a human rights issue and should be the underlying principle when delivering services*'.

The dignity model detailed in Figure 2.1 below provides a framework of best practice for healthcare practitioners to help them to ensure that patient dignity is maintained in their practice setting and that the care that is delivered is person-centred.

Another initiative that set out to improve the dignity and care of older people was the Champions for Older People Programme (Hindle, 2008). This evolved out of a need to address Standard 4 'General Hospital Care' in the NSFOP and was implemented across every acute hospital in the West Midlands (DH, 2001a). The programme included provision for 'older people champions' to attend an intensive two-day workshop and then to cascade the themes from the workshops to their colleagues. In addition, they were tasked with undertaking evaluation of their care environments, promoting dignity, and implementing positive change via action plans. Box 2.1 offers some examples of champions' action plans taken from their service evaluation.

See Chapter 7 for more on medication management.

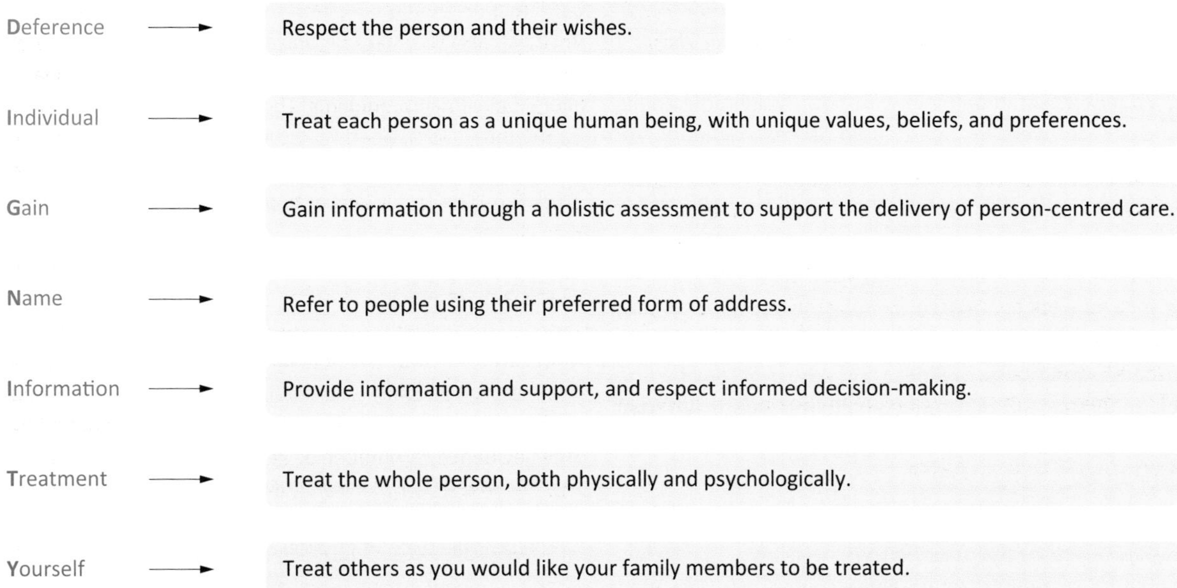

Figure 2.1 The dignity model.

Box 2.1 Examples of champions' action plans taken from their service evaluation

- **Communication**—Poor documentation and poor communication with patients regarding care plan.

  Action plan: Undertake a monthly audit looking at documentation, progress to documenting in one set of notes, and raise awareness of hearing problems.
- Pain management—There is currently no assessment of pain relief or management or use of tools.

  Action plan: To introduce education for staff on pain management, make more referrals to the pain nurse, and have monthly monitoring of the use of pain assessment tools.
- Values and attitudes—Nurses not always using preferred name to address patients.

  Action plan: To improve communication with patients, to act as a role model, and to be advocates. Senior nurses to educate junior staff at handover—for example, patient aged 90 with heart failure will feel exhausted.
- Medicines—Elderly patients are not always able to take on new information regarding their medication.

  Action plan: Dosette boxes have been used increasingly in the community to aid medication concordance by prompting patients to remember to take medication each day. In view of this increased usage, it was decided that Dosette boxes should be provided on the ward before discharge in order to assess a patient's ability to use them, provide an opportunity to develop the habit of using the Dosette system, and thereby promote the patient's independence.
- Mental health support—Poor emotional and psychological support from medical and nursing staff, because focus is very much on the physical illness. Lack of awareness of depression in older people.

  Action plan: Use the education/teaching board to cascade information and establish psychiatric link nurse on the ward. Include depression scoring for each patient, implement psychological/mental healthcare plan and re-evaluation, and involve patient and family in this.
- Incontinence/toileting—Continence not being maintained.

  Action plan:
  - Implement 'behind closed doors' audit.
  - Ensure continence assessment tool is available in all wards.
  - Education for staff regarding continence—identification, and how to assess and manage via specialist nurse.
  - Launch staff awareness to increase patient choice.
  - Improved signage.
  - After toileting, staff to ensure environment is clean.

(Hindle, 2008).

Adult protection and elder abuse

With dignity comes respect, compassion, and esteem—but the loss of dignity is one of many factors that can lead to the development of abuse and abusive practice. Nurses have an important role in safeguarding vulnerable adults, as well as in the prevention and detection of abuse.

Widely accepted definitions of both 'vulnerable adults' and 'abuse' were included in *No Secrets: Guidance on Developing and Implementing Multi-agency Policies and Procedures to Protect Vulnerable Adults from Abuse* (DH, 2000).

A 'vulnerable adult' was said to be:

A person who is aged 18 or over who is or may be in need of community care services by reason of mental or other disability, age or illness and who is or may be unable to take care of him or herself against significant harm or exploitation.

(DH, 2000)

'Abuse' was defined as *'a violation of an individual's human and civil rights by any other person or persons'*.

The UK charity Action on Elder Abuse (AEA) sees elder abuse as having at its heart the violation and/or exploitation of the expectation of trust in a relationship. It defines 'elder abuse' as:

A single or repeated act or lack of appropriate action, occurring within any relationship where there is an expectation of trust, which causes harm or distress to an older person.

(AEA, 2010)

Abuse can take many forms and occur anywhere, including:

- in someone's own home;
- in a carer's home;
- in a day centre or social care setting;
- in a care home; and
- in different types of NHS/health settings, such as within a hospital, a community or intermediate care setting, or a mental health unit.

Both older men and women are at risk of being abused. The abuser is usually well known to the person being abused—for example, a partner, child, or relative, a friend or neighbour, a care worker, a volunteer, or a healthcare professional.

In a study reviewing the prevalence of abuse, it was found that:

Overall, 2.6% of people aged 66 and over living in private households reported that they had experienced mistreatment involving a family member, close friend or care worker (i.e. those in a traditional expectation of trust relationship) during the past year.

(O'Keeffe et al., 2007: 4)

Fifty-one per cent involved a spouse or partner; 49 per cent involved another family member; 13 per cent involved a care worker; and 5 per cent, a friend.

Older people may also be abused by the person for whom they care (Homer and Gilleard, 1990). Some forms of abuse can have a significant negative impact on an older person's mental health and well-being.

The main forms of abuse are described as being physical, psychological or emotional, financial or material, sexual, or neglect, each of which is briefly explored below.

Physical abuse

Physical abuse may be a crime, but is not always prosecuted because of a lack of evidence or the unwillingness of a person to take action. Very often, when people are asked to describe elder abuse, they will talk about physical injuries. However, it can also include the prescription or administering of medication that is not licensed for the purpose used, which can have a traumatic effect.

The possible signs of physical abuse include:

- any injury, such as bruising, cuts, burns, fractures, or unexplained marks, which may be new or untreated, and with which the person's explanation may not equate;
- signs of being restrained; and
- the inappropriate use of medication either by overdosing or underdosing.

Psychological or emotional abuse

Psychological or emotional abuse can include threatening or denying access to older people and may also relate to the older person having to comply with threats or demands, or being isolated from others. Not surprisingly, older people subjected to such abuse may feel trapped, threatened, and humiliated.

The possible signs of psychological abuse can include:

- depression;
- denial of a situation;
- withdrawal or a unwillingness to communicate;
- loss of sleep or appetite;
- implausible stories;
- disorientation or confusion;
- sudden changes in behaviour or unusual behavior; and
- unexplained fear and anxiety.

If the signs indicated above are detected, then this does not mean that abuse is taking place—but it should raise the index of suspicion and lead to further assessment or enquiry by the professional.

Financial or material abuse

As with physical abuse, financial or material abuse may be a crime, but it is not always prosecuted. There are a number of reasons for this, which may include a reluctance on the part of a competent individual to report to matter to or pursue it further with criminal justice agencies. Examples of financial or material abuse can include exploitation and the theft of cash by family members, fraud and deception, and possible misuse of lasting powers of attorney (LPAs).

See Chapter 4 for more on LPAs and the law.

The possible signs of financial or material abuse include:

- a loss of money and unexplained withdrawals of large sums of money;
- uncertain signatures on cheques or documents;
- additional names on bank accounts;
- the misappropriation of property and possessions;
- the sudden appearance of previously uninvolved relatives in the older person's financial affairs;
- unpaid bills, disconnections, or eviction notices; and
- a lack of basic amenities.

Sexual abuse

Sexual abuse of older people can be opportunistic or planned, or may also be found in situations of domestic violence, which continues into old age. Where sexual abuse is suspected, it is vital that forensic evidence is not lost, thus it may be appropriate to avoid washing the older person or their clothing. Contacting the police at the first opportunity is advised.

The possible signs of sexual abuse include:

- bruising, particularly around the breasts or genital area;
- unexplained vaginal or anal bleeding;
- venereal disease or infections; and
- difficulty in walking or standing.

Neglect

Neglect can include intentional neglect by an individual or the practices of an institution, or passive neglect—for example, where a carer is unable to manage the situation or is not getting adequate help.

The possible signs of neglect include:

- people left in poor hygiene and a lack of personal care—for example, dirt, faeces, or urine left on the person;
- rashes, pressure ulcers, and/or lice;
- over-sedation or withholding medication;
- untreated medical problems, including depression and confusion; and
- malnutrition or dehydration.

Legislation

Several pieces of law assist in the recognition and prevention of abuse of vulnerable adults in the UK. These are accompanied by a range of policies across the UK.

For more on these policies, see the Online Resource Centre that accompanies this book

In England, the following key policies apply.

No Secrets

No Secrets provided a framework with which local agencies could develop strategies to tackle abuse, with the local authority being the lead agency (DH, 2000). In 2008–09, there was a review of the policy guidance, which included a consultation at national level about what changes might be necessary to the policy guidance in order to enable society to empower vulnerable adults to keep safe from abuse or harm. This included consideration of whether new legislation was necessary.

The government response to the review, issued in January 2010, was to indicate that it would, within time:

- **Establish an Inter-Departmental Ministerial Group on Safeguarding Vulnerable Adults**
- **Plan legislation to strengthen the local governance of safeguarding by putting Safeguarding Adults Boards on a statutory footing**
- **Launch a programme of work with representative agencies and stakeholders to support effective policy and practice in safeguarding vulnerable adults.**

(DH, 2010b)

The Vetting and Barring Scheme

The Protection of Vulnerable Adults (POVA) List was replaced in 2009 by a Vetting and Barring Scheme under the Protection of Vulnerable Groups Act 2006, which aims to safeguard the most vulnerable members of society, including vulnerable older people. The Independent Safeguarding Authority (ISA) makes all decisions on who should be barred from working with vulnerable people. Employers need to check in advance whether employees or volunteers are barred from working with vulnerable groups, in addition to undertaking the Criminal Records Bureau (CRB) checks that are routinely made in health and social care employment practices. Individuals will also have to register with the ISA when taking up employment in these areas of work (in which there is regular contact with vulnerable individuals). See http://www.isa-gov.org.uk/ for more information.

The Mental Capacity Act 2005

The Mental Capacity Act 2005 applies in England and Wales. This Act enables those people who lack 'capacity' to be at the centre of the decision-making process, safeguarding them and the professionals who work with them. Under this Act, new offences of mistreatment and wilful neglect of people lacking decision making capacity (for example, people with severe dementia) were introduced. New statutory forms of advocacy were also introduced.

See Chapter 4 for more on the law relating to mental capacity.

The Deprivation of Liberty Safeguards (DoLS)

The Deprivation of Liberty Safeguards (DoLS) were introduced into the Mental Capacity Act 2005 through the Mental Health Act 2007 to provide a legal framework in relation to deprivation of liberty. The DoLS resulted from the *Bournewood Case*, in which an individual with learning disabilities was taken to a mental hospital because of the way in which he was behaving; despite his carers wishing him to be returned home, he was kept in hospital. The case was brought before the courts.

See the Online Resource Centre that accompanies this book for more on the Bournewood Case.

Safeguards are provided for vulnerable people who lack capacity to make decisions relating to their care or treatment in hospital and care homes, or care homes with nursing. The aim of the safeguards is to protect the interests of the most vulnerable service users and to:

- **ensure people will be given the care they require, but in the least restrictive regimes**
- **prevent arbitrary decisions that may deprive vulnerable people of their liberty**
- **provide additional safeguards for vulnerable people**
- **provide individuals subject to the safeguards with rights to challenge unlawful detention**
- **avoid any unnecessary bureaucracy**

(DH, 2008a).

NURSING PRACTICE INSIGHT: RAISING CONCERNS OF SUSPECTED ABUSE

The nurse has a responsibility to raise concerns about suspected abuse or neglect, and to ensure the safety and protection of vulnerable adults.

He or she must:

- be aware and familiar with local adult-safeguarding policies and procedures;
- know who the lead person is within their organization for adult safeguarding;
- discuss any issues of potential abuse and/or neglect with a line manager in the first instance, and liaise with the lead for adult safeguarding;
- maintain clinical and professional competence, providing high standards of care;
- always take time to listen to the older person or the carer of the older person;
- maintain accurate written records; and
- practice zero tolerance of any abuse and be prepared to 'blow the whistle' around managers, colleagues, and wider teams.

Person-centred care

The terms 'patient-centred care', 'personalized care', and 'individualized care' consistently feature within government documents for health and social care services. Within the *Essence of Care*, the term 'person-centred' is used to signify '*activities that are based on what is important to a person from their own perspective*' (DH, 2001b).

'Person-centred care' has been defined as treating people as individuals and enabling them to make choices about their care (DH, 2001b). Figure 2.2 illustrates a number of concepts that support the achievement of care that is person-centred.

- **Communication** relates to a two-way process that involves exchanging information; it is important for the sender of the information to establish that the receiver understands the message and that it is communicated in a way that meets any individual communication needs that the receiver may have.
- An **advocate** is a person who intercedes on behalf of another person in a bid to ensure that their best interests are communicated and met.
- **Involvement** is the inclusion or engagement of the patient and, within the context of health care, can relate to communicating with patients regarding their planned care or treatment.
- **Participation** takes involvement a step further, and relates to taking a more active role and sharing. In the context of health care, this can relate to the healthcare practitioner actively engaging the person in the development of their care or therapy plan.
- **Trust** relates to having confidence in another person—that is, to having faith that they are reliable and honest.
- A **partnership** involves working together for a shared purpose and, within the healthcare practitioner–patient relationship, can relate to, for example, jointly developing a plan of care and agreeing how both parties will work

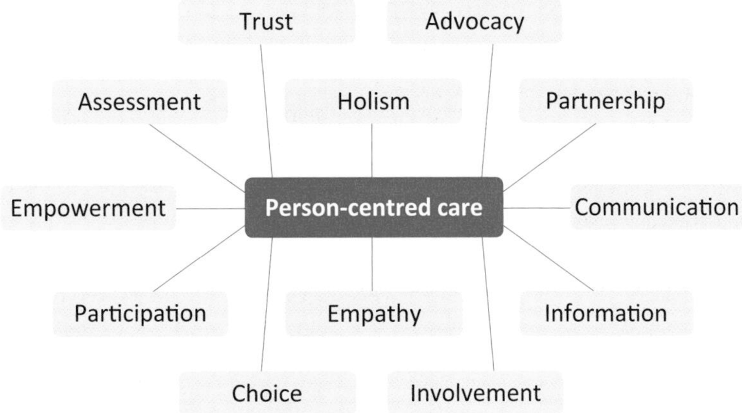

Figure 2.2 Concepts central to person-centred care

together collectively to achieve the outcomes to which they agree.

- To **empower** is to give or delegate power or authority to and, in the context of health care, entails letting the person take responsibility for their consequences.
- **Empathy** involves the healthcare practitioner considering the situation of the person and imaginatively entering into their feelings.
- **Choice** involves providing the person with alternatives from which to choose and goes one step further in respecting the decision that is made, as far as possible.
- **Holism** refers to the practice of considering the person as a whole, addressing their physical and psychological needs collectively, rather than seeing them as two separate entities.
- **Assessment** needs to be undertaken at a level commensurate with patient need and must address patient values, needs, and preferences, as a foundation for the achievement of care that is person-centred.

At the beginning of the patient journey, it is important for the nurse to undertake a holistic assessment to identify the person's needs and personal preferences. These can then be addressed in the care plan, ongoing evaluation of care, and patient outcomes.

See Chapter 8 for more on personalized care planning in primary care.

Case study

Mr Oliver is a 70-year-old man admitted to hospital with a chest infection. He worked as a farmer for over forty years and gets up at 5 a.m. every morning. The ward routine is that lights are not switched on until 7 a.m. in the morning. Mr Oliver wakes up at 5 a.m. the following morning, rings his call bell, and requests a cup of tea. The health care support worker (HCSW) who answers his call bell informs him that it is too early and tells him to go back to sleep.

In this example, the general routine of the clinical area was prioritized and the patient was expected to fit in. In institutions, it is necessary to have routine and also to address the needs of other patients; it is also important to recognize individuality and to address specific needs. Perhaps, in this situation, the patient could have been provided with the drink that he requested and could have been nursed in an area of the ward in which his preference to get up at 5 a.m. would have minimal or no impact on his fellow patients? A holistic assessment of the activities of daily living and personal preferences could have identified Mr Oliver's lifestyle and proactive steps could have been taken to address his need.

The Essence of Care (EoC)

The *Essence of Care* (EoC) benchmark was developed to support the fundamentals of care and to ensure quality of service provision within health care (DH, 2003). The benchmarking process contained within the EoC allows practitioners to take a structured approach to sharing and comparing practice, enabling them to identify best practice and to develop action plans to improve practice where appropriate. Privacy and dignity comprises one of ten EoC benchmarks. Dignity is defined within the benchmark as *'being worthy of respect'*, respect as *'freedom from intrusion'*, and modesty as *'not being embarrassed'*.

Table 2.1 details the benchmarks of best practice for each of the seven areas contained within this benchmark.

Caring

'Caring' is a concept that is central to nursing; encompassing care, compassion, and comfort. *Confidence in Caring* focuses on the relationship between nursing and caring, and

Table 2.1 Essence of Care benchmarks for privacy and dignity

Agreed patient-focused outcome Patients benefit from care that is focused upon respect for the individual	
Factor	**Benchmark of best practice**
1. Attitudes and behaviours	Patients feel that they matter all of the time
2. Personal world and personal identity	Patients experience care in an environment that actively encompasses individual values, beliefs, and personal relationships
3. Personal boundaries and space	Patients' personal space is actively promoted by all staff
4. Communicating with staff and patients	Communication between staff and patients takes place in a manner that respects their individuality
5. Privacy of patient—confidentiality of patient information	Patient information is shared to enable care, with their consent
6. Privacy, dignity, and modesty	Patients' care actively promotes their privacy and dignity, and protects their modesty
7. Availability of an area for complete privacy	Patients and or carers can access an area that safely provides privacy

Source: DH (2003).

provides best practice guidelines and a framework within which to improve patient confidence in nursing care (DH, 2008b). The framework includes five core issues that are important to patients:

- a calm, clean, safe environment;
- a positive, friendly culture;
- good teamwork and working relationships;
- well-managed care with efficient delivery; and
- personalized care for every patient.

It also includes 'means', 'ways', 'skills and will', and 'overall outcome and performance measures', together with simple rules for staff such as '*anticipate and act without being asked*' and '*do what you say you will do—keep promises*'. The framework also highlights the importance of involvement at all levels of the care system, from organizational to individual level.

Supporting dignity in care

There are a number of ways in which healthcare practitioners can promote and achieve dignified care.

Leadership

Staff can demonstrate leadership regardless of their seniority and role in the organization, and healthcare practitioners can act as champions for older people either informally or in a more formally nominated role. Being a 'champion' relates to supporting and defending a cause; in the context of this chapter it relates to ensuring the delivery of privacy, dignity, and person-centred care. The champion role entails acting as a role model, respecting older people as individuals, and ensuring that they receive high standards of care. It also includes challenging negative perceptions and poor practice.

The care environment

The environment in which care is delivered has a significant impact on achieving dignity, and there are factors at both the organizational level and the individual service/practitioner level that can be implemented to ensure the achievement of dignified care. The provision of single-sex accommodation was identified earlier in the chapter as a priority for older people—but single-sex accommodation is often more difficult to achieve in more specialist areas, such as intensive care. Within such areas, dignity needs to be a key priority and staff should implement best practice guidelines, such as those produced by the NHS Institute for Innovation and Improvement (2008).

Other environmental aspects that support dignified care include:

- a well-maintained and well-decorated clinical area;
- dignity curtains—that is, curtains with a printed dignity message or sign attached to them;
- a private room in which to discuss personal, sensitive, or confidential information; and
- segregated washroom and toilet facilities for male and female patients they are fitted with patient safety locks.

Care delivery

A key aspect of the dignity equation relates to the care delivery process in which individual healthcare teams and practitioners can directly influence the standard of dignified care that is achieved on a day-to-day basis.

Interventions can include:

- completing person-centred assessments;
- involving patients in all aspects of their care and treatment;
- respecting closed curtains/doors and seeking permission prior to entry;

- taking steps to ensure safe staffing levels;
- explaining procedures prior to undertaking them; and
- covering patients during personal care activities and ensuring appropriate dress.

Case study

Following an assessment by her community matron, Mrs Jones was admitted to her local community hospital with a chest infection. Mrs Jones became increasingly confused and was diagnosed as suffering from delirium. She had a high temperature and became restless, throwing off the bedclothes and uncovering herself. Lightweight female pyjamas were provided for Mrs Jones to ensure that her dignity was maintained.

In a situation such as this, it can be difficult to ensure that the patient's dignity is maintained at all times. The provision of female pyjamas is a simple and effective way in which to reduce the risk of a patient exposing themselves when they are in a confused state.

The healthcare team

Each and every member of the healthcare team has a responsibility to main privacy and dignity, and, in addition to their own practice, they must act as the patient's advocate and remind or challenge colleagues should they fail to practise the same standards.

Case study

Staff Nurse Lloyd was inserting a urinary catheter on Mrs Ellis, a 75-year-old lady who had developed retention of urine. Just as Nurse Lloyd was about to insert the catheter, a doctor popped her head around the curtains. 'Oh, sorry', said the doctor and proceeded to ask Nurse Lloyd a question, to which she responded.

In this situation, the doctor failed to respect the privacy of the patient and made no attempt to gain permission to enter the bed space. Equally, the nurse failed to challenge the doctor and act as the patient's advocate by letting the doctor know that this practice is unacceptable.

Monitoring and evaluating the achievement of dignity in care

It is important to measure patient outcomes in order to monitor the standard of care delivery achieved, to address any shortfalls that may be identified, and to look at how the outcomes achieved can be further improved. The healthcare practitioner can draw upon a number of strategies, both informal and more formalized, to establish the standards that are being achieved within their practice setting. Strategies can include: professional judgement; evaluating care plans with the patient; completing EoC benchmarks; accessing and reading patient complaints; undertaking patient experience surveys; accessing patient evaluations that are posted on the intranet, such as on the NHS Choices website; and accessing the results of national patient satisfaction surveys—for example, those published by the Care Quality Commission (CQC).

The CQC coordinates the completion of a number of national surveys to reveal patients' evaluations of their recent experiences of health care. Surveys coordinated include, amongst others, in-patient, outpatient, accident and emergency, and maternity. Some surveys, such as the adult in-patient survey, are completed on an annual basis and others less frequently. These surveys enable NHS care providers to benchmark their services against the standard that is achieved nationally.

The *Adult In-patient Survey 2008* included more than 72,000 respondents from 165 acute and specialist NHS trusts in England (CQC, 2009). Table 2.2 provides the results for some of the areas contained within the survey that relate to dignity. The survey results reveal that 79 per cent of patients reported that they were always treated with dignity and respect during their in-patient stay. Conversely, 3 per cent of patients reported that they were not treated with dignity and respect, with a further 18 per cent reporting that they were sometimes treated with dignity and respect. These results reveal that further work is needed to realize the government's target that patients will be treated with dignity and respect in all care settings, all of the time.

In addition to the national report, reports for individual acute and specialist trusts are also published on the Internet that allow the benchmarking of results against those achieved by the 20 per cent that are the best-performing trusts, 60 per cent that are average-performing trusts, and 20 per cent that are the worst-performing trusts.

NURSING PRACTICE INSIGHT: TREATING PEOPLE AS INDIVIDUALS

Always treat each and every person as an individual by:

- **completing an assessment to establish their values and beliefs, and to identify their personal preferences;**
- **establishing and respecting their preferred form of address;**
- **involving them in all decisions about their care;**
- **providing them with choices, and respecting their preferences and decisions;**
- **using a biographical approach for patients who experience memory loss;**
- **promoting independence in everyday activities;**
- **promoting independent living within the community;**

Table 2.2 Adult In-patient Survey Results 2008

Question	Yes, definitely	Yes, to some extent	No	Yes
When you were first admitted to a bed on a ward, did you mind sharing a sleeping area, for example a room or bay, with patients of the opposite sex?			68%	32%
Were you given enough privacy when being examined or treated?	88%	10%	2%	
Were you given enough privacy when discussing your condition or treatment?	70%	22%	8%	
Were you involved as much as you wanted to be in decisions about your care and treatment?	52%	37%	10%	
Overall, did you feel that you were treated with respect and dignity while you were in the hospital?	79%	18%	3%	

Source: CQC (2009).

- **acting as a role model and advocate, and challenging any instances in which the achievement of person-centred care is compromised; and**
- **having a listening ear, a kind word, and a smile.**

Conclusion

Older people need to be cared for holistically and to achieve this their psychological, social, and physical needs must be addressed. Completing a person-centred assessment enables the healthcare practitioner to identify the person's individual needs and preferences in order to inform their plan of care. The practitioner also needs to recognize and respect diversity, and to deliver care that is culturally sensitive to individual needs. The patient needs to be central to the care delivery process, and the healthcare practitioner must actively seek to engage and involve them in decision making at all stages of their patient journey. Lastly, dignity needs to be a core value and embedded in practice.

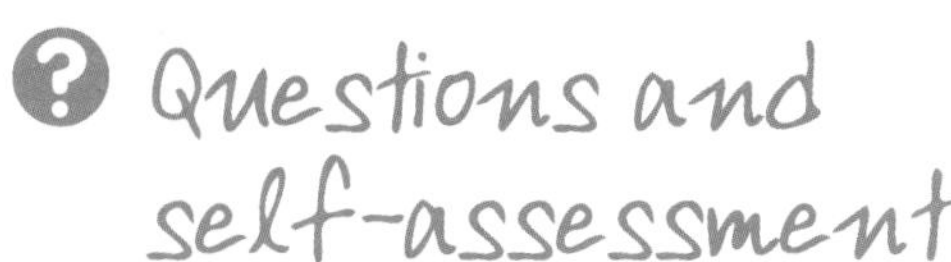

Now that you have read the chapter, answer the following questions.

- What is meant by 'ageism' and how does this impact on care delivery?
- Reflect on a recent clinical experience when working with an older adult. How did you and others involved in care-giving convey dignity and respect to that person?
- Review the EoC benchmarks for privacy and dignity, and consider the degree to which this identified best practice is prevalent within a recent practice setting.
- Talk to one or more of your patients to establish their evaluations and perceptions of the degree to which their privacy and dignity have been maintained.
- Who is the adult-safeguarding lead in your organization and how can you contact them?
- Access a patient survey on the CQC website http://www.cqc.org.uk/—ideally one that relates to your employing organization or, alternatively, to a local healthcare institution.

Self-assessment

- Having read the chapter, how will you change your practice?
- Consider the role of the 'champion', as discussed within the chapter. Reflect upon your own practice, and assess the extent to which you act as a role model in caring for and supporting older people.
- Identify up to three areas relating to dignity in care in which you need to develop your knowledge and understanding further.
- Identify how you are going to develop this knowledge and understanding, and set deadlines for achieving these.

Further suggested tasks to complete

- **Privacy and dignity within my practice setting**
  - Reflect on the standards of privacy and dignity that are achieved within your practice setting.
  - Consider how far the patient perceptions and national survey findings relate to your personal reflections regarding the standards achieved.
  - Consider what you and your colleagues could do to address any areas that require development or could be further improved upon.
  - Discuss your reflections and suggestions with your colleagues and manager, as appropriate.
  - Invite the safeguarding lead to a team or unit meeting to provide updates on new policies and procedures.
- **Being a champion for older people**

  A healthcare practitioner can be a formal or informal champion, and support and defend the provision of privacy, dignity, and person-centred care for older people.
  - Think about the opportunities that are available to you to provide best practice and to encourage your colleagues to do the same.
  - You may wish to join the Department of Health's Dignity in Care Champions Network, information about which is available online at http://www.dh.gov.uk/en/SocialCare/Socialcarereform/Dignityincare/DH_065407

References

Action on Elder Abuse (2010) 'What is elder abuse?', available online at http://www.elderabuse.org.uk/About%20Abuse/What_is_abuse%20define.htm.

Age UK (2010) *Poor-quality Care Services: The Big Q*, available online at http://www.ageuk.org.uk/get-involved/campaign/poor-quality-care-services-big-q/.

Care Quality Commission (2009) *National NHS Patient Survey Programme: Survey of Adult Inpatients 2008,* London: CQC, available online at http://www.cqc.org.uk/usingcareservices/healthcare/patientsurveys/hospitalcare/inpatientservices.cfm.

Centre for Social Care Inspection/Audit Commission/Healthcare Commission (2006) *Living Well in Later Life, London: Commission for Healthcare Audit and Inspection*

Dean, M. (2003) *Growing Older in the 21st Century,* Swindon: Economic and Social Research Council

Department of Health (2000) *No Secrets: Guidance on Developing and Implementing Multi-agency Policies and Procedures to Protect Vulnerable Adults from Abuse, available online at* http://www.dh.gov.uk/en/Publicationsandstatistics/Publications/PublicationsPolicyAndGuidance/DH_4008486.

Department of Health (2001a) *National Service Framework for Older People*, London: DH.

Department of Health (2001b) *The Essence of Care: Patient-focused Benchmarks for Clinical Governance*, London: HMSO.

Department of Health (2003) *The Essence of Care: Patient-focused Benchmarks for Clinical Governance*, available online at http://www.dh.gov.uk/prod_consum_dh/groups/dh_digitalassets/@dh/@en/documents/digitalasset/dh_4127915.pdf.

Department of Health (2006a) *A New Ambition for Old Age: The Next Five Years*, London: DH.

Department of Health (2006b) *The Dignity in Care Campaign*, available online at http://www.dhcarenetworks.org.uk/dignityincare/DignityCareCampaign/.

Department of Health (2007) Mental Capacity Act 2005 Deprivation of Liberty Safeguards Code of Practice, available online at http://www.dh.gov.uk/en/Consultations/Responsestoconsultations/DH_085353.

Department of Health (2008a) *High-quality Care for All: NHS Next-stage Review Final Report,* available online at http://www.dh.gov.uk/en/Publicationsandstatistics/Publications/PublicationsPolicyAndGuidance/DH_085825.

Department of Health (2008b) *Confidence in Caring: A Framework for Best Practice,* available online at http://www.dh.gov.uk/en/Publicationsandstatistics/Publications/PublicationsPolicyAndGuidance/DH_086387.

Department of Health (2009) *The National Health Service Constitution for England,* available online at http://www.dh.gov.uk/en/Publicationsandstatistics/Publications/PublicationsPolicyAndGuidance/DH_093419.

Department of Health (2010a) *Robert Francis Inquiry Report into the Mid-Staffordshire NHS Foundation Trust,* available online at http://www.dh.gov.uk/en/publicationsandstatistics/publications/publicationspolicyandguidance/dh_113018.

Department of Health (2010b) *Government Response to the Consultation on Safeguarding Adults: The Review of the No Secrets Guidance,* London: HMSO, available online at http://www.dh.gov.uk/en/Publicationsandstatistics/Publications/PublicationsPolicyAndGuidance/DH_093419.

Doe Consortium (2005) *Dignity and Older Europeans: A Multidisciplinary Workbook*, available online at http://medic.cardiff.ac.uk/archive_subsites/_/_/medic/subsites/dignity/resources/Educating_for_Dignity.pdf.

Gender, A.R. (2002) 'Administration and Leadership', in S.P. Hoeman (ed.) *Rehabilitation Nursing: Process, Application and Outcomes,* St Louis, MI: Mosby.

Healthcare Commission (2007) *Caring for Dignity: A National Report on Dignity of Care for Older People While in Hospital,* London: Healthcare Commission.

Hindle, A. (2008) 'Champions for Older People Programme', *Ageing & Health* [Journal of the Institute of Ageing and Health West Midlands] 16: 20–3.

Homer, A.C. and Gilleard, C. (1990) 'Abuse of elderly people by their carers', *British Medical Journal*, 301:1359–62.

Independent Safeguarding Authority *(2009) Vetting and Barring Scheme*, available online at http://www.isa-gov.org.uk/.

Manthorpe, J., Clough, R., Cornes, M., Bright, L., Moriaty, J., Iliffe, S., and Older People Researching Social Issues (2007) 'Four years on: The impact of the National Service Framework for Older People on the experiences and views of older people'; *Age and Ageing,* 36(5): 501–7.

NHS Institute for Innovation and Improvement (2008) *Privacy and Dignity: The Elimination of Mixed Sex Accommodation*, Coventry: NHS Institute for Innovation and Improvement.

O'Keeffe, M., Doyle, M., McCreadie, C., Scholes, S., Constatine, R., Tinker, A., Manthorpe, J., Biggs, S., and Erens, B. (2007) *UK Study of Abuse and Neglect of Older People: Prevelance Study Report,* London: National Centre for Social Research, available online at http://www.kcl.ac.uk/content/1/c6/02/96/45/Natcenresearchfindings.pdf.

Royal College of Nursing (2000) *Sexuality and Sexual Health in Nursing Practice,* London: RCN.

Royal College of Nursing (2008) *Defending Dignity: Challenges and Opportunities for Nursing,* London, RCN.

Social Care Institute for Excellence (2006) *Adult Services Practice Guide: Dignity in Care,* London: SCIE.

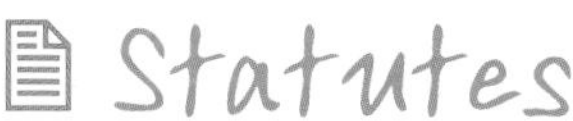

Mental Capacity Act 2005

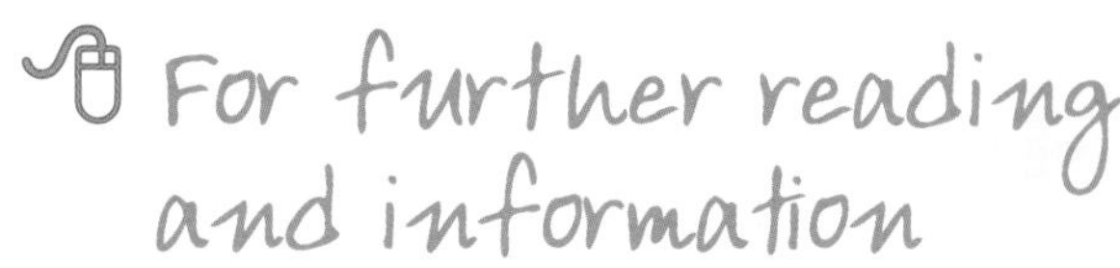

Independent Safeguarding Authority: http://www.isa-gov.org.uk/.

NHS Choices: http://www.nhs.uk/Pages/homepage.aspx

Nordenfelt, L. (2009) *Dignity in Care for Older People*, Oxford: Wiley-Blackwell.

Nursing and Midwifery Council (2009) *Guidance for the Care of Older People,* London: NMC.

Royal College of Nursing 'Dignity' page: http://www.rcn.org.uk/dignity.

Online Resource Centre

You can learn more about dignity, values attitudes, and person-centered care for older people at the Online Resource Centre that accompanies this book: and care http://**www.oxfordtextbooks.co.uk/orc/hindle/**

Hearing and sight loss

Andrew Hindle, Debbie Lynch, and Darren McHale

Learning outcomes

By the end of this chapter, you will be able to:

- understand the prevalence and impact of hearing loss;
- identify how communication skills can be improved;
- understand the practical support that nurses can offer a person with hearing loss;
- demonstrate knowledge of aids that are available to help people with a hearing loss;
- understand and respond to the needs of people with sight loss;
- recognize common causes of sight loss;
- understand the practical support that nurses can offer a person with sight loss; and
- have an increased awareness of what it might feel like to live with a sight loss.

Introduction to hearing and sight loss

Sensory loss (that is, hearing and/or sight loss) is prevalent in older people. The impact that this can have on quality of life can be immense and can result in difficulties, with communication leading to isolation and impaired psychosocial functioning. The loss of either hearing or sight can lead to many challenges for individuals, and for their families and carers. This can be further complicated where there are co-morbidities, and particularly if both sight and hearing are impaired. People who have combined sight-and-hearing loss suffer from high levels of psychological stress (Pavey et al., 2009). Specialist support is required and charities such as SENSE play an important role. (Its website provides helpful information and advice, see http://www.sense.org.uk/.)

This chapter provides an introduction to the anatomy and physiology of the ear and eye, and explores the age-related changes. There is an overview of medical conditions that can arise and the management of these. The experiences that older people face are discussed, along with the strategies, skills, and practical insights that can help nurses to communicate and support people with sensory loss.

Given that older people are the main users of health services in the UK—for example, two-thirds of hospital beds are utilized by older people (DH, 2001)—it is obvious that nurses will come into contact on a daily basis with people with some degree of sensory impairment. Yet their main reason for utilizing health services is usually secondary to their sensory loss, and consequently may not receive the focus and attention that they require. It is also important to note that many older people believe sensory problems are inevitable, and thus avoid seeking medical assessment and assistance (Grue et al., 2009).

The chapter is written by experts in the specialist fields of supporting and treating people with sensory loss. We hope that our philosophy of care will prove insightful to the reader and that nurses will have a heightened awareness of the needs of people with sensory impairment, as well as improve their skills, standards of care, and address the specific needs for this client group. This will enable older people to increase their opportunities to engage socially.

Section one: Hearing loss

Introduction to hearing loss

'Old age does not come alone' is a phrase commonly used by patients in audiology clinic. Hearing loss, deteriorating sight, and poorer cognitive ability all contribute to significant sensory deprivation that is associated with the ageing process. There is a correlation between sensory and cognitive function decline in those over the age of 80 (Baltes et al., 1999), and it is a combination of these factors that can result in social isolation and exclusion from healthcare services. Launching the report at the Strategies for an Ageing Population conference in June 2009, Jackie Ballard, Royal National Institute for the Deaf (RNID) Chief Executive, identified that:

Around 4 million people in the UK could benefit from wearing a hearing aid. We find it staggering that it still takes people around 10 to 15 years before they address their hearing loss, compared to around three years for sight problems.

Age is a major predictor of hearing impairment: as the population ages, more people will be affected (DH, 2007). Hearing loss is the most common disability among older people, affecting one in two people over the age of 60 (RNID, 2009).

Approximately one in five adults in the UK has hearing loss in both ears, which has an impact on their communication ability. In people aged 55–74, 12 per cent have a hearing problem that causes moderate or severe worry, annoyance, or upset (Davis et al., 2007). The severity of hearing loss is significantly associated with reduced quality of life in older adults (Dalton et al., 2003). Clearly, nurses have a role to play in being aware of the extent of the problem, being vigilant to its consequences, and applying theoretical knowledge to limit the impact of hearing loss on the lives of older people.

Definitions

People suffering from hearing loss or deafness identify themselves in different ways, but there are four main categories:

- the **hard of hearing**—likely to have useable hearing, may use a hearing aid, and have normal speech;
- the **deaf**—may not use speech as first language and may use sign language;
- the **deafened**—likely to have become deaf having previously had full hearing; and
- the **deafblind**—different degrees of hearing and sight, may use Braille, and may use manual alphabet or block letters written on the hand.

Acoustics

The physical properties of sound can be measured in terms of amplitude: the higher the amplitude of the sound wave, the higher the intensity—that is, the louder the sounds. The intensity of sound is measured in decibels (dB). To be more precise, it is measured in Decibels of Sound Pressure Level (dBSPL).

A sound of higher frequency will have a shorter wavelength (cycle). The number of cycles per second is measured in hertz (Hz). The range of frequency heard by the human ear is 20–20,000 Hz. Speech sounds generally occur in the range of 200–8,000 Hz.

An important concept of physics and acoustics is the 'inverse square law'. When you call a patient from a waiting room or from the end of a bed space, the sound comes from a focal point, then radiates out from you into a big open space. The further the patient is away from you, the more the sound spreads and reduces in intensity. This means that sound intensity is inversely proportional to the distance from the sound source.

NURSING PRACTICE INSIGHT

Be mindful of the effect of distance on an older person's hearing ability or you will fail to communicate effectively with your patients.

Anatomy and physiology

The ear (see Figure 3.1) consists of three main sections: the outer ear; the middle ear; and the inner ear. The outer ear is the 'pinna' (sometimes called the 'auricle'). The ear canal (the 'meatus') is approximately 2.5 cm long, generally oval in shape, and has a slight bend (useful to note if examining ears for wax and blockages). The outer third is cartilaginous and the inner two-thirds are bone. The function of the outer ear is to protect the eardrum (the 'tympanic membrane'): it acts as a funnel for the sound to travel into the ear. The pinna can amplify sounds by 6 dB. The pinna also helps with the ability to localize sound. A good example of this is when a cat or dog hears a sound: their ears prick up and turn towards the direction of the sound.

Table 3.1 Examples of sound levels

Threshold of pain	140 dBSPL
Loud speech	70–80 dBSPL
Conversational speech	60–70 dBSPL
Soft speech	35–45 dBSPL

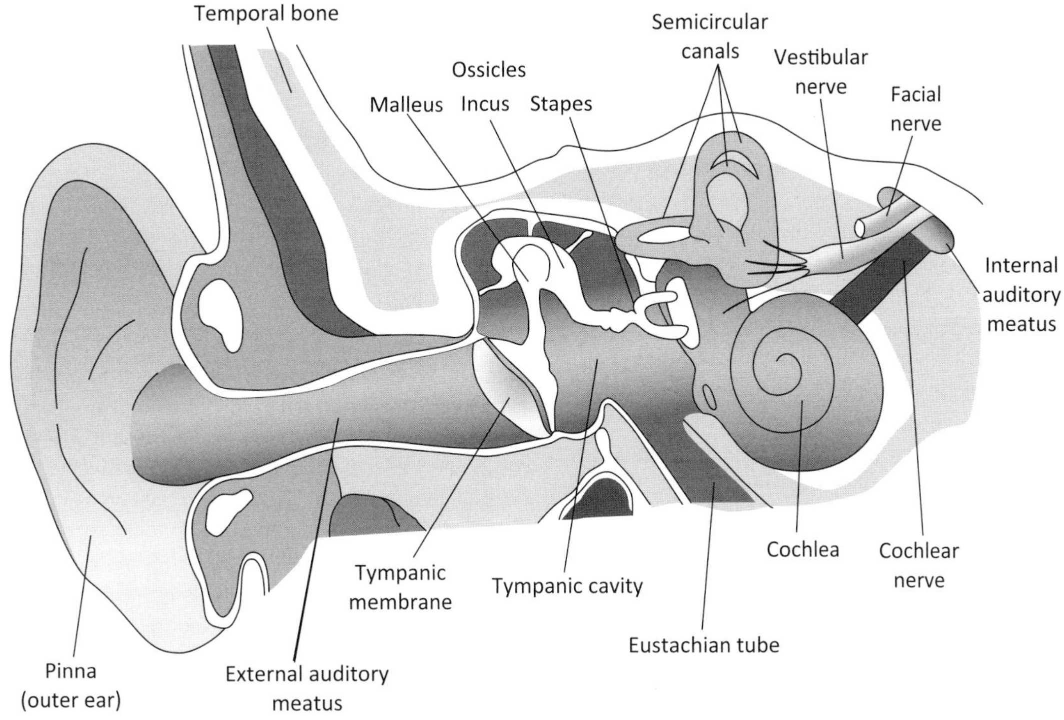

Figure 3.1 The ear.

The pinna (see Figure 3.2) does not have a profuse blood supply. People that have prolonged exposure to sun are at risk of developing cancerous growths on the pinna. A retrospective study of 426 patients with malignant growths in the head and neck area found that 51 patients had carcinoma lesions over the pinna (Ahmed and Das Gupta, 2001).

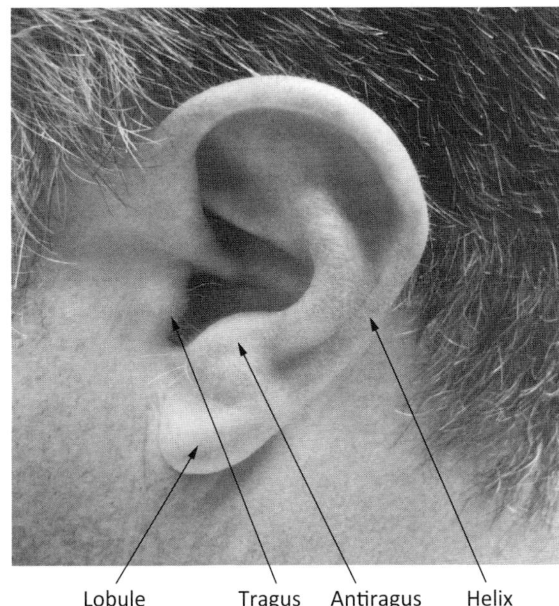

Figure 3.2 The pinna

The middle ear contains the ear drum, or tympanic membrane (see Figure 3.3), which is about 9 mm by 8 mm and contains three layers. The tissue on the lower face of the ear drum is called the 'pars tensa', because it is tight, and the upper part is the 'pars flaccida'.

Attached to the back of the tympanic membrane are the three middle ear bones, or 'ossicles': the hammer (the 'malleus), the anvil (the 'incus), and the stirrup (the 'stapes). The stapes is the smallest bone in your body and is attached to the middle ear cavity by the stapedius muscle. The middle ear has the ability to increase the transfer of energy, so that it is great enough to cause vibration in the fluids of the inner ear. This transfer of energy is possible because the surface area of the eardrum is

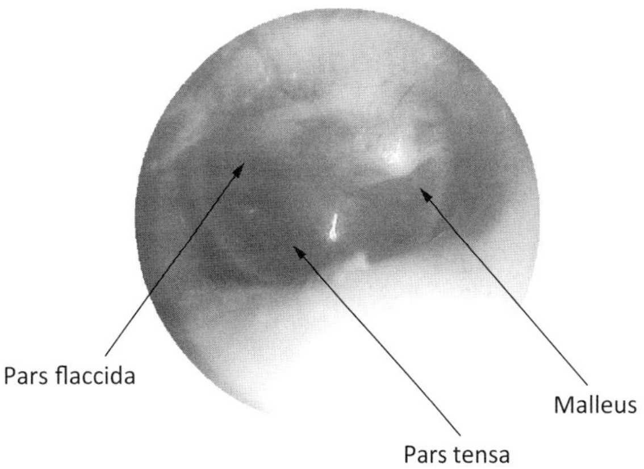

Figure 3.3 The tympanic membrane

much greater than the oval window (that is, the entrance to the cochlea), and so in this way the energy is focused.

The 'Eustachian tube' connects the middle ear to the pharynx. By permitting air to leave or enter the middle ear, the tube equalizes air pressure on either side of the eardrum. When the Eustachian tube is occluded, it can lead to a middle ear infection ('otitis media').

The inner ear has a balance and hearing function. The hearing function is a complex system involving conversion of vibration energy into electrical nerve impulses carrying frequency specific information into the higher centres of the brain. The cochlea converts the sound vibration into electrical signals in the form of nerve impulses. The cochlea is contained in a two-and-a-half turn funnel and in appearance is like a snail shell with three compartments: the 'scala vestibule' and the 'scala tympani', which both contain perilymph fluid, and the inner portion—that is, the 'scala media'—which contains the endolymphatic fluid, which is high in potassium (K^+) and low in sodium (Na^+) ions.

The sensory epithelium of the inner ear is called the 'organ of Corti', and contains outer and inner hair cells. There are approximately 3,500 inner hair cells and 12,000 outer hair cells. The outer hair cells are embedded into a thin gelatinous membrane that stretches across the top of the hair cells. When vibration of the fluid inside the cochlea occurs, then a 'shearing action' across the hair cells takes place, bending the hair cell and creating what is known as a 'transduction channel', which allows the flow of the potassium ions into the hair cells and enables a chemical exchange to take place. This results in an action potential in the neurons in the auditory nerve, so that the nerve impulse stimulates the hearing centres in the brain—primarily, the auditory cortex.

Common ear conditions

Cerumen (ear wax) impaction

The function of cerumen (that is, ear wax) is to cleanse, protect, and lubricate the ear canal. However, it can also build up and cause impaction. Cerumen is the most common hearing problem associated with older people and a fully blocked ear can cause substantial hearing loss. Impacted ear wax is a major cause of primary care consultation and a common problem in older people (Guest et al., 2004). One in five visits to the practice nurse is for ear care (Rodgers, 1994) and 2.3 million people in the UK will need intervention for impacted wax each year (Guest et al., 2004).

Management

Ear wax that has become impacted can be removed by softening ear drops that can be purchased over the counter or prescribed. If this fails to remove the wax, then syringing can be performed by a skilled nurse or doctor.

Perforated ear drum

The eardrum (the tympanic membrane) can be perforated if objects are pushed down the ear canal. If the eardrum is perforated, it no longer acts as an effective drum and therefore does not conduct the sound vibrations further down into the inner ear—hence a problem with sound conduction and a conductive hearing loss. Damage to the tympanic membrane and to the ossicles can cause significant hearing loss. It has been known for people to fracture their middle ear bones (the malleus, incus and stapes) by forcing down a cotton bud.

Management

A perforated eardrum will usually heal by itself within six to eight weeks. When healing does not take place, then a surgical procedure may be required. A tympanoplasty is reconstructive surgery of the eardrum or the small bones of the middle ear.

Otosclerosis

Otosclerosis is a calcification of the joint at the stapes, which attaches to the cochlea. This condition is more common in the younger age groups. However, the condition is a slow, progressive process and in older people it can ultimately cause significant sensorineural hearing loss.

Management

Bilateral hearing aids may be helpful where there is hearing loss. In some cases, a stapedectomy is required. This is a surgical procedure replacing the stapes with an artificial bone.

Acute otitis media

Acute otitis media (that is, ear infection) is caused by a fluid buildup in the middle ear space (as a possible consequence of Eustachian tube dysfunction). This will cause ear pain and a conductive hearing loss.

Management

The majority of cases of acute otitis media clear up within three days without any treatment. Antibiotics may be prescribed if the infection is getting severe. Over-the-counter analgesics may be used to control any pain and fever.

Presbyacusis

Presbyacusis is a progressive condition and the medical term for hearing loss that occurs in some people as they age. The sensory cells of the inner ear (the hair cells) degenerate, leaving the auditory system less sensitive to higher frequency sounds. This is why you get the typical response: 'I am not deaf—there is no need to shout, just speak clearly.' It arises when certain pitches of sound can be heard adequately, but other pitches are no longer within the person's hearing ability. This causes a loss of sensory perception, and hearing loss related to the cochlear and auditory nerve pathway. It is generally termed 'sensori-neural hearing loss', because it is a loss of sensory perception and it relates to the neural pathways.

Management

With mild hearing loss, most people manage well and do not require treatment and speaking clearly will help. When hearing loss increases, then a hearing aid will be required.

Tinnitus

Another common condition is tinnitus, which comes from the Latin *tinnire* meaning 'to ring'. It is a sound heard that has no external stimulus; it might be any sound, or several sounds, not necessarily a ringing. Tinnitus dates back to Egyptian times, when potions were administered to the ear by reed stalks; strange potions in later times included boiled dormouse. There are 4.7 million adults that are affected by tinnitus in the UK and for one in ten it has a severe effect on their quality of life (RNID, 2006).

Management

Typically, patients are told that there is nothing that can be done, and they have to go away and live with it. However, people often find great relief from psychological therapies, tinnitus-retraining therapy, and habituation therapy as a means of reducing the effect and changing the patient's reaction to the tinnitus.

Balance disorders associated with the ears

Common balance disorders are benign paroxysmal positional vertigo (BPPV), which is a short-lived dizziness, typically lasting seconds—for example, when turning over in bed, looking up when in supermarkets, or tipping the head back when having hair washed. This suggests that it is a benign condition, but it can be most disturbing for the individual, and in 80 per cent of cases, it can be treated effectively by an ear, nose, and throat consultant, audiological practitioner, or physiotherapist trained in balance. Population estimates on the frequency of BPPV across various age groups show an increasing prevalence in older people, reaching 10 per cent in people over the age of 80 (Bronstein and Lempert, 2007).

Other related conditions

The outer ear containing the pinna and the meatus is susceptible to ageing conditions of the skin, such as atrophy, loss of elasticity, and dehydration. This can lead to the supporting cartilage collapsing, and can cause problems with fitting ear moulds for hearing aids and discomfort for the patient. It can sometimes lead to inaccurate hearing test results due to collapsing of the ear canal when headphone pressure is applied during a hearing test. If wax or infection blocks the external auditory meatus, then sound is dampened up to 40 dB. Typically, this is known as a 'conductive hearing loss' because there is a problem with sound conduction.

Age-related hearing loss generally should not involve ear pain and the patient should not have any discharge from the ear. If these symptoms occur, then a medical opinion should be sought, because it is unlikely to be solely age-related hearing loss.

Experiences of deaf and hard-of-hearing people

The Royal National Institute of Deaf People (RNID) and the UK Council of Deafness (UKCoD) undertook a survey of 866 deaf and hard-of-hearing groups, and found the following experiences:

- **35% of deaf and hard of hearing people experienced difficulty in communicating with their GP or Nurse**
- **42% of deaf and hard of hearing people who had visited hospital (non emergency) had found it difficult to communicate with NHS staff. This increased to 66% amongst British Sign Language (BSL) users**
- **24% of all respondents had missed an appointment at their GP surgery because of poor communication.**

(RNID/UKCoD, 2004).

The full report is available online at http://www.rnid.org.uk/, and provides stark reading for health professionals and identifies how people with a hearing loss are excluded from obtaining healthcare services.

Table 3.2 Common ear conditions with consequences and type of hearing loss

Common conditions	Outer ear	Middle ear	Inner ear	Consequences and type of loss
Ear wax	✓			Conductive loss of hearing up to 40 dB; can cause discomfort
Ear infection	✓	✓	✓	Conductive hearing loss; discharging ears; can be painful; viral infection of inner ear can cause balance problems
Otitis externa (infection of outer ear canal)	✓			Inflamation of the ear canal
Foreign bodies in the ear, (e.g. cotton bud end)	✓			Conductive loss of hearing; sometimes pain
Perforated ear drum	✓	✓		Conductive hearing loss
Thinning of ear drum, less vascular, rigid		✓		Conductive loss
Meatal atresia (skin changes and atrophy)	✓	✓		Conductive loss
Otosclerosis (calcification of stapes joint)		✓	✓	Conductive component in early stages; can develop into sensory loss in later stages
Ossification/arthritis		✓		Conductive loss
Noise-induced hearing loss			✓	High-frequency hearing loss; sensori neural
Tinnitus			✓	Does not necessarily have associated hearing loss; can have significant psychological impact
Menieres disease			✓	Severe rotational dizziness lasting from minutes to days; progressive hearing loss
Benign paroxysmal positional vertigo (BPPV)			✓	Brief dizziness based on position

Social isolation and the psychological impact of hearing loss

A major consequence for older people of having hearing loss is social withdrawal and isolation. An acquired profound hearing loss will also have a greater psychosocial impact than a milder hearing loss (Hallam et al., 2006). Hearing loss has even been compared to the grieving process and has been seen to involve the stages of bereavement—that is, denial, anger, bargaining, and acceptance (Levene and Tait, 2005). The inability to communicate can limit people's ability to function in the world around them. People with hearing loss can feel isolated from everyday social activities—for example, they may begin to withdraw from social functions, making excuses that their hearing loss will prevent them from being able to participate.

Common problems experienced by people with hearing loss

The following experiences are common among people with hearing loss.

- Typically, patients with hearing loss find it very difficult to follow a conversation if there is background noise—for example, television, radio, or children playing.
- People often find that they can hear television newsreaders, for example, but find that plays and dramas on television are difficult to follow.
- Children are often difficult to hear, because they have softer voices of a higher pitch (typically the range that is difficult to hear).
- The person with a hearing loss may believe that other people are mumbling and not recognize that they have a hearing loss.

- They may stop trying to engage in social situations and suffer from the feelings summarized in Figure 3.4.

Hearing loss and mental health

The impact of hearing loss on mental health in the literature generally points to it having a greater affect on younger adults (Tambs, 2004). This is probably as a consequence of hearing loss in older people being a gradual process, rather than the more sudden onset generally seen in younger adults. The Department of Health (2002) identifies that deaf people of all ages are disadvantaged in trying to access mental health services due to communication difficulties and a lack of services to meet their needs.

Hearing loss in older people may also be mistaken for cognitive impairment (NHS QIS, 2005). The nurse therefore has an important role in distinguishing between any hearing and cognitive impairment, and ensuring that comprehensive and accurate assessment is undertaken.

See Chapter 11 for more on hearing loss in relation to dementia and mental health.

What is it like to have hearing loss as a result of the ageing process?

As identified earlier, the ageing process primarily affects the hair cells in the cochlea—but what does this mean for the person experiencing this deterioration? Difficulty hearing high frequencies is most common, which means that certain sounds become inaudible.

- **Try working out this sentence:**

  Th_/b_y /w _nt /t_ /th _ /sh _p.

The answer of course is: 'The boy went to the shop'. This is the sentence that you would hear if all of the vowels were removed, which are generally the low-frequency sounds. You were probably able to work out the meaning of this sentence, because the most essential parts for meaning were present (that is, heard).

- **Can you understand this sentence?**

  _ _e/_o_/_a_/ o_/_ _e /_ _a_ _

The answer is: 'The dog sat on the grass'. In this case, the consonants are missing, which are the high-frequency sounds. High-frequency hearing loss has a far greater effect on the person's ability to extract the key information. Because of missing key parts of the words, they are unable to understand what is being said and taking part in ordinary conversation becomes difficult.

How to communicate effectively with people who have hearing loss

The exchange of information with others, which is fundamental to everyday life, can be seriously impaired in individuals

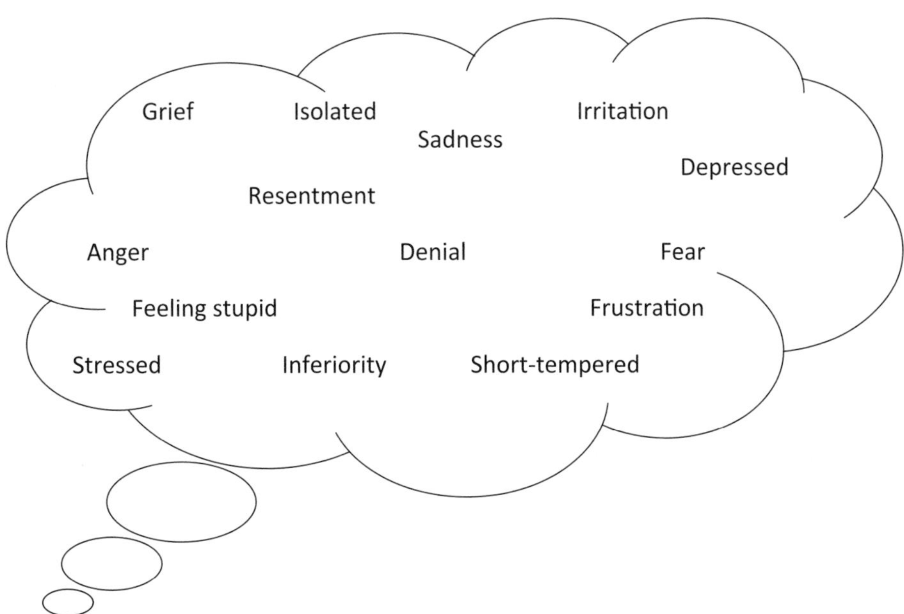

Figure 3.4 Emotions felt by those with hearing loss

with hearing loss (Dalton et al., 2003). Thus, the nurse needs to be proactive in addressing communication difficulties. As previously discussed, background noise is a major barrier to communication for hearing-impaired people and, in particular, people with age-related deafness. The recent emphasis on infection control has led to increased use of vinyl easy-wipe floors and surfaces, which creates very poor acoustic environments, and therefore becomes challenging for those with hearing loss and, in particular, those who wear hearing aids.

Communication involves several processes in addition to auditory processing: visual clues, body posture, and gesture. As demonstrated in the above sentence exercises, not all of the information is always required to understand the context. Therefore, the hearing-impaired person may well use some or all of these additional factors to fill in the gaps. The person that intently looks for facial clues and/or the person that invades your personal space may simply be striving to make sense of what you are saying.

In the same way, barriers to good communication will be things that restrict these processes: for example, poor lighting impairs the ability to see the face of the person speaking and hence loses vital clues from lip-reading. This is especially the case if the light is behind the communicator, because it casts their face into shadow.

Being clear in what you say and how you say it is important. Think before you speak or ask for information, ensuring that your message is clear and checking that you have been understood. This is particularly important in relation to gaining consent from a patient before carrying out a procedure.

NURSING PRACTICE INSIGHT: KEY SKILLS TO MORE EFFECTIVE COMMUNICATION

Noise

- Reduce the background noise.

Distance

- Reduce the distance between yourself and the patient.

Vision

- Consider where you stand in relation to windows and lighting. Sit with the light on your face, so that your expression and lips can be clearly seen.

Clarity

- Alert the person before talking to them.
- Speak clearly and with natural rhythm (that is, do not overexaggerate).
- Speak slowly.
- Rephrase sentences if not understood (rather than simply repeat them louder, which does not help).
- Use short sentences.
- Check understanding. (It is useful to get the person to repeat what it is they think you have said—but be careful not to do overdo this to avoid being patronizing.)

It is paramount that the nurse feels confident enough to raise the issue of hearing loss with patients so that potentially life-changing support can be made available to them.

Aids to communication

There are relatively low levels of hearing-device usage within Western countries (Smith et al., 2005). Only marginal numbers of older people who might benefit from hearing aids own one and even fewer use them (Smeeth et al., 2002). Yet there is a vast range of devices that can be utilized to improve hearing loss and therefore have a positive impact on quality of life.

Hearing aid

A hearing aid is an amplification device and therefore makes things louder. Hearing aids have significantly improved over the last decade, with the introduction of digital hearing aid technology. The hearing aid can be programmed to the individual's hearing loss and most hearing aids are fitted to a prescriptive formula that calculates the amount of amplification needed. The main disadvantage of hearing aids is the problem with background noise. Most hearing aid users find the level of background noise intrusive and distracting. Digital aids are better at dealing with background noise than earlier analogue hearing aids, but still do not remove the noise completely.

For the nurse to communicate with a hearing aid wearer, try to reduce as much of the background noise as possible. A side room with better acoustics is ideal.

A good hearing aid is one that is IN, ON, and WORKING.

Additional aids to communication

- **Text phones**—Enables the person receiving the call to read text.
- **Sign language interpreters**—It is the responsibility of the healthcare provider to ensure that suitable language interpreting services are available.
- **Lipspeakers**—People who are trained to convey the message by lip movement. This is particularly useful in meetings.
- **Loop systems**—Good effective ways of reducing background noise; personal loop systems might be used in a

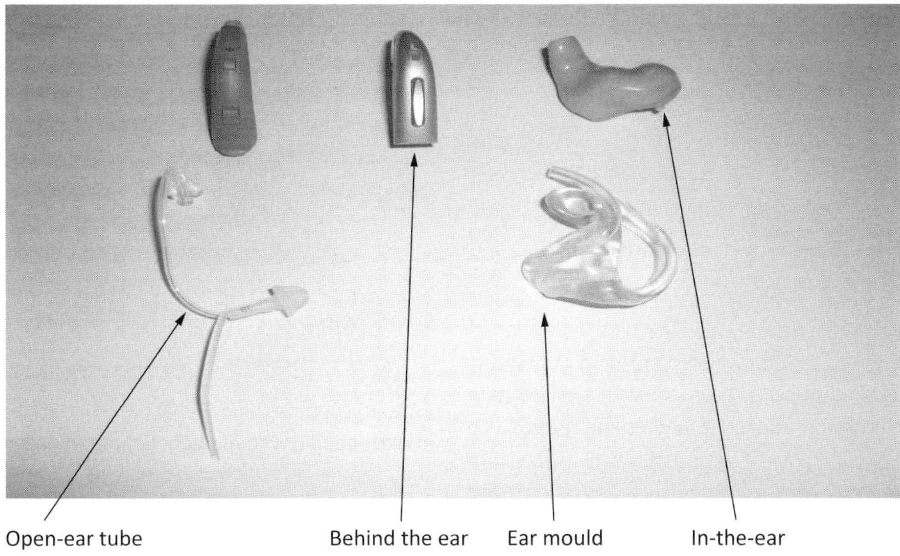

Figure 3.5 Hearing aid formats

ward setting to reduce background noise. Loop systems are beneficial, as the speaker uses a microphone and the wearer (generally for personal loops) wears a neck loop.

Table 3.3 Hearing aid troubleshooting

Fault	Consequence	Solution
Hearing aid incorrectly inserted in the ear (see Figure 3.6)	Hearing aid whistles	Fit the aid correctly
Hearing aid whistles	Patient or nurse turns the volume of the hearing aid down, stops the whistle, but patient cannot hear	Check aid is fitted correctly; check for ear wax
No sound from hearing aid	Patient cannot hear	Change the battery (typically a hearing aid battery lasts two–three weeks if used all day)
No sound from hearing aid despite new battery	Patient cannot hear	Check tubing is not blocked by condensation or wax

Note: Hearing aids should be regularly cleaned to keep them in good working condition, with ear moulds and tubing kept free of debris to ensure optimal hearing results.

- **SMS text messaging**—With mobile phone technology, SMS messaging is an ideal way to communicate important information. (Care is needed to ensure patient confidentiality.)
- **Written material**—Ensure that people are literate before relying on written information

Perspectives of people with hearing loss

The following comments were made by a nurse who has severe hearing loss and works in a hospital ward.

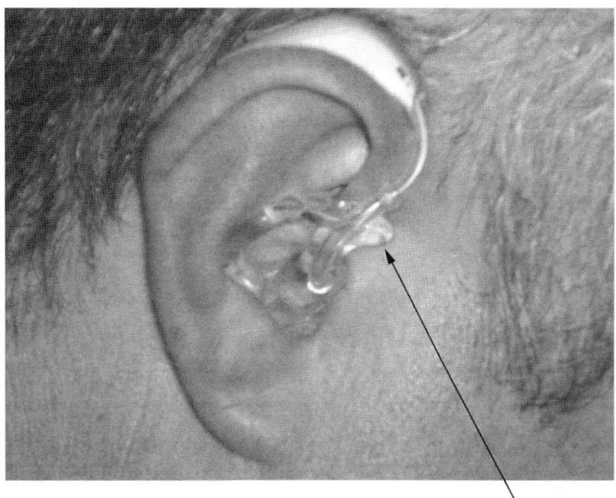

Figure 3.6 Incorrectly fitted ear mould

- On a day to day basis, with lots of different staff about, it is not always passed over about a patient's deafness, therefore creating the patient's first barrier to communication.
- Basic hearing aid knowledge is poor amongst nursing staff.
- We have basic teaching packs to aid communication with patients. This includes: pen and paper; finger spell boards; and picture boards. Sadly, these are not used enough.

The following are comments from an elderly patient who, at the time of writing this chapter, had recently had a six-week hospital stay following surgery. The person is a local hearing aid volunteer and plays an active role in Hearing Concern.

- None of the nursing staff had any idea about hearing aids[...] There should be at least one member of staff trained to deal with hearing aids on each ward and in nursing homes[...]
- My hearing aids were sent down to Audiology as they thought they were faulty. When I was given them back, I was not told what had been the fault, if any.

Both of these perspectives highlight the need to raise awareness of the difficulties faced by people with hearing loss. Improved training and education is needed for all staff, as is access to communication aids.

Case study

Mr Williams is a 61-year-old gentleman who has been admitted to hospital. He has had a fall and now needs hip replacement. He has recently been fitted with a digital hearing aid by his local adult hearing aid service. He was finding his hearing aid useful at home, but since being in hospital, he is struggling to hear other patients on the ward and is finding it particularly difficult to hear the nurses.

Mr Williams' daughter quickly realizes that her father is becoming very upset and appears very anxious. She reports her concerns to you and asks you if there is anything that can be done to help.

- **Why do you think Mr Williams might be experiencing hearing problems in the hospital?**
- **What changes could you make to the ward environment to help to improve Mr Williams' ability to hear?**
- **What changes to your communication skills could you make to improve communication between yourself and Mr Williams?**

In the case study above, the ward is noisier than at home and Mr Williams is likely to be anxious. Mr Williams needs all of his processing powers to follow and process speech, and the noisy busy ward, with so much background noise, challenges this focus. Mr Williams is used to having one-to-one conversation at close quarters; now, he is having conversations at a distance with nurses and other patients in less-than-ideal acoustic conditions.

To improve communication, you must remember: **noise**, **distance**, **vision**, and **clarity**.

Conclusion to hearing loss

Sacks (1990) wrote '*We are remarkably ignorant about deafness* [...] *ignorant and indifferent*', and despite the huge advances in technology in hearing aids, those who cannot hear are still at a disadvantage—often not by the technology, but by people, and health and social care professionals, who fail to use good communication skills. Twenty years on and, sadly, the evidence suggests that this statement still stands.

However, nurses can be far more supportive and improve their communication skills when working with hearing-loss patients by increasing their knowledge and the identification of ear conditions that result in hearing loss, and applying the techniques suggested in this chapter.

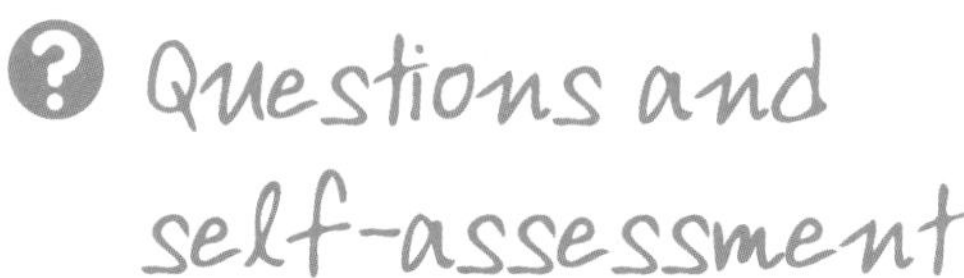

Now that you have worked through section one, answer the following questions.

- What are the main causes of older adult hearing loss?
- What skills should the nurse use when communicating with a person with hearing loss?
- What practical support can nurses offer a person with hearing loss?
- What different types of hearing aid are available for people with a hearing loss?

Self-assessment

- Having read the chapter, how will you change your practice?
- Identify up to three areas relating to hearing loss in which you need to develop your knowledge and understanding further.
- Identify how you are going to develop this knowledge and understanding, and set deadlines for achieving these.

Section two: Sight loss

Introduction to sight loss

There are 1.7 million people over the age of 65 in the UK who have a significant sight loss, and this number is expected to double in the next 25 years due to an ageing population and the increase of diabetes (RNIB, 2006a). Therefore, nurses can expect to come into contact with large numbers of older people with visual impairment.

Vision loss in older people is an independent risk factor for disorientation, disability, loss of independence, and social isolation (Horowitz, 2004). Older people also face difficulties with interacting with those who provide care and services. This is due to a lack of awareness, knowledge, skills, and understanding of the impact of sight loss by health professionals (Campbell, 2005; Smith, 2006).

The first part of the chapter aims to cover the key causes of sight loss, and to help the nurse gain a better understanding of the problems that are incurred and practical solutions that will help them to support people with sight loss. The chapter will then cover support services to help people with sight loss.

The eye is shaped like a ball. The 'cornea' is the very front part of the eye and is transparent. The 'sclera' is the firm, white, fibrous membrane that forms the outer covering of the eyeball, covering the entire eyeball except the cornea. The 'pupil', close to the front, is the opening that allows light to enter the eye. Just behind the pupil is the 'lens', which focuses the light onto the retina at the back of the eye. The 'retina' is a delicate tissue, which converts the light into images and sends them to the brain. The 'vitreous' is a clear, jelly-like substance that helps the eye to keep its shape. The 'iris' is the coloured part of the eye, which helps to control the size of the pupil. The 'macula' helps the eye to see fine detail and colour. The 'optic nerve' connects the eye to the brain.

There are a number of age changes that affect the eye, including:

- the sclera may yellow and lose opacity;
- the cornea becomes thinner;
- the retina and optic pathways lose some of their cells, making it harder for the older person to see detail and colour contrast;
- the size of the pupil diminishes and this decreases the amount of light that can enter the eye, and the eye therefore admits less light to the retina; and
- the lens grows larger and there is less ability to focus on near objects.

Common causes of sight loss

The most common causes of sight loss are:

- age-related macular degeneration (AMD);
- cataract;
- glaucoma;
- diabetic retinopathy; and
- stroke.

AMD, glaucoma, and diabetic retinopathy have all increased in prevalence in England and Wales in the last two decades,

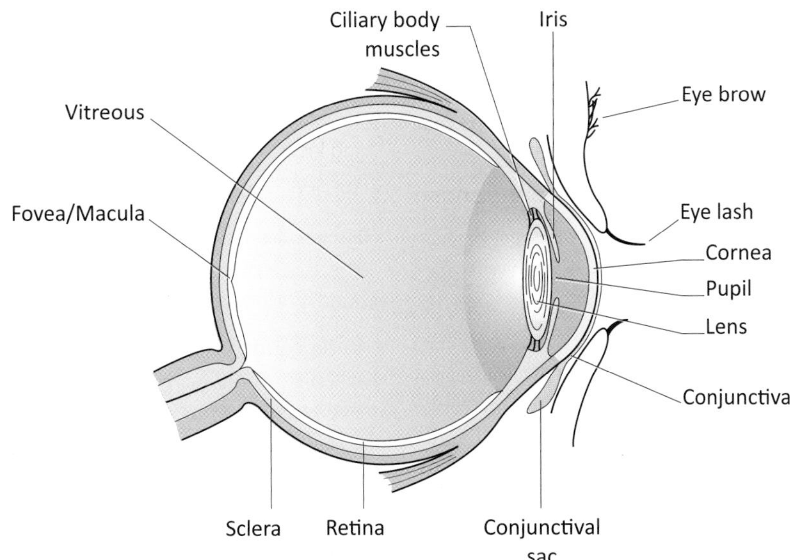

Figure 3.7 The eye

and figures for diabetic retinopathy among the over-65s have more than doubled (Bunce and Wormald, 2006).

See the Online Resource Centre for examples of what life might look like if you had AMD, cataracts, glaucoma, or diabetic retinopathy.

Age-related macular degeneration (AMD)

AMD is the most common cause of sight loss in the UK and it has been estimated that there are over 500,000 people with macular conditions in the UK (Macular Disease Society, 2008). AMD is a chronic degenerative condition characterized by loss of central vision due to diminished functioning of the macular of the retina.

There are two main forms of AMD: wet and dry. Approximately 90 per cent of people will have the dry form and10 per cent the wet form.

- **Non-neovascular (dry, atrophic) AMD** develops slowly, causing gradual loss of central vision. The main features are the yellowish-white spots identified as 'drusen' (that is, tiny yellowish hyaline deposits that develop between the retinal and hyaline epithelium).

  There is currently no treatment for advanced dry AMD. Techniques such as magnifying glasses can help people to live with the condition.

- **Exudative AMD (wet) AMD** has similar clinical features to dry AMD, but can develop quickly and is followed by abnormal leaking blood vessels (that is, subretinal fluid, haemorrhages, exudation), which can lead to severe loss of vision.

  The primary treatment is 'anti-vascular endothelial growth factor' medications (anti-VEGFs). These medications reduce the growth of new blood vessels, slow their leakage and reduce vision loss. Anti-VEGFs are administered as an injection into the vitreous via the scelera.

The Macular Disease Society website http://www.maculardisease.org/ offers further information.

Cataract

Cataract is a very common eye condition associated with ageing. A cataract arises when the lens inside the eye becomes opaque due to the degeneration of the lens fibres and reduces the amount of light able to reach the retina.

Cataracts can also be caused due to injury. They often occur in both eyes, but can affect only one eye at a time.

Cataracts can be treated by a surgical procedure: the cloudy lens is removed and replaced with a clear plastic lens, called an 'intraocular lens implant'. Cataract surgery is not performed on both eyes at once to avoid risk of blindness, such as a severe eye infection.

Glaucoma

In the UK, some form of glaucoma affects about 2 in 100 people over the age of 40 (RNIB, 2008). Glaucoma is the name for a group of eye conditions characterized by damage to the optic nerve, usually due to high intraocular pressure in the eye. In some people, the damage is caused by raised fluid pressure in the eye, which can occur when the aqueous fluid does not drain away properly. In other people, it can be caused because of damage or weakness in the optic nerve. Glaucoma damages a person's peripheral vision.

There are two main types of glaucoma.

- **Primary open-angle glaucoma** is the most common type. It occurs when there is gradual elevated pressure caused by a blockage and the aqueous fluid is unable to drain correctly. The eye pressure rises very slowly, causing the field of vision gradually to become impaired. This form of glaucoma is usually not painful.
- **Primary angle-closure glaucoma** is less common and occurs when the drainage of aqueous fluid is impaired, causing a rapid rise in pressure. This form of glaucoma can be painful and will cause permanent damage if treatment is not given very quickly.

Treatment with eye drops can limit damage to the eye if started at an early stage. The other key treatment procedures are laser surgery or an eye operation called a 'trabeculectomy'. This involves a small section of the trabecular meshwork (that is, the eye's drainage) being removed. This then allows aqueous fluid to bypass the blocked trabecular network, drain more easily, and relieve intraocular pressure.

Diabetic retinopathy

Diabetic retinopathy is a serious eye condition associated with diabetes and a common cause of blindness in the UK. Retinopathy is microvascular leakage or haemorrhaging and occlusion in the blood vessels (that capillaries) of the retina. It can occur over many years in people with diabetes, particularly where there is high blood glucose. Over time, this may become more severe and lead to a loss of central vision, or a total vision loss if undetected and treated.

The three main types of diabetic retinopathy are background, pre-proliferative, and proliferative.

- **Background retinopathy** is the least serious and occurs when small red dots appear on the retina due to minute swellings in the blood vessel walls.

  No treatment is required, but regular monitoring by a GP or ophthalmologist is required.

- **Pre-proliferative diabetic retinopathy** is the early stage of the disease and less severe. This is when vision is obstructed due to swelling of the retina and leakage of blood.

Laser treatment is an option if leakage begins to threaten vision. This will not restore any lost vision, but it can prevent further deterioration.

- **Proliferative retinopathy** occurs when there are new blood vessels growing (that is, neovascularization) and a haemorrhage, causing a scarring of the retina and blurred vision or a sudden loss of vision.

  Laser treatment can burn the abnormal blood vessels and prevent further growth. Eye surgery may be an option if laser treatment has proved ineffective.

Retinopathy is less likely to develop with well-controlled blood glucose levels and when other risk factors, including cholesterol and blood pressure levels, are stable.

The Diabetes UK website http://www.diabetes.org.uk/ offers further information on diabetic retinopathy.

See Chapter 10 for more on diabetes.

Sight loss after a stroke

Visual problems are common following a stroke and can affect up to two-thirds of stroke survivors (MacIntosh, 2003). However, as the brain recovers, visual problems often resolve themselves (Zhang et al., 2006).

Visual disturbance

The four main categories in which visual disturbance occurs are:

- central vision loss;
- visual field loss;
- eye movement problems; and
- visual processing problems.

Central vision loss is the partial or complete loss of vision in one or both eyes.

Visual field loss usually affects both eyes after a stroke. Often, people may lose half of their visual field which relates to seeing with either the right or left half of each eye—known as 'hemianopia.' Treatments include optical aids, such as magnifiers, minifiers (which can enable focus on the remaining area of retained vision), and prisms, which are customized to fit glasses and enable widening the field of view. Training in compensatory strategies can also help to improve awareness of the visual field loss.

Eye movement problems occur as a result of nerve damage following a stroke. This can include:

- impaired eye movements;
- inability to move eyes up or down or sideways, with nerve problems possibly arising, causing blurred vision or diplopia (that is, double vision) impacting on everyday activities;
- impaired depth perception and difficulty locating objects; and
- nystagmus (that is, involuntary and jerky repetitive movements), causing the patient to see objects wobbling and causing much distress.

Treatment options for eye movement problems include:

- exercises to improve eye movements;
- prisms for increasing the field of view; and
- occluding, or patches, applied to one eye in which there is double vision, meaning vision in one eye only (that is, monocular vision). However, this can also cause problems such as reduced depth perception and field of vision, leading to mobility problems.

Visual processing problems refer, for example, to when the recognition of objects, people, colours, or text is impaired following a stroke. Visual neglect is also a common visual processing problem, in which there is a reduced ability to look or make movements towards one half of the environment. It is also more common in people who have suffered a stroke in the right side of the brain affecting the left side of the body.

Treatment can include prisms of occlusion, but the primary treatment is awareness strategies. Support and input from healthcare professionals and carers is needed to promote awareness of the person's affected side.

Care and treatment for a person who has suffered a stroke with vision loss is particularly important, because it can affect the rest of their rehabilitation.

The Stroke Association Factsheet 37, 'Visual Problems after Stroke', is a comprehensive look at the subject and is available online at http://www.stroke.org.uk/

See Chapter 10 for more on stroke.

Supporting people with sight loss

The most important thing that nurses can do is understand that no two people with sight loss are the same. People with sight loss have different needs, which are shaped by a variety of things other than their sight loss. Nurses, therefore, need to consider the person's cultural background, their likes and dislikes, and whether the person also has another disability.

Where there is visual and cognitive impairment, there is a high risk of disability (Whitson et al., 2007). A recent study into the experiences and needs of older people with dementia and visual impairment found that individuals experienced a profound sense of disorientation, and were highly vulnerable to social isolation (Lawrence and Murray, 2009).

Some people will not be able to see anything at all; others may have some useful sight. The golden rule is not to make assumptions: talk to the person and find out what works for them. There are several practical ways in which nurses can ensure that support is provided in a manner that respects privacy and dignity, promotes independence, and reduces isolation:

- psychological support;
- communication strategies;
- information;
- environmental lighting;
- supporting and orientating the older person with sight loss;
- maintaining dignity and independence; and
- referral to low-vision support services.

Psychological support

Social isolation and loneliness is a common experience for people with sight loss, and support needs to come from family, friends and health or social care professionals (Percival and Hanson, 2005; RNIB, 2009). The lack of understanding by professionals can be apparent to families if they are not offered services and support (Douglas et al., 2008). It is also suggested that older people's families are less likely to be offered support (RNIB, 2009), so the nurse has a key role in signposting and referring to appropriate agencies.

The emotional impact of adjusting to sight loss in later life was found to be associated with depression, reduced quality of life, and poorer social functioning (Nyman et al., 2008). Depression is also at least twice as high among those with a visual impairment than among the general population (Burmedi et al., 2002). In addition to listening and finding time to talk to the older person with sight loss, psychological support needs to be addressed by offering and providing services and information, addressing and improving communication issues, practical solutions including low-vision aids, and referral to the wider multidisciplinary team, including psychology and occupational therapy.

Communication

Communication is a critical skill for nurses and even more so when supporting older people with sight loss. It is very easy to unintentionally treat a person with sight loss in an undignified manner. There are many situations that can be embarrassing, frustrating, frightening, and confusing for people with sight loss. The following recommendations will aid communications and help to maintain people's dignity.

- Always introduce yourself by saying your name and saying the person's name so they know you are talking to them.
- Use a gentle touch on a person's arm to let them know you are there.
- Always say the person's name when you begin a conversation so that they know you are there.
- Always talk to the person not to their companion / carer.
- Always consider your position—a person with AMD for example may prefer you to sit or stand at their side because their central vision has been affected by their eye condition. Whereas a person with glaucoma may prefer you be directly in front of them as their peripheral vision has been affected by their eye condition.
- Think about non-verbal communication—older people with sight loss may not be able to see you pointing, may not know you are smiling so may not realize you are joking about something.
- Describe everything you are planning to do before you do it.
- Describe everything you are doing as you do it.
- Think about the language you use—over there' means nothing to a person with sight loss.
- Think about your tone of voice—often statements are softened by a smile which may not be seen by an older person with sight loss.
- Always talk naturally—do not try to avoid terms such as 'I see', 'Do you see what I mean'.
- Describe things in detail. Most older people will have previously had vision so descriptions can stimulate memories for example flowers, colours and scenery.
- Always tell the person you are leaving.

(RNIB, 2001)

Many older people with sight loss may also have hearing loss, which could have a serious impact on their ability to communicate. SENSE, a charity working for deafblind people, estimates that one in 20 people over the age of 75 are likely to be classed as deafblind (SENSE, 2010). Nurses therefore should consider the need to learn about alternative methods of communication, one of which is the manual alphabet (RNIB, 2003), shown in Figure 3.8.

Information

It can be the experience of people with sight loss—particularly in a hospital or institutional care environment—to have information read out in front of other people, which can be embarrassing, degrading, or humiliating.

Difficulty accessing important information can also impact on everyday activities, such as taking medication—for example, in relation to needing to recall for what a medication is prescribed, what to do if a dose is missed, understanding side effects and not being able to read the leaflet to find out.

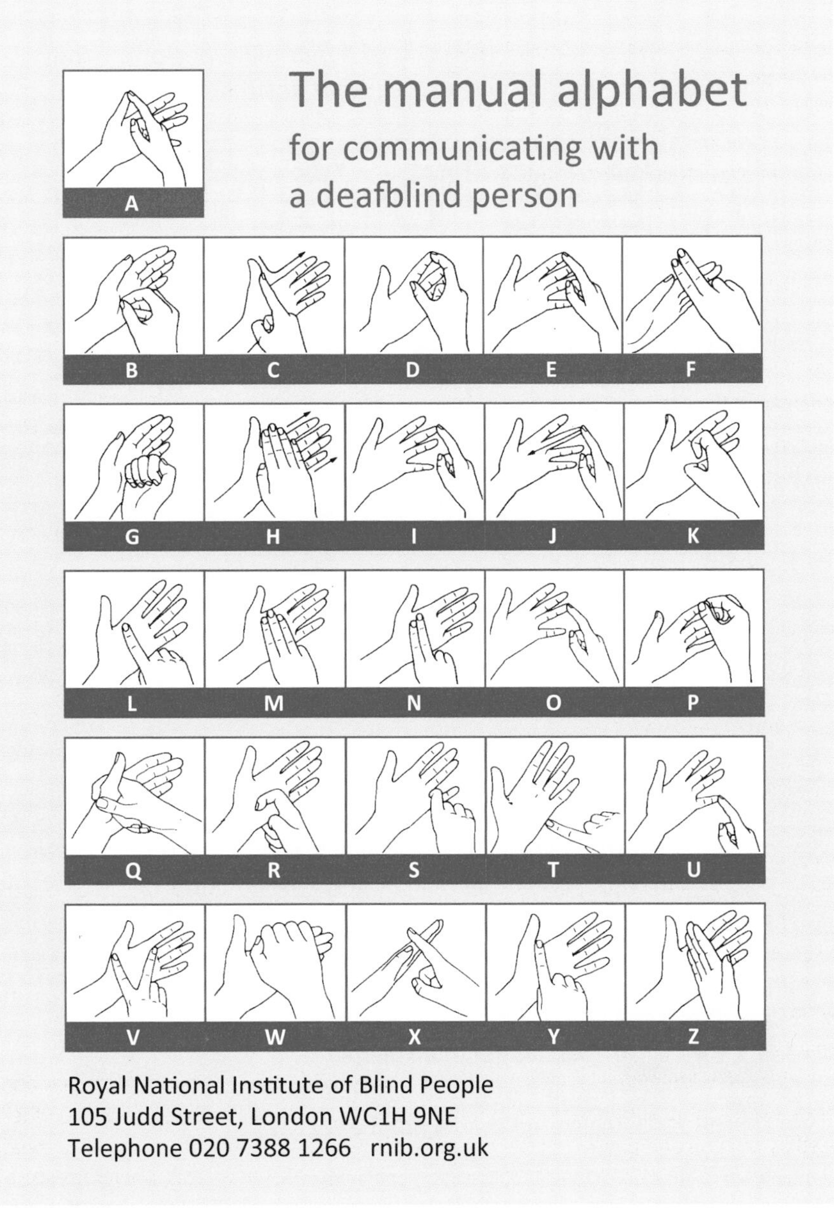

Figure 3.8 The RNIB manual alphabet
Source: From RNIB Deafblind card http://www.rnib.org.uk/shop, with kind permission from RNIB.

NURSING PRACTICE INSIGHT: COMMUNICATING INFORMATION TO THOSE WITH SIGHT LOSS

- Ask the person how they access or read information—for example, large print, Braille, or audio tape.
- Always try to produce any information in the person's preferred format. For example, nurses could write information on a piece of paper in black bold marker pen or use the computer to enlarge the font size.
- Nurses could liaise with patient advisory liaison services, or trust communication and engagement teams, to have relevant information produced in Braille, large print, audio or CD form.
- If sensitive information has to be given verbally, always ask the person if they would like to go to a private room.
- Ensure that optical aids are available for those suffering sight loss, such as magnifying glasses.
- Ensure that menus and key written information is in large print—for example, font size 16—but not all in capitals.
- Display notices in a prominent position.

How to write letters on the palm of a deafblind person's hand
(the lines show the direction and sequence of strokes on the palm)

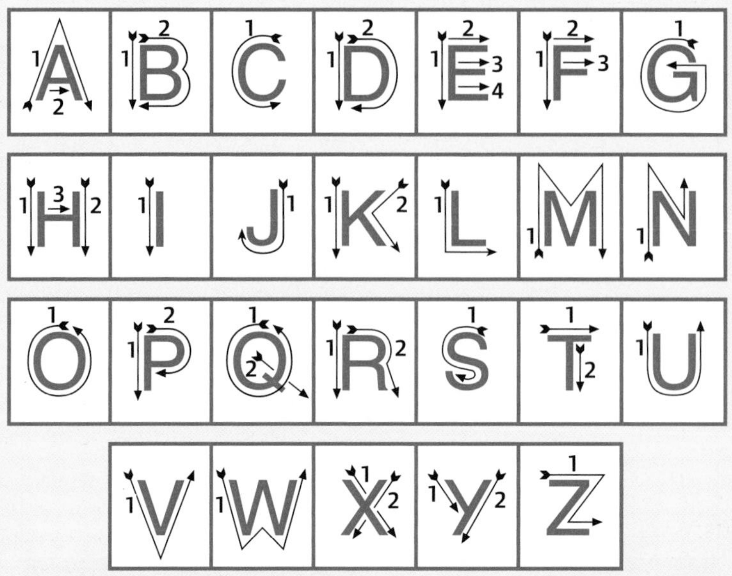

RNIB offers a number of services to people who have a combined sight and hearing difficulty. We can help local authorities to evaluate provision for deafblind children, and provide advice and support. We offer training in deafblind awareness, support work with deafblind people and work in partnership with local authorities to develop and provide services for deafblind adults.

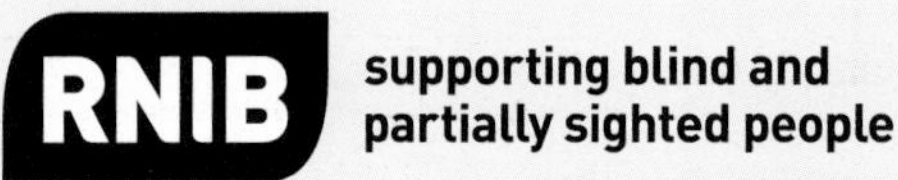

Figure 3.8 *(Continued)* The RNIB manual alphabet
Source: From RNIB Deafblind card http://www.rnib.org.uk/shop, with kind permission from RNIB

Environmental lighting

As stated at the beginning of this chapter, as we get older, less light reaches the retina. Thus, more light is required to aid vision and environmental lighting needs to be considered to enable the person with sight loss to be supported in everyday activities, and particularly to mobilize without risk.

There are a number of practical solutions that can improve the lighting for the older person with light loss, including:

- maximum use of daylight, but avoid glare;
- bright and even lighting throughout the care environment or home;
- avoiding pools of light;
- strip light and dimmer switches;
- replacing bulbs as soon as needed; and
- as well as ceiling and wall lights, someone with low vision could benefit from a task lamp for reading and seeing what is on their plate.

Supporting and orientating the older person with sight loss

The vast majority of older people with sight loss have some residual vision and can mobilize independently with the use of practical aids. However, even for the person with normal vision, admission to a care environment can be disorientating, and careful support and orientation is required. The nurse should first take time to discuss the routines, and establish if the older person with sight loss can move around independently and their level of confidence. Those older people with serious visual impairment will need more support and guidance. Older people with dementia and sight loss are more at risk of disorientation, and require consistency in the physical environment (Lawrence and Murray, 2009).

To support the older person with sight loss and their mobility, the following needs to be addressed.

- Spend time with the person by walking with them to the toilet or other areas, such as the day room.
- Find out what mobility aids the person needs and make sure that they always have access to them.
- Establish how they prefer to be guided.
- Do not hold the person's arm; let them hold your arm at the elbow. Your arm should be by your side. Whilst you are walking, continually talk to the person. Pause before going through narrow doorways, and up or down slopes and kerbs. When going through narrow doorways, check to see if the person is in the right position and that they will not bang any part of their body on the doorframe.
- When you reach the destination, the person may want to sit down. Do not push or pull the person to the seat. Tell the person that you are going to put their hand on the back of the chair, so that they can feel the back and the arms. Then allow the person to sit in the chair independently, offering further guidance if there is any risk of them missing the chair.
- Record the person's need for assistance and their requirements in the care plan.

The correlation between falls and the visually impaired is well documented (Legood et al., 2002; Campbell, 2005). Simple intervention strategies, including regular eye examinations, cleaning lenses, the use of single-lens glasses, and removing hazards that could cause someone to trip or fall, have the potential to prevent falls in older people (Campbell, 2005).

See Chapter 6 for more on the prevention of falls.

Maintaining dignity and independence

For the older person with sight loss, everyday tasks, such as getting washed and dressed, eating, using the telephone, shaving, telling the time, using the toilet, and watching television, can all be problematic and time-consuming. Limited knowledge on how and when to help by family members can result in individuals struggling for independence (RNIB, 2009). Family members can also have concerns over safety and this can lead to placing limits on their relative's activities, resulting in conflict and tension on relationships (Thomas Pocklington Trust, 2008). Sometimes, tasks will need to be carried out for the person; at other times, carers and nurses may simply provide the support necessary to enable a person to carry out the tasks independently.

The following insights will help nurses to provide support in a manner that promotes an older person's independence, and respects their privacy and dignity.

- On arrival to a new care environment, offer assistance to a person with unpacking their belongings. Ask them where they would like them put and show the person where you have put them.
- Never move anything belonging to an older person with sight loss without first asking permission and explaining where it is going to be put.
- Make things **bigger**, **brighter**, and **bolder**. Use a strong-coloured blanket or duvet cover to make sure that it does not look the same as the flooring; put black tape on the edge of the bedside table to make it stand out.
- Always ask the person how they prefer a task to be carried out. Remember that, quite often, people will be worried about being a burden, so a sensitive and understanding approach is needed.
- Always remember that many older people with sight loss will be able to carry out most tasks independently if given a little support.
- When carrying out tasks for people, make sure that you continually explain what you are doing. This will ensure that they are not surprised or frightened by any actions that you take.
- If the person has indicated that they can wash or bathe alone, ensure that they have everything that they need to hand, such as soap, flannel, towels, etc., and a call bell, and leave them to carry out the task in private.
- Similarly, if a person has indicated that they can dress themselves, make sure that they know where their clothes are and that they can reach them easily.
- Use colour and tone contrasts, and arrange crockery that contrasts with the table. For example, if the table is dark brown, a white plate would be easily noticeable. If necessary, a boldly coloured non-slip mat would help.
- Use the clock method for older people with sight loss to indentify where food is on a plate. For example, meat/fish at '6 o'clock', potatoes/rice at '12 o'clock', and vegetables at '3 o'clock' and '9 o'clock', and explain what is on the plate when serving the food.

- Nurses may need to think about using a rimmed plate or a plate guard to help to support an older person to eat in a dignified manner. Ask the person if this would be helpful.
- Always tell the person where the condiments are. They may be a different shape, but if not, nurses could put a rubber band around the salt to help to differentiate.
- When serving drinks, always tell the person where you have put it and what it is.
- If you notice that someone has spilled something on themselves, always tell them as discreetly as possible, so that they can decide whether to change or not.
- If a person has to use a commode, make sure that it has a different coloured seat to the base (for example, black toilet seat, white base).

See Chapter 2 for more on privacy and dignity.

Box 3.1 Imagining that you have sight loss

- Imagine not being able to find something without having to ring for assistance.
- Imagine falling over because someone moved your furniture, or you could not tell where the edge of your bed was, because the cover was a similar colour to the floor.
- Imagine not being able to go the toilet on your own because there are no guide rails.
- Imagine having to ask someone to help every time you want to move around.
- Imagine being helped to move around and banging your head on the doorframe, because the person does not know how to guide properly.
- Imagine having to use a commode in a large ward because people do not know how to guide you.
- Imagine sitting quietly in your bed when some unknown person approaches you, takes hold of your arm, and begins to fasten something on to it.
- Imagine that you are chatting away to a nurse only to realize suddenly that you are no longer getting responses, because they have moved on to the next patient.
- Imagine suddenly being swung into the air because you are being hoisted.
- Imagine someone talking to your relative about the treatment that you are going to receive as if you were not there.

Consider the strategies and practical measures raised in this chapter that you would like to be addressed to assist you in the above issues.

Low-vision support services

Most local authorities or borough councils will have a low-vision support services team, and it is important for the nurse to be aware of what these services provide, where they are located, and how to refer to them in order to support the older person with sight loss—particularly if they have not accessed such services.

A typical low-vision service will provide physical and emotional support with daily living activities, and a full assessment of the needs of the client. Services may include:

- assessment of client needs around communication, daily living skills, personal management, and mobility;
- the issue of equipment (practical aids);
- training and education on any adaptations identified through the needs assessment—for example, magnifiers;
- carers' needs assessment;
- information on statutory concessions and benefits; and
- information and signposts to voluntary agencies, and referrals to local and national associations for the visually impaired.

See the Online Resource Centre for an example of a low-vision services pathway.

Eye clinic patient support workers or liaison officers

Eye clinic liaison workers are emerging new professionals that support people within hospital eye clinics, particularly following a diagnosis of sight loss. The quality of patient care at the time of diagnosis is a significant issue to be addressed (Percival, 2003) and thorough competent guidance is required, with a personal attitude to the blind or partially sighted person (Durham Sight Loss Survey Partnership, 2008). The liaison officer has a specialist knowledge base of services for visually impaired patients. Their role, however, is particularly focused on providing emotional support to patients following a diagnosis of sight loss and to support patients, with their agreement, through the registration process (that is, registration as blind or partially sighted). A consultant ophthalmologist would initially certify as severely sight impaired/blind or sight impaired/partially sighted.

The role also includes supporting patients who are experiencing anxiety, distress, and/or practical difficulties due to their eye condition, and signposting patients, families, and carers to low-vision services, and statutory and voluntary agencies, as appropriate.

Questions and self-assessment

Now you have worked through section two, answer the following questions.

- Reflect on a recent experience of undertaking an assessment of an older person. Were their sight impairment needs assessed and addressed?
- How can the nurse ensure that an older person's sight loss is incorporated into care planning?
- What communication strategies could you use to support the older person with sight loss?
- Why is consideration of the environment so important in caring for people with sight loss?

Self-assessment

- Having read the section on sight loss, how will you change your practice?
- Identify areas relating to sight loss in which you have increased your knowledge and understanding.
- Identify how you are going to develop this knowledge and understanding, and set deadlines for achieving this.

References

Ahmed, I. and Das Gupta, A.R. (2001) 'Epidemiology of basal cell carcinoma and squamous cell carcinoma of the pinna', *Journal of Laryngology & Otology*, 115(2): 85–6.

Baltes, P.B., Staudinger, U.M., and Lindenberger, U. (1999) 'Lifespan psychology: Theory and application in intellectual functioning', *Annual Review of Psychology*, 50: 471–507.

Beck, D. and Sockalingam, R. (2009) 'Audition, cognition, ageing and listening success', *ENT & Audiology News*, 18(4): 101–3.

Bronstein, A. and Lempert, T. (2007) *Dizziness: A Practical Approach to Diagnosis and Management*, Cambridge Clinical Guides, Cambridge: Cambridge University Press.

Bunce, C. and Wormald, R. (2006) 'Leading causes of certification for blindness and partial sight in England and Wales', *BioMed Central Public Health*, 6: 58.

Burmedi, D., Becker, S., Heyl, V., Wahl, H.W., and Himmelsbach, I. (2002) 'Emotional and social consequences of age-related low vision', *Visual impairment Research,* 4(1).

Campbell, S. (2005) *Deteriorating Vision, Falls and Older People: The Links*, Glasgow: Visibility.

Dalton, D.S., Cruickshanks, K.J., Klein, B.E.K., Klein, R., Wiley T.L., and Nondahl, D.M. (2003) 'The impact of hearing loss on quality of life in older adults', *The Gerontologist,* 43(5): 661–8.

Davis, A., Smith, P., Ferguson, M., Stephens, D., and Gianopoulos, I. (2007) 'Acceptability, benefit and costs of early screening for hearing disability: A study of potential screening tests and models', *Health Technology Assessment*, 11(42).

Department of Health (2001) *National Service Framework for Older People*, London: DH.

Department of Health (2002) *A Sign of the Times*, available online at http://www.dh.gov.uk/prod_consum_dh/groups/dh_digitalassets/@dh/@en/documents/digitalasset/dh_4018723.pdf.

Department of Health (2007) *Transforming Adult Hearing Services for Patients with Hearing Difficulties: A Good Practice Guide*, available online at http://www.dh.gov.uk/en/Publicationsandstatistics/Publications/PublicationsPolicyAndGuidance/DH_076884.

Douglas, G., Pavey, S., and Corcoran, C. (2008) *Network 1000: Access To Information, Services and support for Older People with Visual Impairment*, Birmingham: University of Birmingham.

Durham Sight Loss Survey Partnership (2008) *Taking a Blind Bit of Notice in County Durham*, available online at http://www.actionforblindpeople.org.uk/news/a-blind-bit-of-notice-in-county-durham,108,SNS.html.

Grue, E.V., Kirkevold, M., and Ranhoff, A.H. (2009) 'Prevalence of vision, hearing, and combined vision and hearing impairments in patients with hip fractures', *Journal of Clinical Nursing*, 18(21): 3037–49.

Guest, J.F., Greener, M.J., Robinson, A.C., and Smith, A.F. (2004) 'Impacted cerumen: Composition, production epidemiology and management', *Quarterly Journal of Medicine*, 97: 477–88.

Hallam, R., Ashton, P., Sherbourne, K., and Gailey, L. (2006) 'Acquired profound hearing loss: Mental health and other characteristics of a large sample', *International Journal Of Audiology*, 45(12): 715–23.

Herdman, S.J., Blatt, P., Shcubert, M.C, and Tusa, R.J. (2000) 'Falls in patients with vestibular deficits', *American Journal of Otology*, 21: 847–51.

Horowitz, A. (2004) 'The prevalence and consequences of vision impairment in later life', *Topics in Geriatric Rehabilitation*, 20(2): 185–95.

Lawrence, V. and Murray, J. (2009) 'Promoting independent living among people with dementia and sight loss', *Journal of Care Services Management*, 3(3): 261–74.

Legood, R., Scuffham, P., and Cryer, C. (2002) 'Are we blind to injuries in the visually impaired? A review of the literature', *Injury Prevention*, 8(2): 155–60.

Levene, B. and Tait, V. (2005) *Managing Your Hearing Loss: Impairment to Empowerment*, London: Hearing Concern.

MacIntosh, C. (2003) 'Stroke re-visited: visual problems following a stroke and their effect on rehabilitation', *British Orthoptic Journal*, 60: 10–14.

Macular Disease Society (2008) *Facts and Figures about Macular Degeneration and Useful Links*, available online at http://www.maculardisease.org/core/documents/download.asp?id=960.

NHS Quality Improvement Scotland (2005) *Best Practice Statement: Maximizing Communication with Older People Who Have a Hearing Disability*, Edinburgh: NHS QIS.

Nyman, S.R., Gosney, M.A. and Victor, C.R. (2008) 'Assessment of the current provision of psychological support to older people with sight loss', presented at the 37th Annual Conference of the British Society of Gerontology, 'Sustainable Futures In An Ageing World', 6–9 September, University of the West of England, Bristol.

Pavey, S., Douglas, G., Hodges, L., Bodsworth, S., and Clare, I.C.H. (2009) *The Needs of Older People with Acquired Hearing and Sight Loss*, Research Findings No. 23., London: Thomas Pocklington Trust.

Percival, J. (2003) 'Sight loss in later life: A vision for health service intervention', *Nursing Times*, 99(15): 36–8.

Percival, J. and Hanson, J. (2005) '"I'm like a tree a million miles from the water's edge": Social care and inclusion of older people with visual impairment', *British Journal of Social Work*, 35(2): 189–205.

Rodgers, R. (1994) 'Primary aural care', *ENT News*; 3(3): 34–5.

Royal National Institute of Blind People (2001) *Older People and Sight Loss*, London: RNIB.

Royal National Institute of Blind People (2003) *Manual Alphabet Card*, London: RNIB.

Royal National Institute of Blind People (2006a) *Open Your Eyes Campaign Report*, London: RNIB.

Royal National Institute of Blind People (2006b) *See It Right*, London: RNIB.

Royal National Institute of Blind People (2008) *Glaucoma*, available online at http://www.rnib.org.uk/eyehealth/eyeconditions/eyeconditionsdn/pages/glaucoma.aspx.

Royal National Institute of Blind People (2009) *Understanding the Needs of Blind and Partially Sighted People: Their Experiences, Perspectives and Expectations*, London: RNIB.

Royal National Institute for Deaf People (2006) *Facts and Figures on Deafness and Tinnitus*, London: RNID.

Royal National Institute for Deaf People (2009) *Hearing Progress: Ten Years of Biomedical Research*, available online at http://www.rnid.org.uk/information_resources/aboutdeafness/science/.

Royal National Institute for Deaf People/UK Council on Deafness (2004) *A Simple Cure* London: RNID, available online at http://www.rnid.org.uk/.

Sacks, O. (1990) *Seeing Voices*, New York: Harper Perennial.

SENSE (2010) 'How many deafblind people are there?', available online at http://www.sense.org.uk/media_centre/Facts+and+figures/deafblind_population.

Smeeth, L., Fletcher, A.E., Ng, E.S., Stirling, S., Nunes, M., Breeze, E., Bulpitt, C.J., Jones, D., and Tulloch, A. (2002) 'Reduced hearing, ownership and use of hearing aids in elderly people in the UK: The MRC trial of the assessment and management of older people in the community—A cross-sectional survey', *The Lancet*, 359(9316): 1466–70.

Smith, C. (2006) 'Making the link: Ageing and sight loss', *Journal of Integrated Care*, 14(3): 32–8.

Smith, J.L., Mitchell, P., Wang, J.J., and Leeder, S.R. (2005) 'A health policy for hearing impairment in older Australians: What should it include?', *Australia and New Zealand Health Policy*, 2: 31.

Tambs, K., (2004) 'Moderate effects of hearing loss on mental health and subjective well-being: Results from the Nord-Trondelag hearing loss study', *Psychosomatic Medicine*, 66(5): 776–82.

Thomas Pocklington Trust (2008) *The Experiences and Needs of People with Dementia and Serious Visual Impairment: A Qualitative Study*, London: Thomas Pocklington Trust.

Whitson, H.E., Cousins, S.W., Burchett, B.M., Hybels, C.F., Pieper, C.F., and Cohen, H.J. (2007) 'The combined effect of visual impairment and cognitive impairment on disability in older people', *Journal of the American Geriatric Society*, 20(2): 185–95.

Zhang, X., Kedar, S., Lynn, M.J., Newman, N.J., and Biousse, V. (2006) 'Homonymous herianopia in stroke', *Journal of Neuro opthamlmology*, 26: 180–3.

For further reading and information

http://www.actionforblindpeople.org/

http://www.diabetes.org.uk/

http://www.maculardisease.org/

http://www.pocklington-trust.org.uk/

http://www.rnib.org.uk/

http://www.stroke.org.uk/

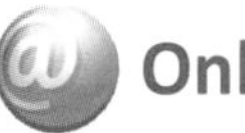

Online Resource Centre

You can learn more about hearing and sight loss at the Online Resource Centre that accompanies this book: **http://www.oxfordtextbooks.co.uk/orc/hindle/**

The law and the older person

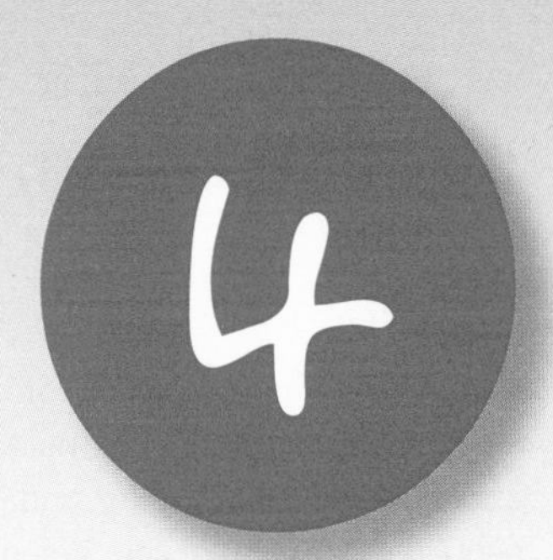

Herman Wheeler

Learning outcomes

By the end of the chapter, you will be able to:

- **demonstrate an understanding of how different sources of law impact on older people;**
- **define the concepts of advanced directives (ADs), living wills, and lasting powers of attorney (LPAs); and**
- **demonstrate an understanding of end-of-life issues in relation to older people, including resuscitation and 'not for resuscitation' (NFR) issues, withdrawal of medical treatment, permanent vegetative state, and assisted suicide.**

Introduction

It is important that nurses have an understanding of the law as it relates to older people—but it is important to note straight away that there is no single body of law that deals uniquely with older people, or sets them apart from others on the basis of age. The way in which the law deals with the older person is similar to the way in which it deals with younger adults. However, there are some areas of law that have particular relevance for older people and these areas are the central focus of this chapter:

- ageism, age discrimination, and abuse;
- legal assertions and their implications;
- ethics, sources of law, and the older person's right to care;
- confidentiality;
- informed consent;
- anticipated and actual lack of capacity to consent; and
- the law and end-of-life issues for the older person.

The legal cases referred to in this chapter have been identified as helping the reader to understand how the principles of law have been applied in healthcare settings.

As the older population increases in size, nursing in the twenty-first century is challenged to provide high-quality care within a legal and professional framework. Nurses should be familiar with the Nursing and Midwifery Council (NMC) *Guidance for the Care of Older People* (2009), in which essential principles of caring for older people are identified against standards set out in The Code (2008). Being older does not reduce the person's need for quality care or information about legal issues relating to their health care. Inability to deliver nursing care to the older person within a sound legal and professional framework will leave nurses legally and professionally culpable, and potentially open to litigation suits.

Some areas of law have particular relevance to older people and these areas will be discussed in this chapter so that all nurses will be able to respond positively and successfully when working with older adults.

Ageism, age discrimination, and abuse

Ageism

Ageism is the most common form of discrimination in the UK (Age Concern, 2007). Help the Aged (2002) defines 'ageism' as prejudging, stereotyping, and making assumptions against people on the basis of age. Age discrimination is institutionalized in official policies and in everyday health and social care practices (Norman, 1985; Roberts, 2000; McDonald and Taylor, 2006). Older people are the highest consumers of acute services in the National Health Service (NHS) and nurses must be aware of issues that can have an impact on how treatment is given. Negative attitudes may, for example, have an influence on:

- resource allocation;
- terminal illnesses;
- making wills and advanced directives (ADs);
- lasting powers of attorney (LPAs);
- mental incapacity; and
- older people's property and possessions.

These issues are by no means confined to the older adult, but they are prominent in their lives. Amidst these realities, nurses need to be aware of older people's unquestionable right to health and social care services irrespective of age.

Age discrimination

There is no law that introduces a 'cutoff point' for medical and nursing care for the older adult, and medical and nursing care cannot be withdrawn on the basis of age. European Council Directive 2000/78 establishing a general framework for equal treatment in employment and occupation made age discrimination in employment illegal. This objective was implemented in the UK in 2006 under the Employment Equality (Age) Regulations 2006. These regulations apply only to employment and vocational training, and presently only up to the age of 65, after which a worker may be dismissed in line with procedures within the regulations. However, employees have the right to request working beyond the age of 65 and employers have a duty to consider such a request. Nurses may be faced with the possibility of lending a listening and sympathetic ear to those affected—perhaps with reassuring them of their employment rights under the law. Nurses may even be able to guide the unemployed person who is still seeking employment towards local employment and voluntary work agencies.

Abuse

Age UK (2010b) points out that older people without mental capacity are particularly vulnerable to abuse and ill treatment, including:

- financial abuse;
- not being informed about medical treatment;
- being given treatment without consent; and
- being admitted to and detained in hospitals without proper safeguards or deployed policies in respect to their human rights.

The last of these was seen in the *HL v UK* (2004) ECHR 720—known as the *Bournewood Case*—in which the European Court of Human Rights (ECtHR) concluded that a patient with autism, who lacked mental capacity and who was admitted informally to hospital out of 'necessity' (that is, for his own benefit, in his 'best interest'), had been deprived of his liberty. He had not been detained under the Mental Health Act 1983 (MHA) and could therefore not benefit from its safeguards pertaining to liberty, such as appealing against his detention to the Mental Health Review Tribunal. Instead, he was detained under common law powers of 'necessity'. He brought a claim that he was unlawfully detained. The ECtHR agreed that his liberty under Article 5 of the European Convention on Human Rights (ECHR) had been breached.

Nurses and student nurses need to know that there are other, more common forms of older adult abuse from which patients may suffer, including physical cruelty, and sexual and psychological abuse. Under the Public Interest Disclosure Act 1998, nurses can 'whistle-blow'—that is, report or expose—any form of abuse of the older adult, without the risk of detrimental treatment or victimization. Besides, Article 5 of the ECHR accords rights, liberty, and security to individuals, including older people.

Under the Human Rights Act 1998, older people, like younger people, have the following rights:

- a right to life (Schedule 1, article 2);
- a right not to be tortured or subjected to inhuman and/or degrading treatment (Schedule 1, article 3);
- a right to private and family life (Schedule 1, article 8);
- a right to freedom of thought, conscience, and religion (Schedule 1, article 9);
- a right to freedom of expression (Schedule 1, article 10);
- a right not to be subjected to discrimination (Schedule 1, article 14);
- a right to freedom from abuse of their rights (Schedule 1, article 17); and
- a right to the protection of their property (Schedule 1, article 18).

These articles lay the basis for the student to detect and whistle-blow on older patient abuse.

See Chapter 2 for more on the abuse of older people.

> **Reflection point**
>
> Make sure that you are familiar with your area of work's policies and procedures. Students should follow the policies of the organization in which they are working and inform the appropriate person if they suspect that abuse is taking or has taken place.

Legal assertions and their implications

> **Box 4.1** Legal definitions (in England and Wales)
>
> - **Capacity**—Competence to make an agreement.
> - **Civil law**—The law of the state (or country); derived from Roman law. It is established in written codes generated by Parliament, such as statutes.
> - **Common law**—Judge-made law, which is derived from court decisions, as opposed to laws created by statute. In common law, a case sets a precedent that is followed by subsequent cases.
> - **Contract**—An agreement that the law will enforce; by making the contract, the parties undertake obligations to each other, and confer rights upon each other that these obligations will be fulfilled and rights, upon failure to do so, to enforce the obligations at law.
> - **Statute**—Also known as an 'Act of Parliament', a document that sets out legal rules, normally passed by the House of Commons and the House of Lords.
> - **Statutory instruments**—A form of law delegated to statutory bodies.
> - **Tort**—The law of tort is mainly concerned with providing compensation for personal injury and property damage caused by negligence.

Mental capacity

The law asserts that older people have the capacity to make personal decisions. The law can help vulnerable individuals who are capable or incapable of taking personal healthcare decisions. The law's assumption that older people have the mental capacity to take personal decisions means that family and friends carry no legal responsibility for the older adult—a fact that all nurses need to be aware. However, any person, including a relative, who agrees to undertake the role of attorney under a lasting power of attorney (LPA)—that is, a personal formal legal undertaking to look after the property, possession, and personal welfare of an older person, should the person later lack capacity to do so—has a legal obligation and a duty of care to that person in making decisions on their behalf under the Mental Capacity Act 2005.

In Scotland, the Mental Capacity Act 2005 does not apply; the Adults with Incapacity (Scotland) Act 2000 is its equivalent.

In Northern Ireland, there is no equivalent legislation, but legislation is currently being considered and you can keep up to date with developments online at http://www.northernireland.gov.uk/index.htm

> **Reflection point**
>
> There is a presumption of capacity in the Mental Capacity Act 2005. This means that family and friends carry no automatic legal responsibility for the older adult.

Contract, tort, and compensation

Although a relative normally has no legal responsibility for, or obligation towards, an older relative, a nurse or other healthcare professional who enters into a professional caring relationship with a patient has a duty of care, and a combined legal, professional, and ethical responsibility and obligation to provide the highest standard of care for that patient. Failing to do so—and, moreover, damaging the patient through negligent practice—would entitle the patient to seek legal redress.

This legal redress could be pursued under the civil law of contract (if the patient has a formal contract with the healthcare professional) or, more commonly, under the civil law of the tort (here meaning a civil wrong, not an intentional criminal wrong done to another person) of negligence (see 'Common law' below).

A right to sue for compensation (that is, damages) is not unique to older people; a patient of any age can sue in negligence or contract, whichever applies.

Ethics, sources of law, and the older person's right to care

Every older person has a legal (and ethical) right to health and social care. It would be unethical to discriminate against the older adult, since any nursing and social care relationship should aim to:

- promote what Beauchamp and Childress (2008) describe as the '*ethics of beneficence*'—that is, doing good to benefit the patient;
- respect people's rights to autonomy and independence—that is, self-power, self-reliance, self-determination, and independence;
- practise non-maleficence—that is, to do the patient no harm; and
- promote justice—that is, fairness, equity, and absence of prejudice, discrimination, and abuse within health and social care.

Moreover, the State's obligation to provide health and social care is based on needs, disability, and mental health status. Thus care intervention is rooted in '*the general law*' (McDonald and Taylor, 2006: 2). Both the older adult and those who care for them need an understanding of the law, in terms of rights, duties, and obligations. This way, older people can exercise their rights, and healthcare professionals, their obligations.

As healthcare professionals, our statutory obligations to provide health care to older people come mainly from the National Health Service Act 1977. This is a statute (that is, written law) enacted by Parliament. It imposes powers and duties on health authorities and NHS trusts, and consequently on nurses as employees. Furthermore, the NHS was founded on the premise that it would provide care on the basis of need, not ability to pay.

Continuing NHS care

People who receive hospital treatment in the NHS have always been statutorily entitled to free treatment, and any incidental personal care and accommodation required. The law requires, in given circumstances, that such services must be provided free wherever they are delivered, whether in a private nursing home or otherwise. However, leading cases such as *Coughlan* (1999), brought to light that not all people were being provided with this entitlement.

See the Online Resource Centre that accompanies this book for more on Coughlan and Grogan.

The outcomes from both cases were that policies and guidelines were to be reviewed to reflect the legal position on who should be eligible for 'continuing NHS care'. 'Continuing care' means care provided over an extended period of time to a person aged 18 or over to meet the physical and mental health needs that have arisen as the result of a disability, accident, or illness. 'Continuing NHS care' means a package of continuing care arranged and funded solely by the NHS.

The *Grogan* judgment had major implications for nursing, because most single assessment documents will now include continuing NHS care as part of a specialist assessment.

See the Online Resource Centre that accompanies this book for an assessment tool and reflective exercises.

Social care provision

In terms of social care provision, local authority social services gain their powers, duties, and obligations essentially from the Local Authority Social Services Act 1970. However, statutes can be complex and difficult to translate into operational provisions. Therefore, governments often produce statutory instruments, which set out detailed rules, regulations, and operative procedures to help with implementing a statute. To achieve uniformity of health and social care policy implementation, for example, the Secretary of State for Health issued the Community Care Assessment Directions 2004, (DH, 2004) requiring local authorities to establish partnerships with service users and carers in assessments. In respect of the *National Service Framework for Older People* (NSFOP) (DH, 2001), the Department of Health issued implementation guidance in the form of health service circulars (HSCs).

Further information can be found on the Age Scotland website http://www.ageconcernandhelptheagedscotland.org.uk/ and the Age UK websites http://www.ageuk.org.uk/

Common law

There are other legal issues affecting the care of older people that come under the common law (that is, the law decided by the courts). Judges make decisions on the basis of the material evidence of each case, relating to established principles arising from earlier similar cases (known as 'legal precedence'). Patients can sue under tort of negligence only if they have been harmed; alternatively, they can sue for non-performance of a contract. Patients who have been harmed can sue for the harm received; in contract, they can sue for negligent performance of the contract if there is a contractual relationship. They can sue if they are third parties for whom the contract was put in place, so can sue for non-performance of the contract or negligent performance. Patients without rights under a contract can sue under various torts, or can sue for breach of statutory duty if a relevant duty exists or can be implied from the statute.

The nurse, as an employee of a NHS trust, has a duty to take reasonable care, exercise reasonable skill and competence, and follow reasonable orders from the employer. If, in caring for the patient, a nurse breaches the terms of employment, they can be disciplined. This may include suspension from duty, demotion, being formally warned, or (in extreme cases) being dismissed by the employer. Therefore, as a nurse caring for the older patient, it is important that you take the utmost care to exercise skill and competence in delivering care to the highest standard possible. Nurses owe it to their patients and their employers to deliver safe care.

An NHS trust or employer has two forms of liability in negligence:

- **vicarious liability**—also known as 'indirect liability'—involves the employer being responsible for the faults of the employee;
- **direct liability** involves the employer itself being at fault.

A patient who is in a contractual relationship with a health professional and who is harmed could sue the professional directly. However, in the NHS, patients who are harmed in care tend to sue under vicarious liability. This should not be taken to mean that the employer may not attempt to recover from the employee the money paid out vicariously. Employers such as an NHS trust, a private hospital, or a general practitioner (GP) employing their own staff, or even a company, can be sued for negligent care. Employers have more economic muscles than individual nurses to settle negligence claims, and so it makes sense for patients to sue employers even where an individual employee's practice was negligent.

Nurses consequently need to have protective indemnity insurance just in case they are ever sued directly, or their employers decide to recover from them money paid out on negligence claims under vicarious liability.

For clarity on the principles relating to sound legal and professional standards of care, the student is advised to read *Bolam v Friern Barnet HMC* [1957] 2 All ER 118; 1 WLR 528. A later case of critical importance is *Bolitho v City & Hackney HA* [1997] 3 WLR 115, which has further scrutinized professional practice standards by ensuring that health professionals deliver the most up-to-date care, taking into consideration logical expert evidence and weighing all risks in the delivery of care.

Mental capacity and consent

Sections 2 and 3 of the Mental Capacity Act 2005 identify 'mental capacity' as the cognitive ability to make decisions, to understand information for decision-making, to recall information as and when required, to believe in that information, to weigh up the information in arriving at a decision, and to communicate that decision. All social and healthcare professionals, and informal carers of older people, need to be aware that the Mental Capacity Act 2005 supports the key principles below and, by implication, requires health and social care professionals and informal carers to respect these principles.

(1) The following principles apply for the purposes of this Act.

(2) A person must be assumed to have capacity unless it is established that he lacks capacity.

(3) A person is not to be treated as unable to make a decision unless all practicable steps to help him to do so have been taken without success.

(4) A person is not to be treated as unable to make a decision merely because he makes an unwise decision.

(5) An act done, or decision made, under this Act for or on behalf of a person who lacks capacity must be done, or made, in his best interests.

(6) Before the act is done, or the decision is made, regard must be had to whether the purpose for which it is needed can be as effectively achieved in a way that is less restrictive of the person's rights and freedom of action.

(Mental Capacity Act 2005, section 1).

Every adult of sound mind has a right to self-determination and autonomous decision-making, to consent or refuse to consent to treatment, to determine who touches their body, to decide whether or not to take medication, food, and water, to decide whether or not to accept admission to hospital, or to discharge themselves against medical advice. Although it is perhaps more likely to find a higher incidence of mental incapacity in the older rather than the younger population due to, for example, higher incidences of dementia, the law nevertheless assumes that every older person has the requisite mental capacity to make decisions for themselves (Mental Capacity Act 2005, section 1(2)). Nurses must assume that the patient has mental capacity until proven otherwise, and must remember that the ageing process in itself does not remove mental capacity for self-decisions and that the older mentally competent person's decision about whether to accept care is final.

NURSING PRACTICE INSIGHT: THE RIGHT TO REFUSE TREATMENT

As nurses, we may feel that we want to persuade the patient to have the treatment that best evidence indicates would benefit the patient. However, that mentally competent older person has the right to refuse treatment and cannot be forced to accept treatment simply because professional staff believe that they should.

Lack of capacity

If the older patient is found not to have the prerequisite mental capacity and does not make an advanced decision whilst possessing capacity, then all decisions taken on their behalf must be in their 'best interest' (Mental Capacity Act 2005, section 5). An 'advanced decision' (AD) is not like a simple will that one makes, declaring, for example, how one's property should be shared out at death; rather, an AD is a formal, written, and witnessed decision that the individual makes, setting out a clear refusal of medical treatment should they later suffer mental incapacity. For example, the person may not wish to be resuscitated if that need arises, or they may refuse in advance other treatment that they personally regarded as futile. (See 'Advanced decisions' later in this chapter).

Under section 2 of the 2005 Act, a lack of capacity cannot be established merely with reference to a person's age and a two-stage functional test needs to be used to establish if a person lacks capacity. The Code of Practice Mental Capacity Act 2008 provides guidelines for determining mental capacity:

Stage 1. Is the person suffering from an impairment of, or a disturbance in the functioning of the mind or brain?

Stage 2. If yes does the impairment of the disturbance cause the person to be unable to make a decision when he needs to?

If a person is unable to make their own decision, then it must be for one or more of the following reasons:

- they do not understand the information;
- they cannot remember the information;
- they are unable to weigh up the information; and
- they cannot communicate the decision.

Every effort must be made to find ways in which to communicate with the person, and carers, family, and other professionals should be involved. Records should record how the decision was reached.

NURSING PRACTICE INSIGHT: THE MENTAL CAPACITY ACT 2005

The NMC has issued advice on the Mental Capacity Act 2005 and nurses should read the advice sheet available online at http://www.nmc-uk.org/Nurses-and-midwives/Advice-by-topic/A/Advice/Mental-Capacity-Act-2005/

Confidentiality

The law regards the older person as entitled to confidentiality, privacy, and dignity. Statute law—such as the Data Protection Act 1998, article 8 of the Human Rights Act 1998, and the Access to Medical Report Act 1988—grants rights of confidentiality. Nurses owe the older patient a duty to maintain confidentiality, which strengthens the nurse–patient relationship through trust. Confidentiality is owed under the NMC's Code, statutes such as the Data Protection Act 1998, the contract of employment, and the ethical principles of consent, confidentiality, justice, beneficence, non-maleficence, autonomy, and right of the patient to disclose or not to disclose. Breach of confidence can be punished professionally, legally, and through an employer's disciplinary code.

NURSING PRACTICE INSIGHT: CONFIDENTIALITY

The NMC has issued advice on confidentiality and nurses should read the advice sheet on available online at http://www.nmc-uk.org/Nurses-and-midwives/Advice-by-topic/A/Advice/Confidentiality/

When confidentiality can be broken

Under certain conditions, however, confidentiality may be legally broken, such as by an authority of the court in the public interest. Under section 3(1) of the Access to Health Records Act 1990, an older patient has the right to demand that, in certain given situations, their health records must not be accessed after their death. Nurses need to apply this in any situation: for example, if insurance companies attempt to locate dead patients' records against the express and formal wishes of the dead person when they were alive. It may also be broken under the Road Traffic Act 1988, section 11 of the Prevention of Terrorism Act 1988, and the Public Health (Control of Disease) Act 1984.

With respect to the Road Traffic Act 1988, as a nurse, if you know that one of your patients has been involved in a road traffic accident—for example, they may have been driving one of the vehicles involved—and someone was hurt, if the police ask you to disclose that patient's identity, you are obliged by law to do so. In other words, patient's privilege does not apply here. Equally, under the Prevention of Terrorism Act 1988, if you have information that you reasonably believe could help to prevent terrorism, you are obliged in law to pass it on to the police. For example, if, when working in accident and emergency (A&E), you find that you have reason to believe that a patient's wound was caused by a terrorist act, then you should inform senior staff, and they will take the appropriate action and contact the police.

Under the Public Health (Control of Disease) Act 1984, a medical practitioner is duty-bound to report 'notifiable diseases' (including cholera, diphtheria, smallpox, plague, and typhus) to the Medical Officer of Health. Where public interest is at serious risk, the courts can force you to disclose information about your patient without their permission.

Informed consent

By 'informed consent', it is meant that the patient is provided with adequate information about procedures and risks in such a way that they understand and are therefore able to make an informed decision. Under section 3(2) of the Mental Capacity Act 2005, a person is not to be regarded as unable to comprehend information relevant to a decision if they are able to understand an explanation given in an appropriate format—for example, in simple language, which might include use of written or audio-visual aids. Therefore every person must be individually assessed to determine their mental capacity to consent to or refuse treatment.

Older people with the requisite capacity are no different under the law from younger mentally competent adults in relation to informed consent and confidentiality. A general principle common law is that a mentally competent adult has the right to consent or refuse consent to medical treatment. As a nurse, you have no legal right, except under the doctrine of necessity—that is, of taking the perceived best course of action on the unconscious (mentally incompetent) person's behalf, to save life and limb—to touch a patient without their consent. If the older person is touched without giving consent, they may sue for trespass of their person (that is, battery); if threatened to be touched, this is assault. Informed consent negates a claim of trespass. Refusal to consent can be for good, bad, or no reasons at all.

Consent is valid if given by a mentally competent patient, voluntarily without undue pressure, duress, or fraud. It can be in writing, it may be verbal, or it may be implied from action, such as the older patient offering their arm to have their blood pressure taken. Failure to inform the patient can lead to a claim of negligence should they suffer injury from the treatment, or simply to a claim of battery or 'trespass to the person' if there is treatment—even touch—without prior consent even if there is no injury. In certain circumstances, refusal to consent may be overridden—for example, under the Mental Health Act 1983 (as amended by the Mental Health Act 2007) and section 5 of the Mental Capacity Act 2005.

NURSING PRACTICE INSIGHT: CONSENT

The NMC has issued advice on consent and nurses should read the advice sheet on available online at http://www.nmc-uk.org/Nurses-and-midwives/Advice-by-topic/A/Advice/Consent/

Anticipated and actual lack of capacity to consent

In an emergency in which the older patient is brought into hospital unconscious and there is no evidence of their wishes to the contrary, they can still be treated legally without their consent under the doctrine of necessity.

Anticipated lack of capacity to consent

Older patients can decide in advance how they would like to be treated—and in particular, what treatment they will refuse. Yet planning for mental incapacity is something that some older people are reluctant to do (McDonald and Taylor, 2006). Age UK encourages people to anticipate possible incapacity and take appropriate action—for example, setting up ADs or advance statements, often known as 'living wills' (Age UK, 2010a).

Advanced decisions (ADs)

ADs and living wills are formal means of expressing refusal of some form of medical treatment in the future should incapacity prevail, and are means by which individuals express their wishes about how they would like to be treated if they become mentally incapacitated. An advanced decision does not have to be written, but if verbal, a senior member of the medical team should be a witness. Written decisions help avoid confusion.

Further information and advice on ADs and living wills can be found online at http://www.direct.gov.uk/en/government citizensandrights/death/preparation/dg_10029683

Under common law, a nurse or a doctor must respect the competent patient's wishes to refuse treatment, such as a blood transfusion (*Re T (An adult: refusal of medical treatment)* [1992] All ER 649). An AD cannot rule out the basic nursing care of an incapacitated patient or demand illegal treatment.

Lasting power of attorney (LPA)

Under the Mental Capacity Act 2005 and the Adults with Incapacity (Scotland) Act 2000, an older mentally competent person can set up an LPA regarding medical treatment, property, personal possessions, and personal welfare. The donor (that is, the person setting up the LPA) can give the donee the power the right to make decisions on their behalf with respect to property, affairs, and personal welfare. The former enduring power of attorney (EPA) could give only delegated decisions in relation to property and affairs; the new LPA can give delegated powers to make decisions relating also to personal welfare. As of 1 October 2007, an EPA could no longer be set up; however, those set up prior to this date can remain in use.

With an LPA relating to property and affairs, the donee can act even whilst the donor still possesses capacity. In relation to personal welfare, however, the donee can carry out the delegated obligation only when the donor lacks the requisite capacity. Both LPAs and EPAs are forms of ADs or living wills. With an LPA involving life-saving treatment for the donor of the power, refusal of treatment (by the donee) on behalf of the donor is effective only if specified. In respect of life-saving decisions, the donee's power cannot be used with the aim of causing the donor's death. This would be a breach of the duty of care, making the donee a possible party to murder, or guilty of murder itself—especially in the UK where euthanasia (that is, the active ending of life) is illegal.

With respect to personal welfare, the attorney's power can extend (unless expressly prohibited) to consent to medical treatment, access to medical records, and to securing community care.

NURSING PRACTICE INSIGHT: ADs AND LPAs IN PRACTICE

So what would this look like in practice? Can the nurse simply trust a verbal assertion?

The first point that could be made here is that nurses will, from time to time, welcome patients' legal representative(s) who come to visit patients in hospital. Sometimes, patients even ask nurses to ring their legal adviser on their behalf to pass on a message—for example, asking the adviser to visit the patient.

What nurses should not do is sign legal documents such as LPAs and ADs, because this could compromise their position. If asked to do so, you should politely refuse, explaining that you are not allowed to do so, and pass the information to the hospital managers or senior nurse. Beware of the person who comes into the ward brandishing a document, saying: 'I am Mrs Smith's son. Please can you persuade her to sign these papers, so that her house can be sold and the money kept in a bank to look after her when she is discharged from hospital?'

If you have reasons to think that your patient who lacks capacity is being abused by anyone, relatives included, it is your responsibility and professional obligation to act. You must advocate on your patient's behalf by pointing out the irregularity to a senior member of staff. If you are in doubt about the credibility of a document in the patient's notes that says this patient is not to be resuscitated, then question it. All questionable documents are worth questioning!

As a student, your duty of care and responsibility to the patient is no less than that of the qualified nurse. You are not justified in saying: 'I'm only a student nurse'. It must be reiterated that a patient is not allowed to use an AD to refuse basic nursing care when they lose mental capacity.

Court of Protection and the older person

Under the Mental Capacity Act 2005, a new Court of Protection has been set up with jurisdiction to make decisions about personal welfare, as well as property and finance. The former Court of Protection could make decisions only in respect of property and affairs. The 2005 Act also makes it possible for independent mental capacity advocates to be appointed when necessary: for example, where serious medical treatments are indicated, accommodation decisions are to be made, and the patient lacks the requisite capacity and had hitherto not set up the appropriate LPA. In these circumstances, an independent mental capacity advocate must be appointed to report on the best interest of the patient. This should also happen when a patient is being transferred from hospital back home or into residential care.

NURSING PRACTICE INSIGHT: ASSESSMENT OF CAPACITY

So with whom would the nurse liaise? The assessment of capacity rests with the person delivering treatment or care. Therefore, in the case of nursing care, nurses can make decisions. If there is significant doubt, then the nurse should discuss this with senior staff.

What matters are the patient's individual needs and disposition, and their express wishes with regard to their care. They cannot demand specific treatment—certainly, they cannot demand illegal treatment—but they can, if they possess capacity, refuse medical treatment.

The NMC (2007) has issued advice on the covert administration of medication, which provides guidelines for nurses to work within in certain clinical situations, and nurses should read the advice sheet on available online at http://www.nmc-uk.org/Nurses-and-midwives/Advice-by-topic/A/Advice/Covert-administration-of-medicines

The law and end-of-life issues for the older adult

'Do not resuscitate' (DNR) or 'not for resuscitation' (NFR)

In 2007, a joint statement from the British Medical Association (BMA), the Resuscitation Council (UK), and the Royal College of Nursing (RCN) set out guidance on when a patient may not be resuscitated. Key to the decision-making process is that each decision should be made on an individual basis and that decisions should not be based on factors such as age (BMA, 2007).

To decide on a 'not for resuscitation' (NFR) or a 'do not resuscitate' (DNR) measure on the basis of chronological age would be discriminatory and illegal.

Withdrawal of treatment and permanent vegetative state

As the case of *Airedale NHS Trust v Bland* [1993] 1 All ER 821 demonstrates, medical interventions may be withdrawn when the patient's prognosis is hopeless.

Case study

Tony Bland had survived the Hillsborough Football Stadium disaster of 15 April 1989. This was an FA Cup semi-final between Liverpool and Nottingham Forest at Hillsborough Stadium (the home of Sheffield Wednesday Football Club). Too many fans entered the ground and a crowd surge forward led to 96 deaths (all Liverpool fans). Bland was severely injured and, although he could breathe and digest food, he could not hear, see, taste, communicate, or smell; he was 'brain dead' and had no chance of recovery. He remained in an unconscious 'permanent vegetative state', although he did not require a ventilator.

When the case was brought before the House of Lords, the Law Lords ruled that artificial feeding and hydration could be withdrawn in the patient's long-term best interest. His quality of life was judged poor and his outcome hopeless. No distinction was made between the withdrawing of food or water and other life-sustaining treatment. Withdrawing of medical intervention in cases of permanent vegetative state does not amount to deprivation of life under Schedule 1, article 2, of the Human Rights Act 1998 (*An NHS Trust v M; AN NHS Trust v H* [2001] 2 FLR 367).

Nurses should familiarize themselves with *Airedale NHS Trust v Bland* [1993] 1 All ER 821 and understand its key principles, since it is one of those landmark cases that will keep cropping up—particularly in relation to whether or not treatment can be safely and legally withdrawn from patients who are brain dead, and who therefore have a very poor outlook and a hopeless prognosis.

Has an old person a right to die by assisted suicide?

The issue of assisted suicide has long been one of public concern, interest, and debate in the UK. As UK law stands, euthanasia (so-called 'mercy killing', in which a person or persons take the life of another) is illegal. Taking the life of another would, under UK law, leave the life-taker liable to the charge of murder or manslaughter. The penalty for those who aid, abet, counsel, or procure the suicide of another carries a maximum prison sentence of 14 years under section 2(1) of the Suicide Act 1961.

In launching an interim policy on prosecuting cases of assisted suicide in September 2009, the Director of Public Prosecutions (DPP) stated:

> **Assisting suicide has been a criminal offence for nearly fifty years and my interim policy does nothing to change that. [...] There are also no guarantees against prosecution and it is my job to ensure that the most vulnerable people are protected whilst [...] giving enough information to those people, like Ms Purdy, who want to be able to make informed decisions about what actions they may choose to take**
>
> (CPS, 2009)

So what led the DPP to issue, in September 2009, an interim policy statement regarding prosecutions in cases of assisted suicide?

Mrs Debbie Purdy, a sufferer from progressive multiple sclerosis, had argued in the High Court of Justice, in October 2008, before Lord Justice Scott Baker and Mr Justice Aikens, that the DPP infringed her human rights by failing to clarify the law relating to assisted suicide. She wanted to know if her husband Omar Puente assisted her suicide—for example, by helping her to travel to Switzerland to the Dignitas clinic to die—he would be prosecuted. If he would be prosecuted by so doing, Mrs Purdy said that she would make the journey sooner, unassisted. Both the High Court and the Court of Appeal gave no clear ruling in favour of Mrs Purdy, but stated instead that it was up to Parliament to change the law relating to prosecutions for assisted suicide.

In July 2009, at an appeal hearing in the House of Lords, five Law Lords unanimously backed Mrs Purdy's call for a clear policy statement from the DPP on when someone might be prosecuted for helping a loved one to end their life abroad. Until that time, many UK citizens had escorted loved ones and friends to Switzerland to end their life in the Dignitas clinic without facing prosecution. The Law Lords thought that there needed to be legal clarification and ordered the DPP to end the uncertainty. This resulted in the DPP interim guidelines being published in September 2009 and a final policy statement in February 2010.

Fundamentally, the *Purdy* case has not changed the law, nor has the DPP's policy, which has failed to decriminalize the offence of encouraging or assisting suicide. This policy has not opened the door to euthanasia; to aid or encourage someone to commit suicide is therefore still a serious criminal offence:

> **Nothing in the policy can be taken to amount to an assurance that a person will not be prosecuted if he or she does an act that encourages or assists the suicide or the attempted suicide of another person.**
>
> (DPP, 2010)

In fact, the BMA (2010) notes that:

the law on attempted suicide has not changed. Helping or encouraging another person to end his or her life remains a criminal offence and all cases are referred to the Crown Prosecution service.

It is also an offence to encourage suicide by disseminating such encouragement via media. It is interesting to note, too, that the BMA points out that among the DPP guidelines on public-interest factors in favour of prosecution for assisting suicide are circumstances under which the person accused of assisting or encouraging suicide '*was acting in his or her capacity as a medical doctor, nurse [or] other healthcare professional*' (BMA, 2010).

The NMC reminds nurses that assisted suicide is illegal; nurses must make patients the centre of care, always practising within their code of conduct and within the context of national laws. The NMC position is also that: '*the law on assisted suicide has not changed*'.

You are advised to read the DPP policy guidelines on possible prosecution in cases of assisted suicide, which spells out the discretionary powers of the Crown Prosecution Service (CPS) to prosecute, taking into account the set of circumstances involved in each individual case. The policy also lists factors that could mitigate against prosecution: for example, where the victim had reached clear, voluntary decision to commit suicide, and the suspect was wholly motivated by compassion, and reported the suicide to the police and fully assisted enquiries. This is perhaps a factor influencing whether or not loved ones who escort their relative to Dignitas clinics in Switzerland to end their life are prosecuted.

There are some 16 factors in favour of prosecution for assisted suicide, which are worth reading, including where victims are aged under 18, or where suspects are paid or stand to gain from their act. The issue of whether the victim had terminal illness, incurable physical disability, or severe degenerative physical illnesses will no longer mitigate against prosecution. The guidelines now focus more on the motives of the suspect and less on the health of the victim.

For moral and legal reasons, doctors, nurses, and other healthcare professionals must avoid actions that might be interpreted as helping, assisting, encouraging, or facilitating suicide. The BMA states that doctors must not tell patients what constitutes a fatal dose of any drug in relation to a planned overdose, nor recommend the option of committing suicide abroad, nor write reports that specifically favour assisted dying abroad. These pieces of advice also apply to nurses.

In summarizing this section, it must be noted that nurses and other healthcare professionals need to be aware that, in the UK, no individual has a legal right to secure the death of another. Whilst Schedule 1, article 2, of the Human Rights Act 1998 affirms a right to life, the House of Lords in an earlier landmark case (*Pretty v DPP* [2002] 1 All ER 1) and the ECtHR in a later European ruling (*Pretty v UK* [2002] 2 FCR 97) stated that a 'right to life' does not mean a right to die by assisted suicide. By implication, just as Diane Pretty's husband could have been tried for murder or manslaughter had he assisted his wife to die, so too can nurses or doctors who *deliberately* assist patients to die. Whilst the DPP guidelines since *Purdy* are a little clearer than they were at the time of Diane Pretty, fundamentally the law has not changed.

Case study

Mrs Diane Pretty, a mentally alert woman, suffered from motor neurone disease, a progressive degenerative illness, from which she would never recover. She faced the prospect of a distressing death and therefore sought to take steps to end her life peacefully at the time of her choosing. She hoped to ask her husband, Brian, to aid her death—effectively, to kill her. He was willing to do so, but sought legal assurance that, if he did, he would not be prosecuted under section 2(1) of the Suicide Act 1961 for aiding and abetting her suicide. The DPP would not give the assurance.

Mrs Pretty petitioned the British courts right up to the House of Lords, but failed to get the assurance that she needed. Eventually, she petitioned the ECtHR in Strasbourg, which ruled that she did not have the right to have her husband end her life. As stated above, clearly, if her husband had helped her end her life, he would, in all probability, have been tried for murder or for aiding someone to commit suicide. By reiteration, whilst the DPP guidelines after *Purdy* may be clearer, they have not changed the law.

Caring competently, compassionately, diligently, and sensitively for a dying patient must be the nurse's first consideration. The law on assisted suicide and the DPP guidelines do not mean abrogating professional nursing and medical responsibility to give the best care to a dying person. As a healthcare professional, one must do nothing to hasten a patient's death. If professional care—for example, pain-relieving drugs—indirectly, but unintentionally, hastens the patient's death, this is not the same as deliberately helping the patient to commit suicide. If a patient is competent, albeit severely disabled, the hospital or care home cannot prevent the patient from going abroad for euthanasia, although they may have a duty to ask the courts to confirm that the person has the mental capacity to take such a decision and that they are not being put under any duress to end their life abroad.

Conclusion

The growing number of old people in our society indicates that there is a critically important role for nurses working with older people to work within the remit of the law. The evidence shows that there is no specific body of law that defines older people, nor is there a specific age point that determines the health and social care interventions available for older people. Human rights legislation, including ECHR Article 14 and the Employment Equality (Age) Regulations 2006, prohibits age discrimination.

As indicated in the chapter, nurses need to work with patients and their significant others, social services, and other health and social care agencies within the NMC Code (2008) and within its *National Service Framework for Care of Older People* (2009) to care effectively for older people on the basis of needs, not age. A number of legal instruments and specific age discrimination legislation are paving the way for older people to be treated fairly and not discriminated against. It is crucial that nurses understand how the law influences nursing practice—particularly in relation to anticipating lack of capacity and around end-of-life issues.

Questions and self-assessment

Now that you have worked through the chapter, answer the following questions.

- The Mental Capacity Act 2005 addresses the concept of capacity and incapacity. Imagine that you are about to ask an older patient to consent to a nursing treatment or procedure, but think that the patient lacks capacity to understand what you are about to do and the risks involved. Identify the legal issues involved and what action you should take.
- You are working in a ward specifically designated to care for older adults with dementia. What would you do as a nurse to promote favourable attitudes, a positive philosophy, and the right ethical values that would benefit your patients?
- Whilst you are giving a terminally ill older patient their pain-relieving drugs, the patient pleads with you to increase the dosage substantially to relieve him permanently of his pain and end his life. What actions would you take and why? Use professional and legal arguments to address this question.

Self-assessment

- Identify two areas in which you have increased your knowledge and understanding, and how this will improve your practice.
- Identify how knowledge of the law and ethics relates to the NMC Code (2008).

References

Age UK (2010a) *Legal Issues*, available online at http://www.ageuk.org.uk/money-matters/legal-issues/living-wills/.

Age UK (2010b) *Safeguarding Older People from Abuse*, available online at http://www.ageuk.org.uk/health-wellbeing/relationships-and-family/protecting-yourself/?paging=false.

Beauchamp, T.L. and Childress, J.F. (2008) *Principles of Biomedical Ethics*, 6th edn, Oxford: Oxford University Press.

British Medical Association (2007) *Decisions Relating to Cardiopulmonary Resuscitation*, available online at http://www.bma.org.uk/images/DecisionsRelatingResusReport_tcm41-147300.pdf.

British Medical Association (2010) *Comment on Director of Public Prosecutions' Final Guidance on Assisted Dying*, available online at http://www.bma.org.uk/ethics/.

Crown Prosecution Service (2009) 'DPP publishes interim policy on prosecuting assisted suicide', available online at http://www.cps.gov.uk/news/press_release/144_09/.

Department of Health (2001) *National Service Framework for Older People*, London: DH, available online at http://www.dh.gov.uk/prod_consum_dh/groups/dh_digitalassets/@dh/@en/documents/digitalasset/dh_4071283.pdf.

Department of Health (2004) *Community Care Assessment Directions 2004*, available online at http://www.dh.gov.uk/en/Publicationsandstatistics/Publications/PublicationsLegislation/DH_4088476.

Department of Public Prosecutions (2010) *Assisted Suicide*, available online at http://www.cps.gov.uk/.

Help the Aged (2002) *Age Discrimination in Public Policy: A Review of the Evidence*, London: Help the Aged.

McDonald, A. and Taylor, M. (2006) *Older People and the Law*, Bristol: Policy Press.

Norman, A. (1985) *Triple Jeopardy: Growing Old in a Second Homeland*, London: Centre for Policy in Ageing.

Nursing and Midwifery Council (2007) *Covert Administration of Medicines: Disguising Medicines in Food and Drink*, available online at http://www.nmc-uk.org/Nurses-and-midwives/Advice-by-topic/A/Advice/Covert-administration-of-medicines/.

Nursing and Midwifery Council (2008) *The Code*, available online at http://www.nmc-uk.org/Nurses-and-midwives/The-code/The-code-in-full/.

Nursing and Midwifery Council (2009) *Guidance for the Care of Older People*, London: NMC, available online at http://www.nmc-uk.org/General-public/Older-people-and-their-carers/Care-and-respect-every-time-new-guidance-for-the-care-of-older-people/.

Office of the Public Guardian (2008) *Code of Practice: Mental Capacity Act 2008*, available online at http://www.publicguardian.gov.sg/pdf/COP%20guide.pdf.

Roberts, E. (2000) *Age Discrimination in Health and Social Care*, London: Kings Fund.

Statutes

Information about the statutes referred to in this chapter (see list below) can be obtained online at http://www.opsi.gov.uk/about/index.htm

Access to Health Records Act 1990

Access to Medical Report Act 1988

Adults with Incapacity (Scotland) Act 2000

Data Protection Act 1998

Human Rights Act 1998

Local Authority Social Services Act 1970

Mental Capacity Act 2005

Mental Health Act 1983 (as amended by the Mental Health Act 2007 and by the Mental Capacity Act 2005)

National Health Service Act 1977

Prevention of Terrorism Act 1988

Public Health (Control of Disease) Act 1984

Public Interest Disclosure Act 1998

Road Traffic Act 1988

Suicide Act 1961

Statutory instruments

Employment Equality (Age) Regulations 2006

European legislation

European Council Directive 2000/78 of 27 November 2000 establishing a general framework for equal treatment in employment and occupation [2000] OJ L303/16.

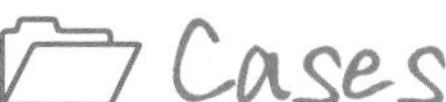

Cases

Airedale NHS Trust v Bland [1993] 1 All ER 821

An NHS Trust v M; An NHS Trust v H [2001] 2 FLR 367

Bolam v Friern Barnet HMC [1957] 2 All ER 118; 1 WLR 528

Bolitho v City & Hackney HA [1997] 3 WLR 115

Coughlan v North & East Devon Health Authority [1999] EWCA Civ 1871

HL v UK (2004) ECHR 720 (the *Bournewood Case*)

MB (Adult: refusal of medical treatment), Re [1997] 2 FLR 426

Pretty v DPP [2002] 1 All ER 1

Pretty v UK [2002] 2 FCR 97

T (An adult: refusal of medical treatment), Re [1992] All ER 649

Online Resource Centre

You can learn more about the law and older people at the Online Resource Centre that accompanies this book: **http://www.oxfordtextbooks.co.uk/orc/hindle/**

Carers, families, and single householders in the community

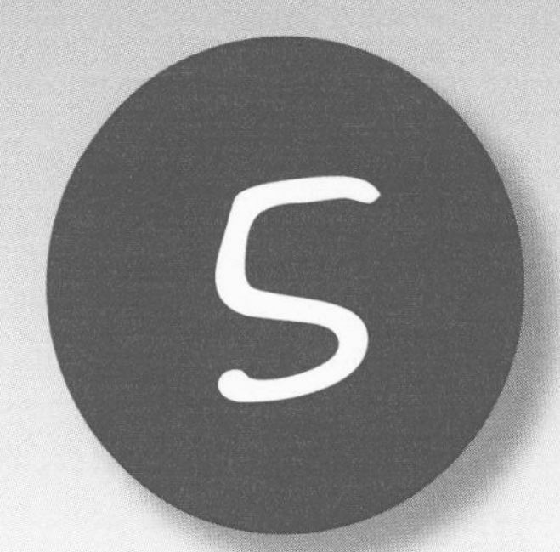

Andrew Hindle

Learning outcomes

By the end of the chapter, you will be able to:

- understand the reasons why loneliness can become a reality, the implications, and some of the interventions for preventing or managing loneliness.
- understand the role of families and the importance of support for carers;
- define a carer and what their role can entail;
- understand the importance of an assessment for carers and what the assessment should include; and
- have some knowledge of support and interventions for carers.

Introduction

The ageing population has major implications for the organization of support and care for older people. This chapter will focus on some of these implications relating to the impact on the support of single householders, families, and carers. The *National Service Framework for Older People* (DH, 2001) highlights the need for all older people and their carers to be treated with respect, dignity, and fairness. Yet it is too often the experience of carers that support is not provided, that their needs are not listened to, and that they are not included in care planning. The *National Carers Strategy* (DH, 2008a) has now raised the important contribution of carers and sets out the vision for support for carers over the next ten years.

Single householders

Since the Second World War, there have been dramatic increases in the number of older people living alone in the UK and across Europe; at the same time, there has been a decrease in the numbers of multigenerational households. The reasons for the increase in independent living among older people are multifold, but include the prevalence of divorce, changes in attitudes towards living in communal dwellings, better financial independence, and possible improvements in health.

The UK Office for National Statistics (ONS) publication *Focus on Older People* (ONS, 2005) stated that 60 per cent of women and 29 per cent of men aged 75 and over live alone. This gives cause for concern regarding the availability of family support and the alternatives of care provision for frail older people who require care. Whether or not an older person lives alone or not is primarily affected by marriage, the incidence of divorce, and widowhood. Older men are more likely to be married than older women, with two-thirds of men over the age of 75 living with a spouse, compared to three in ten of women aged 75 and over (ONS, 2005). The reasons for this include the tendency for men to marry younger women and the higher life expectancy of women. Older Asian people are also less likely to live alone compared with white, black, and other mixed ethnic groups (ONS, 2005).

Older gay, lesbian, and bisexual people

Given that male homosexuality only became legal in the UK in 1967, it is not surprising that many gay men kept their sexuality a private issue, and that older men from this generation still fear discrimination and prejudice. Concannon (2009) argues that there is unique oppression and marginalization faced by older lesbians, gay men, bisexual, and transgendered citizens. When older gay men and lesbians experience illness or the death of a partner, their potential lack of family or friendship network can result in loneliness and isolation. The importance of friendships and relationships is a source of social support, reducing loneliness, and contributing to better physical and mental health (Grossman et al., 2000).

Studies have indicated that many gay men and lesbians do not disclose their sexuality to healthcare and social services, because of anxieties and fears about differing treatment (Fitzpatrick et al., 1994; Jacobs et al., 1999). This can extend to gay and lesbians avoiding even routine health care due to their perceptions of health services as unwelcoming places. Such issues are taken up by Glover (2006) and Concannon (2009), who advocate a shift in policy to address more inclusion, and access to appropriate and open levels of care, with non-judgemental and supportive services.

Older people and loneliness

Older people who live alone, and particularly those that are housebound or have a disability, are at increased risk of experiencing loneliness and social isolation. Where there is little social or family support, this risk is even higher. The absence of social relationships can have a detrimental influence upon the quality of life of older people (Victor et al., 2004). There is increasing recognition that loneliness and social isolation can also have an adverse impact on health and well-being. Findings from a review of research into loneliness indicated that it has strong associations with depression and appears to have a significant impact on physical health, due to raised blood pressure, reduced sleep, and worse cognition over time in the elderly (Luanaigh and Lawlor, 2008).

Older women report more loneliness than male peers, and the experience of loneliness in older women is influenced by social and cultural factors (Beal, 2006).

Assessing loneliness

Specialized scales for assessing loneliness have been developed, including the UCLA scale and the de Jong Gierveld scale. Yet asking overt questions of an older person being interviewed can affect their answers because they may wish not to reveal their feelings and attract the social stigma of loneliness (Victor et al., 2004). Self-report scales are therefore suggested as the most appropriate for older people (Holmen and Furukawa, 2002).

It is important that nurses undertake an assessment of their older clients or patients for loneliness and, where appropriate, discuss interventions. The single assessment process will generally include questions that will help to identify loneliness or social isolation. Under a heading of 'emotional well-being', for example, there maybe questions on whether the older person enjoys their life to the full, whether they have worries, and also whether they have support from family or other carers.

See the Online Resource Centre that accompanies this book for more on scales for assessing loneliness.

Interventions

Interventions that promote social contact, encourage creativity, and use mentoring are more likely to positively affect health and well-being. Ekwall et al. (2005) highlight the need for nurses to identify those at risk of loneliness and poor social networks, and to help them to create or maintain better networks—particularly before there is deterioration in a person's health status, because illness and disability can make social contacts even more difficult.

A study that evaluated practical interventions for addressing social isolation in older people via an 'upstream healthy living centre' indicated a range of psychosocial and physical health benefits (Greaves and Farbus, 2006).

A close friend or relative can be a key preventive factor in avoiding isolation, and having a confidant has been identified as a protective factor for loneliness (Grenade and Boldy, 2008).

A study in Holland evaluated the outcomes of an Internet-at-home intervention experiment among chronically ill and physically handicapped older adults. It found that email facilitated social contact, and that the computer and Internet were often used to pass the time, taking people's minds off their loneliness and improving people's self-confidence (Fokkema and Knipscheer, 2007).

The Social Care Institute for Excellence website (http://www.scie.org.uk/) has a practice guide that identifies factors that cause social isolation, and provides practical guidance to support service providers and practitioners in the development of their practice.

Families

Whether older people have family support can affect both living arrangements and care provision. Older people who have many children are less likely to live alone than those with fewer children.

Older people born in the 1920s are characterized by high levels of childlessness when compared with those born in the 1930s and 1940s (Tomassini et al., 2004). Older people who co-reside with relatives can receive informal support at home and thus are at less risk of institutionalization.

Family contact was included in the ONS report on older people, which found that 55 per cent of men and 63 per cent of women aged 75 and over met with their children at least twice weekly; 83 per cent and 90 per cent aged over 75 would speak on the phone to their children each week (ONS, 2005). The interesting dimension was that mothers had more contact with children than fathers, supporting previous studies that women are more likely to maintain family networks.

To enable better understanding of the relationships in the later life and family life experiences, Jerome (1993) identifies several areas of change in relation to the family and intergenerational support over the last hundred years.

- Demographic—Falling rates of fertility and mortality, reduced family size, age at marriage, and the number of children born to each family has contributed to the reduction in families' provision to support parents and wider social support.
- Technological—The increased numbers of women that joined the workforce, particularly in mid-life, further reduces the availability of women to provide support.
- Legal—New legislation regulating marriage, divorce, and civil partnerships has affected the structure of the family, with a higher number of families that are divided and less conventional than in previous generations.
- Ideological—There has been, in recent decades, a move away from institutional to community care. Changing ideologies of marriage and parenthood have also introduced conflicts into family life.
- Economic—Improved pension and welfare provision, coupled with the rise in affluence in society, have provided wider choice in families, and thus ties between older parents and their adult children are no longer those of obligation, but rather those of sentiment.

The influence of family history, including the sibling position and the relationship with parents and other siblings, can affect the provision of support. This theme was considered by Schofield (1999), who suggests that ageing parents can be affected by the siblings' motivation, socialization, affiliation, and aggression. Parents can also favour certain siblings and have expectations that can influence relationships in later life.

The nurse should understand and take into account that there can be complexities in family histories that may be under the surface of family tensions when care and support is required for older people.

Who is a carer?

A 'carer' is someone who looks after a person with a disability, long-term illness, mental health difficulties, or who is old and frail.

Carers UK defines a carer as:

Someone of any age whose life is restricted because they are looking after a relative, friend, partner or child who cannot manage without help because of illness, age or a disability of any kind.

The *National Carers Strategy* proposes a pan-governmental definition of the term 'carer':

A carer spends a significant proportion of their life providing unpaid support to family or potentially friends. This could be caring for a relative, partner or friend who is ill, frail, disabled or has mental health or substance misuse problems.

(DH, 2008a).

Carers are also referred to as 'informal carers' to differentiate between those who are paid to give care and those who are not—although some carers consider that this term undervalues their role. Carers may increasingly be paid for some of their caring, through personal budget approaches to community care, but most will remain in a largely unpaid role. 'Family carers' is another term that is used, but it should be noted that carers may also be caring for friends or neighbours.

The amount, impact, and duration of caring can vary enormously. There are approximately 1.3 million people caring for 50+ hours per week (ONS, 2003). The 'carer job description' produced by Carers UK (see Figure 5.1 below) was created as an example of what the role of the carer often entails. This is a tall order for anyone—but, in old age, caring can be particularly stressful and exhausting.

NURSING PRACTICE INSIGHT: PUTTING YOURSELF IN THE SHOES OF A CARER

- Most carers wish to carry out some level of caring. Many see caring as a duty, or even a privilege, with many positive aspects.

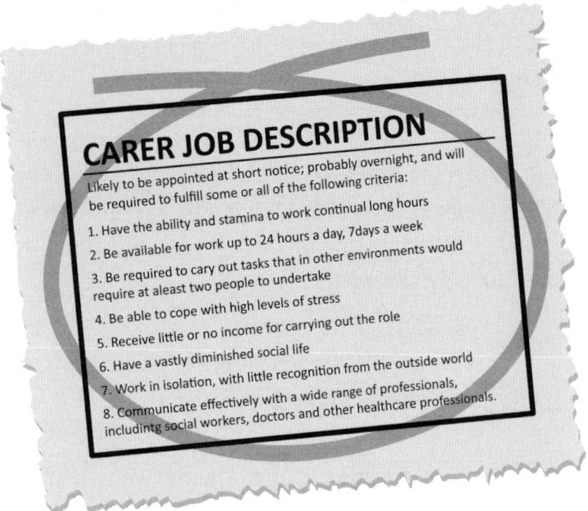

CARER JOB DESCRIPTION

Likely to be appointed at short notice; probably overnight, and will be required to fulfill some or all of the following criteria:

1. Have the ability and stamina to work continual long hours
2. Be available for work up to 24 hours a day, 7days a week
3. Be required to cary out tasks that in other environments would require at aleast two people to undertake
4. Be able to cope with high levels of stress
5. Receive little or no income for carrying out the role
6. Have a vastly diminished social life
7. Work in isolation, with little recognition from the outside world
8. Communicate effectively with a wide range of professionals, includintg social workers, doctors and other healthcare professionals.

Figure 5.1 Carer's job description
Source: Reproduced with permission from *carers UK*

- Caring should be an informed choice, not an obligation. Many carers feel that they have limited choices when it comes to caring. Many would like to spend less time caring. They can feel that a higher level of health support or better quality of care would be needed for this to happen.
- Carers can find themselves carrying out medical, physical, or emotional caring tasks for which they feel ill-equipped or under-supported.
- Changes to the home environment can include hospital beds, hoists, commodes, and a variety of other unusual equipment. These can make the difference between caring being sustainable and the need for someone to enter residential care. But they can be quite disruptive, and even distressing for both patient and carer alike, as they try to maintain the atmosphere of home rather than a hospital ward.
- When several people from the multidisciplinary team are involved (in addition to friends and family), there can be the feeling of a busy train station with a constant ringing of the doorbell. Remember that the care setting is the family's home.
- Carers can feel as if they are the visitor when staff 'take over' or take a call about someone else. Carers wish to be recognized as (in the words of the *National Carers Strategy*) 'expert care partners'.
- Alternatively, carers may have to stay in for people who do not turn up or are late.
- Carers may be suffering actual loss in terms of income, time with their family, and social lives.
- Think also about how the carer will feel when the person for whom they care dies or when they cannot provide care any more.

Key conditions that require care of the older person

Nearly any long-term condition or disability can require the need for a carer. However, there are conditions that more commonly require the support from a carer. These include neurological conditions—particularly Parkinson's disease, which affects one in a hundred older people—strokes, disabilities, and mental health—particularly dementia.

See Chapter 12 for more on key health conditions in the elderly.

See Chapter 13 for more on mental health and the ageing process.

The value and contribution of unpaid caring to the health economy

It has been estimated that, every day, 6,000 new people take on caring responsibilities in the UK and a high percentage of carers are over the age of 65 (DH, 2008a). In the future, older people's lives will usually include at least one episode of caring. There are approximately 1.5 million people aged 60+ providing unpaid care and over 8,000 carers are aged 90+. Some 4,000 of these very aged carers provide 50 or more hours of care each week.

The support that carers provide to health and social care services is immense, and it has been estimated by Carers UK that the monetary value of 'informal care' in the UK is £87bn a year. Yet it often costs the carer dearly in terms of their health, finances, and independence.

Why are family and carers so important to the health of older people?

The capability and willingness of a carer and families to provide care for people who would otherwise need alternative support from the State or other agencies is pivotal to the organization of care provision. The economy simply could not afford the care that is provided informally by carers and families. It is thus not surprising that the government is recognizing the crucial role that carers provide and the need to ensure that they are supported.

It is important for the nurse to be aware of the support that is required for the carer and to ensure, as part of normal good practice, that a carer's assessment is undertaken—particularly by colleagues in the community—and reviewed every six months or when the caring situation changes.

Older people as care-givers

The spouse is usually the primary source of care, so being married at an old age can have particular issues. Older couples often see caring for each other as a natural part of their lives, and of being together 'in sickness and in health'. For some, the caring role can come on gradually, with time to adjust; for others, it may be quite sudden.

Either way, it can manifest in a reluctance to seek assistance and can ultimately lead to a breakdown in the older carer's health. It can also result in a loss of social life and friends, and changes to families. In some cases, older people may still be in employment and thus it might also lead to a loss of income. Studies have also shown that carers often neglect their own health and that health services can be inaccessible to carers, who may need respite care to leave the house. The breakdown of a carer's health can lead to the collapse of the caring role, so support for carers to stay healthy is doubly beneficial.

National policy and legislation

The Carers (Recognition & Services) Act 1995 gave carers over the age of 16 the right to an individual assessment of their needs if they provide 'regular and substantial' care to a person undergoing a social care assessment.

The assessment was extended to all other carers in the Carers & Disabled Children Act 2000, including people caring for someone who has declined a social care assessment. The Act also highlighted that authorities must recognize the impact of caring.

Following the 1999 *Carers' Strategy* (DH, 1999), carers are now included in most, if not all, key social and health government White Papers.

The Carers (Equal Opportunities) Act 2004 was intended to ensure better practice by councils and the health service. This includes placing a duty on local authorities to ensure that all carers know that they are entitled to an assessment of their needs and to consider a carer's outside interests (work, study, or leisure) when carrying out an assessment.

The White Paper *Our Health, Our Care, Our Say* (DH, 2006b) announced a new deal for carers made up of four parts:

- *'a comprehensive national information service'*, comprising a single telephone number and website, to assist carers directly or refer them onto more appropriate support, was launched in Spring 2009;
- a training programme for carers called 'Caring with Confidence' was to provide training to carers, empowering and enabling them in their caring role, informing them of their rights and the services available to them, providing information, and also developing their advocacy skills and their ability to network with other carers to support their needs;
- *'emergency care cover'* via additional funding to local authorities; and
- *'a major review of the Carer's Strategy'*.

In 2007, the government announced a new Standing Commission on Carers, which would have a key role in the implementation of the *Carers' Strategy*, as well as a responsibility to advise the government on matters that it feels are relevant to carers in the longer term. It was also to ensure that the voice of carers is kept at the very heart of government and external stakeholders.

The Department of Health, in conjunction with other government departments, produced a key strategy entitled *Carers at the Heart of 21st-century Families and Communities* (DH, 2008a), which was shaped by carers and their advocates, families, the National Health Service (NHS), local government, and the voluntary and independent sector. This sets out the changes that need to be made to meet the needs of carers over the next ten years. The vision is that carers will be universally recognized and valued as being fundamental to strong families and stable communities. Support will be tailored to meet individuals' needs, enabling carers to maintain a balance between their caring responsibilities and a life outside caring, whilst enabling the person whom they support to be a full and equal citizen.

By 2018, carers will be:

- respected as expert care partners and will have access to the integrated and personalized services that they need to support them in their caring role;
- able to have a life of their own alongside their caring role;
- supported so that they are not forced into financial hardship by their caring role; and
- supported to stay mentally and physically well, and treated with dignity.

Other strategic drivers include the following.

The *Stroke Strategy* (DH, 2006a) promotes support for carers and has a number of quality markers for NHS bodies, which includes:

- offering people who have had a stroke, and their relatives and carers, access to practical advice, emotional support, advocacy, and information throughout the care pathway and throughout their lives;
- involving individuals and their carers in developing and monitoring stroke services;
- making a range of services locally available to support the individual long-term needs of people who have had a stroke and their carers; and
- assessing and reviewing the needs of people affected by stroke.

The assessment and review requirements specify that people who have had strokes, and their carers, will be offered a review from primary care services of their health and social care status, and secondary prevention needs, within six weeks of discharge and again before six months after leaving hospital.

The *End-of-Life Care Strategy* (DH, 2008b) sets out three key principles about how carers should be involved and supported during end-of-life care:

- carers are central to the team that cares for someone at the end of their life, and should be treated as co-workers within the health and social care team;
- carers have their own needs and are entitled to a community care assessment; and
- the condition of the person who is cared for should not affect how the carer is treated, or the services that the carer may be able to access.

Practically, carers should be:

- better informed and communicated with, including information about a person's condition and services that are available;
- involved in care delivery, including decision-making training in their caring role;
- recognized in relation to their own needs; and
- offered practical and emotional care and support during and after the person's life.

The *National Dementia Strategy* (DH, 2009) recognizes that families are the '*most important resource*' in providing care to someone with dementia. With nearly one in nine UK carers looking after someone with dementia, this is a significant group for whom care needs must be addressed, including practical and psychological support.

See Chapter 11 for more on dementia.

Carers as experts

Carers are increasingly being recognized across health and social care as being experts, with a wealth of experience of caring for someone with a disability or chronic illness. Even a person new to caring will have spent more time observing the person than the nurse has had time or opportunity to do. Because carers are so often the primary provider of care, they are increasingly invited to be representatives on boards, groups, forums, and committees. Their input is regarded as paramount when developing and redesigning new services. The nurse should listen and ask the carer what they think, use their knowledge, and value their opinion.

Carers' assessments

One of the most important ways in which caring can be made easier is to ensure that the carer is involved appropriately in care planning for the person requiring care. Their involvement is dependent on that person's wishes, which should be ascertained, but it should be noted that no care plan can be put together that relies on assumptions about a carer's contributions that have not first been checked with the carer.

Caring may be a positive experience that many people will take on willingly and easily. Others, however, want to provide care, but find themselves overwhelmed by the situation in which they find themselves. Nurses are in a front-line position to assess the needs of carers and to refer them onto appropriate agencies for help. This, more often than not, is at time when the primary focus of assessment and care is on the patient. Thus the carer's needs must not be overlooked—particularly because, as previously noted, the majority of care that is provided is by family carers. Furthermore, it will be beneficial to the patient that the carer is having their needs assessed.

Carers have a right under the Carers (Equal Opportunities) Act 2004 to an assessment of their needs, and anyone who provides a regular and substantial amount of care for someone aged 18 or over can ask their social services department in their local council for a carer's assessment. Carers' assessments are intended to ascertain the level of caring that the person wishes, and is able, to carry out and what support they need in order to do so. People also have a right to assessment if they intend to look after someone—for example, someone who is about to be discharged from hospital and who will require care.

The person carrying out the assessment should not assume that the carer wants to take on a caring role or continue caring. There are many tasks in caring that are difficult and may not come easily to the carer, such as intimate tasks involving assisting with hygiene needs, manual handling, and stress in coping with challenging behaviour.

Box 5.1 identifies factors that might impact on the carer that should be considered during the preparation of an assessment. It is also helpful if both the carer and the person being cared for are involved in the assessment, and therefore have a discussion beforehand about which points to raise.

Box 5.1 Factors that might impact the carer

Health

- Do you get enough sleep?
- Is your health affected by caring?
- Does the person for whom you care have health problems with which you find it difficult to deal?

Input

- How many hours a week do you provide care?
- Is the help during the day or night, or both?

- What does the care provided include? (For example, manual handling, housework, shopping, laundry, bathing, toileting, pensions, medications, and taking them to hospital.)
- Does anyone else help? Who and for how long?
- Can you leave the person whom you are looking after on their own?

Social

- Are you worried about having to give up work or social activities?
- Do you get enough time for yourself?

Housing

- Are you living apart from or in the same household as the person for whom you are caring? Does this create difficulties?
- Are there any mobility issues in the home, such as access to stairs, that need adaptations?

Emergencies and unplanned events

- Do you have a plan should you become ill or have an emergency?
- Do you know who to contact in the event of an emergency?

An assessment is usually carried out by a member of social services, but it is part of the nurse's role to ensure that the carer is referred for an assessment and to ensure that this has being carried out. Where a lot of work is being delivered by the carer, the nurse and/or general practitioner (GP) should also be involved.

The primary aim of a carer's assessment is to focus on an individual's needs; following an assessment, a care plan should be developed that will include the support and services that the person has been assessed as needing. Should the caring situation be ongoing, then a review date should be set to ensure that any support provided is meeting the needs. Many carers are willing to provide the bulk of the care as long as they are offered a break. It is also important to note that, with the increasing pressures that local authorities are facing, the support provided for carers is often limited. Carers who are assessed as being at a 'critical' level of need are entitled to support. In other cases, councils have the power to support rather than a duty, but most provide a range of support and breaks services.

An example of a carer's action plan is supplied in Figure 5.2 below.

See the Online Resource Centre that accompanies this book for an example of a full carer's questionnaire.

Support for carers

Local authorities

Most, if not all, local authorities and metropolitan borough councils (MBC) have a carers' support service that is often underpinned by a strategy. This is often delivered by one or more third-sector (that is, voluntary, not-for-profit, non-government) organizations.

A typical service will comprise the following elements.

- A third sector carers' centre will identify carers and provide information, emotional support, and a range of activities. There are many such centres in the network of the Princess Royal Trust for Carers—http://www.carers.org/. Many carers' centres provide services located in GP surgeries, hospital wards, and other settings.
- A breaks service will provide respite care. There are many such services provided by the Crossroads Care network—http://www.crossroads.org.uk/
- In-house provision will involve carers' specialists, who will lead on carers' assessments and the commissioning of support services.

It is worth a nurse's while to contact their local carers' service and familiarize themselves with the support, services, and information that it provides. This local background knowledge will be particularly beneficial in undertaking assessments.

Primary care trusts (PCTs)

Many primary care trusts (PCTs) also have a carers' lead or coordinator, who will focus on carers with health needs and supporting healthcare staff. They will work closely with the local authority's carers support service, but also carry out many of the functions listed above. Many PCTs circulate information on carers via their Patient Advice and Liaison Service (PALS).

Expert Patient Programme for Carers ('Caring with Confidence' or 'Looking After Me')

All PCTs are now running the Expert Patient Programme, which is a training programme that aims to improve quality of life by developing the confidence and motivation of people to use their own skills and knowledge to take effective control over life with a long-term health condition. It provides opportunities to people, including parents, young people, and their carers, who live with long-term illness to meet other people with similar conditions, and to develop new skills and support networks to manage their condition better within the community.

Name of Carer: ....

Name of Assessor: .... Contact no: ....

Please complete this form for each relevant section.

Need	Action agreed to meet need	Who's responsible	Target date
1. Information about the needs of the person cared for			
2. Information on what to do and who to contact in a crisis			
3. Advice on income, housing, education, and employment			
4. Short term breaks for Carer			
5. Social support including access to carers support groups			
6. Information about appeals or complaints procedure			
7. Planning for the future			
8. Other needs			

Can this information be shared With the person you care for? Yes ☐ No ☐

Date of next review: ....

Signature of Carer: ....

Signature of Assessor: .... Date: ....

Figure 5.2 Carer's action plan (to be completed after assessment)
Source: Reproduced with permission from Dudley Metropolitan Borough Council.

This is now being extended to a specific programme for carers called 'Caring with Confidence', which is available in some areas of England.

Hospitals

Similar to PCTs, some hospitals will have a lead for carers, but there are professionals, such as 'discharge liaison nurses' or 'employees of carers' centres' who will have skills in undertaking carers' assessments and who will act as a resource for the wider multidisciplinary team.

Carers' assessments in hospitals are particularly important because this is often the first time that the carer's needs come to light. It frequently coincides with an increase in the needs for support following deterioration in a person's condition. In some cases, the reason for the admission to hospital is the carer becoming ill. A further example is a crisis situation in which the carer has had no or limited support—particularly if the person is diagnoses dementia.

A study of an intensive intervention programme set in a psychiatric unit in Sydney, Australia, provided carers with training and coping skills to care for relatives with dementia. It found that the programme can reduce the psychological morbidity of the carer and delay the placement of the patient in an institution (Brodaty and Gresham, 1989).

See Chapter 11 on dementia, mental health, and the older adult.

Carers UK

Carers UK coordinates national campaigns to promote carers and their rights, including 'Carers' Rights Day' in September and also 'Carers' Week' in June.

The Princess Royal Trust for Carers

The Princess Royal Trust for Carers is a UK network of carers' centres supporting some 350,000 carers of all ages, including around 20,000 young carers.

Crossroads Care

Crossroads Care is the UK's leading provider of support for carers. It works with over 35,000 individuals and their families, helping carers to make a life of their own outside caring.

Ethnicity

The 2001 Census estimates that, overall, 4 per cent of the population aged over 65 define themselves as belonging to minority ethnic groups (ONS, 2003). This statistic is likely to change in future years, as the population of people who moved to the UK in the 1950s and beyond begins to age. This will be most significant in some of the large cities, where there are well-established concentrations of minority ethnic groups. Many of these people from older minority ethnic groups are disadvantaged and are thought to have double discrimination on account of their age and minority status (Blakemore and Boneham, 1994). The needs of those from ethnic minority groups may get overlooked, or assumptions may be made that they have their own networks of support and thus do not require the help of other services (Gunaratnum, 1993). However, it is important that support for such groups is addressed and that all means possible are used to engage with them—including, for example, producing carers' leaflets in a variety of languages, and ensuring that these are visible in health practices and libraries.

When considering carers, we also need to be aware of the significant numbers of carers who do not identify themselves as such. For example, cultural concepts of caring are not universally shared throughout communities in the UK: many people from other countries do not have experience of a 'welfare state' and therefore, among a whole range of concepts, would not understand the concept of a 'carer'. This is highlighted by the National Black Carers and Carers Workers Network (2008), in that it has been unable to find a word in Gujarati, Urdu, Punjabi, or Bengali that translates as 'carer'.

There are many older people from minority communities whose first language may not be English and who may be unaware of support services. The nurse needs to be aware of local interpreting services and how to access them, or how to signpost and utilize carers and relevant carers' groups.

Student activity

Mr Sampson is a 75-year-old whom you have been asked to visit for a blood pressure check on behalf of the GP. During the initial assessment, you are made aware that Mr Sampson cares for his wife, who has severe dementia. They have no children.

- What would be your first steps to assess Mr Sampson's needs as a carer?
- Which further assessments might need to take place?
- To which support agencies would you consider referring Mr Sampson?
- What interventions could be offered?

NURSING PRACTICE INSIGHT: CARING FOR CARERS

- The nurse needs to appreciate that a person (carer) may be about to provide care for the first time. They may therefore be apprehensive, frightened of doing something wrong, confused, and thus needing reassurance and a contact to call should they need it.
- A relative might not be willing and/or able to provide care. Taking on caring should be an informed choice. A local carers' support service can help the carer to understand the range of options open to them before taking on a caring role.
- Nurses must check that the carers have the information that they need (that is, they must undertake a carer's assessment).
- Patients should not be told 'you can go home now' without first checking that the carer can manage and carrying out a full carer's assessment.
- Health professionals also must not accept the statement 'my daughter/son/husband/wife will look after me' at face value. They should remember, however, not to ask the carer if they can manage in front of the patient or service user, but rather to ensure that they have a private conversation with the carer.

- Nurses need to treat carers as partners are able to contribute expertise and observations on the person's condition.
- Information to the carer is 'central' and it is important to ensure that this is not only provided, relevant, and jargon-free, but also understood by the carer. In the same way as nurses receive training, so carers should be offered training and support (see 'Caring with Confidence' above).
- Remember that many carers have their own health problems and that their health needs have to be addressed. (Who cares for the carers?)

Conclusion

Caring is universal but also very personal, with carers experiencing many different emotions and having different capabilities, needs, and wishes. Many carers say that the recognition of their role is often the most important 'service' that professionals can provide. Nurses need carers and we need their expertise, which is why we should value them as true partners in care.

Questions and self-assessment

Now that you have worked through the chapter, answer the following questions.

- Why might loneliness become a reality for many older adults and how might you, as a nurse, help to facilitate greater social contact for an older adult?
- How can carers' expertise be respected and integrated into care planning?
- Think back to a recent placement in which you were working with an older adult and their carer. Were the carer's needs assessed and, if so, how were their needs met?

Self-assessment

- Having read the chapter, how will you change your practice?
- Identify up to three areas relating to carers' support in which you need to develop your knowledge and understanding further.
- Identify how you are going to develop this knowledge and understanding, and set deadlines for achieving this.

For further reading and information

http://www.ageuk.org.uk/

http://www.alzheimers.org.uk/

http://www.carersuk.org/

http://www.crossroads.org.uk/

http://www.direct.gov.uk/en/caringforsomeone

http://www.scie.org.uk/

The Princess Royal Trust for Carers supports:

- adult carers at http://www.carers.org/
- young carers at http://www.youngcarers.net/
- carers' professionals at http://www.carers.org/professionals/ (including an *Action Guide for Primary Care*, produced in association with the Royal College of General Practitioners)

References

Beal, C. (2006) 'Loneliness in older women a review of the literature', *Issues in Mental Health Nursing*, 27(7): 795–813.

Blakemore, K. and Boneham, M. (1994) *Age Race and Ethnicity*, Buckingham: Open University Press.

Brodaty, H. and Gresham, M. (1989) 'Effect of a training programme to reduce stress in carers of patients with dementia', *British Medical Journal*, 299: 1375–9.

Concannon, L. (2009) 'Developing inclusive health and social care policies for older LGBT citizens', *British Journal of Social Work*, 39(3): 403–17.

Department of Health (1995) *Carers (Recognition & Services) Act: Policy Guidance*, London: DH, available online at http://www.dh.gov.uk/en/publicationsandstatistics/index.htm.

Department of Health (1999) *Caring about Carers: A National Strategy for Carers*, London: DH.

Department of Health (2001) *The National Service Framework for Older People*, London: DH, available online at http://www.dh.gov.uk/en/publicationsandstatistics/index.htm.

Department of Health (2006a) *A Strategy for Stroke*, London: DH, available online at http://www.dh.gov.uk/en/publicationsandstatistics/index.htm.

Department of Health (2006b) *Our Health, Our Care, Our Say*, London: DH, available online at http://www.dh.gov.uk/en/publicationsandstatistics/index.htm.

Department of Health (2008a) *Carers at the heart of 21st-Century Families and Communities: A Caring System on Your Side—A Life of Your Own*, London: DH, available online at http://www.dh.gov.uk/en/publicationsandstatistics/index.htm.

Department of Health (2008b) *End-of-Life Care Strategy*, London: DH, available online at http://www.dh.gov.uk/en/publicationsandstatistics/index.htm.

Department of Health (2009) *The National Dementia Strategy*, London: DH, available online at http://www.dh.gov.uk/en/publicationsandstatistics/index.htm.

Ekwall, A.K., Sivberg, B., and Hallberg, I.R. (2005) 'Loneliness as a predictor of quality of life among older caregivers', *Journal of Advance Nursing*, 49(1): 23–32.

Fitzpatrick, R., Dawson, J., Boulton, M., McLean, J., Hart, G., and Brookes, M. (1994) 'Perceptions of general practice among homosexual men', *British Journal of General Practice*, 44: 80–2.

Fokkemer, T. and Knipscheer, K. (2007) 'Escape loneliness by going digital: a quantitative and qualitative evaluation of a Dutch experiment in using ECT to overcome loneliness among older adults', *Aging & Mental Health*, 11(5): 496–504.

Glover, D. (2006) 'Overcoming barriers for older gay men in the use of health services: A qualitative study of growing older, sexuality and health', *Health Education Journal*, 65(1): 45–52.

Greaves, C.J. and Farbus, L. (2006) 'Effects of creative and social activity on the health and well-being of socially isolated older people: outcomes from a multi-method observational study', *Journal of the Royal Society for the Promotion of Health*, 126(3): 134–42.

Grenade, L. and Boldy, D. (2008) 'Social isolation and loneliness among older people: issues and future challenges in community and residential settings', *Australian Health Review*, 32(3): 468–78.

Grossman, A.H., D'Augelli, A.R., and Hershberger, S.L. (2000) 'Social support networks of lesbian, gay, bisexual adults 60 years of age and older', *Journal of Gerontology*, 55B(3): 171–9.

Gunaratnum, Y. (1993) 'Breaking the silence: Asian Carers in Britain', in J. Bornat, C. Pereria, D. Pilgrim, and F. Williams (eds) *Community Care: A Reader*, Basingstoke: Macmillan.

Holmen, K. and Furukawa, H. (2002) 'Loneliness, health and social network among elderly people: A follow-up study', *Archives of Gerontology and Geriatrics*, 35(3): 261–71.

Jacobs, R.J., Rasmussen, L.A., and Hohman, M.M. (1999) 'The social support needs of older lesbians, gay and bisexuals', *Journal of Gay and Lesbian Social Services*, 9(1): 1–30.

Jerome, D. (1993) 'Intimate Relations', in J. Bond, P. Coleman, and S. Peace (eds) *Ageing in Society*, London: Sage.

Luanaigh, C.O. and Lawlor, B.A. (2008) 'Loneliness and the health of older people', *International Journal of Geriatric Psychiatry*, 23(12): 1213–21.

National Black Carers and Carers Workers Network, The (2008) *Beyond We Care Too: Putting Black Carers in the Picture*, London: Afiya Trust.

Office for National Statistics (2003) *Census 2001: National Report for England and Wales*, London: HMSO, available online at http://www.statistics.gov.uk/hub/index.html.

Office for National Statistics (2005) *Focus on Older People*, London: DWP, available online at http://www.statistics.gov.uk/hub/index.html.

Schofield, I. (1999) 'Relationships, Communication and Social Support', in H. Heath and I. Schofield (eds) *Healthy Ageing: Nursing Older People*, London: Mosby.

Tomassini, C., Glaser, K., Wolf, D., Broese van Groenou, M., and Grundy, E. (2004) 'Living arrangements among older people: An overview of trends in Europe and the USA', *Population Trends*, 115: 24–34.

Victor, C.R., Scambler, S.J., Bond, J., and Bowling, A. (2004) 'Loneliness in Later Life', in A. Walker and C. Hagan Hennessy (eds) *Growing Older: Quality of Life in Old Age*, Maidenhead: Open University Press.

Statutes

Carers and Disabled Children's Act 2000

Carers (Equal Opportunities) Act 2004

Carers (Recognition and Services) Act 1995

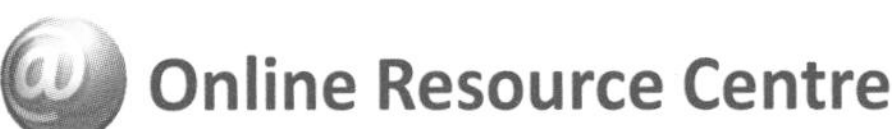

Online Resource Centre

You can learn more about carers and older people at the Online Resource Centre that accompanies this book: **http://www.oxfordtextbooks.co.uk/orc/hindle/**

Part 2

Patient safety

Mobility and falls

Andrew Hindle

Learning outcomes

By the end of the chapter, you will be able to:

- identify why falls are so debilitating for health;
- identify risk factors associated with falls;
- understand the principles of nursing and medical assessments; and
- recognize key components of falls prevention programmes.

Introduction

Mobility for the older person is important for independence, interacting with the environment, contact with others, and socializing. Maintenance of mobility further supports a person's dignity and can impact on their privacy, and is part of a safety net against accidents, as identified by Maslow's hierarchy. Nurses working in a variety of settings have a critical role in ensuring optimum mobility for the older person. It is thus an integral part of assessment to describe the older person's mobility. This can lead to the use of tools such as risk assessment and a management plan.

In this chapter, there is a focus on the impact of falls on older people and the paramount importance of maintaining mobility for the older person. Understanding risk factors, prevention, and the importance of a holistic assessment need to be core skills for the nurse, because these can have a hugely positive impact on the well-being of the older person.

A fall can have a devastating impact on an older person's life. Many people die each year as a result of a fall, and for thousands of other older people, a fall can lead to an admission to a nursing or residential home.

Falls are not an inevitable consequence of old age but can be attributed to one or more underlying risk factors, which include intrinsic and extrinsic factors, or a combination of both (see Tables 6.1 and 6.2 later in the chapter). Around a quarter of a million people over the age of 75 seek medical assistance in an accident and emergency (A&E) department every year as a result of a fall at home. Even a minor fall can have a serious impact on well-being and quality of life, with both physical and psychological consequences.

Definition of a fall

A fall is defined as an event whereby an individual comes to rest on the ground or another lower level with or without loss of consciousness.

(American and British Geriatrics Societies, 2001)

Facts about falls

- About a third of all people over the age of 65 fall each year, with higher rates among those over the age of 75.
- Falls represent over half of hospital admissions for accidental injury—particularly hip fracture (Help the Aged, 2005).
- Half of those with hip fracture never regain their former level of function and one in five die within three months (Help the Aged, 2005).

- '*A hospital setting is not a safe place for elderly people but is actually associated with an increases risk of falls*' (Fonda et al., 2006).
- Research has shown that half of the individuals who have fallen will fall again within one year (Close et al., 1999).
- Of those older people who enter a falls prevention programme, most do so only after they have fallen, by which time they may have suffered serious consequences.
- In an average primary care trust (PCT) (that is, one serving a population of 300,000), there will be 360 hip fractures per year (DH, 2009).
- Falls and instability account for 40 per cent of nursing home admissions.
- In care homes, falls account for around 90 per cent of reportable injuries to residents.
- Some 10–25 per cent of institutional falls result in fracture, laceration, or the need for hospital care.
- Most common sites of fracture are the hip, the wrist, and the spine.
- Many slips, trips, and falls in care environments are preventable.

Hip fractures in the UK

- Healthcare costs associated with fragility fractures amounts to £2bn a year, with hip fractures the most frequent fragility fracture caused by falls (RCP, 2007).
- Some 80 per cent of people who fracture their neck or femur never regain their previous level of mobility.
- Half of hip fracture patients lose the ability to live independently (Eddy et al., 1998).
- Around 30 per cent of hip fracture patients die within a year of their fracture.

Hip fractures have serious consequences in terms of reduced function, increased disability, and increased dependence, as well as a significant increase in mortality (Cooper et al., 1993). The loss of mobility and independence that can arise from falling is a genuine fear for older people. Salkeld et al. (2000) found that 80 per cent of women who were surveyed would rather die than experience loss of independence and quality of life, combined with admission to a nursing home, following a bad hip fracture.

Fractures rarely occur spontaneously: a person has to fall with enough force to break their bone. However, in the very elderly, vertebral fractures can occur with little force being applied.

Causes of falls

Falls in older people tend to be caused by a combination of intrinsic events (see Table 6.1) and extrinsic events (see Table 6.2).

Fonda et al. (2006) discovered that, in a new environment, we are all slightly out of our depth: we do not know where things are; hospitals are large and disorientating; and we will have little or no clue as to what may be dangerous within this environment. Often, an older person will have their home environment set up so that they feel safe and supported: for example, all of the things that they need are close at hand. In contrast, in a hospital, it is often the simple things that cause problems, such as sliding toilet doors. The nurse can make an older person feel a lot less anxious about their new environment by taking time to show them around and how things work.

National Service Framework for Older People Standard 6: Falls

The prevention and management of falls in older people was a key government target in reducing mortality and injury. This is outlined in Standard 6 on falls in the *National Service Framework for Older People* (NSPOP), which states:

Every health system should, in partnership with councils, agree and implement local priorities to reduce the incidence of falls, and to reduce the impact which a fall can have on health, well-being and independence, including appropriate interventions and advice to prevent osteoporotic fracture.

(DH, 2001)

A successful falls prevention service is one in which there is good leadership (such as a falls coordinator), joint working across agencies, and multidisciplinary teams.

Figure 6.1 illustrates a falls care pathway from the NSFOP Standard 6—that is, a pathway of care from when an older person either falls or is at risk of falling, through to assessment, treatment, rehabilitation, specialist programmes, and review.

Multifactorial falls risk assessment

The most effective intervention found to prevent or reduce the incidence of falls in older people is a multifactorial risk assessment and management programme (Gillespie et al., 2003; Chang et al., 2004; NICE, 2004).

The National Institute for Health and Clinical Excellence (NICE) Guidelines (2004) state that older people presenting to a healthcare professional because of a fall, or reporting recurrent falls in the past year, or who demonstrate abnormalities

Table 6.1 Intrinsic risk factors include age-related changes

Intrinsic factors	Assessment and management
Mobility and balance impairment Unsteadiness on feet, particularly associated with neurological conditions such as Parkinson's disease and with stroke.	Refer to physiotherapist for assessment, and identify use of walking aid and/or referral to approved falls exercise programme.
Functional impairment Affecting mobility, transfers, and activities of daily living.	Refer to moving and handling assessors, physiotherapist, and occupational therapist for assessment of aids, and check that aids are at appropriate height and within reach of patients.
Visual problems **(see also Chapter 3 for sight loss)** Age-related changes in the eye can increase the risk of falls due to a failure to see obstacles or a changed environment.	Ensure regular eye tests. Surgical interventions. Environmental modifications. Staff awareness that older people take longer to adjust to changes in light intensity. If in hospital, then help and guidance should be given to support the person to move around.
History of previous falls.	Full assessment and refer to GP, falls clinic, physiotherapist, and occupational therapist.
Postural hypotension Unsteady or giddy when first stands up.	Refer to GP. Undertake medications review.
Cognitive impairment Agitation, poor judgement, and poor awareness of risk and safety.	Refer to GP, mental health team, physiotherapist, and occupational therapists for aids. Monitor safety, particularly bed rails.
Medications Sedatives, antihypertensives, strong analgesics, and diuretics that lead to dehydration can cause side effects of unsteadiness, dizziness, confusion, sedation, blurred vision. This can also be exacerbated when commencing a new medication and at night-time.	Discuss medication with GP or prescriber. Medication withdrawal if needed. Possible non-pharmacological interventions.
Chronic medical conditions Stroke, arthritis, cognitive impairment, depression, neurological conditions such as Parkinson's disease.	Assessment by clinicians. Review by physiotherapists and occupational therapist for implementation of aids and exercise programmes.
Acute medical conditions Chest infections/pneumonia, urinary tract infections, vertigo and dizziness, labrynthitis, transient ischaemic attacks (TIAs), cardiac conditions such as ventricular tachycardia, hypothermia, and delirium can lead to unsteadiness and falls.	Urgent review by GP and acute medical care.
Osteoporosis (see section 5)	Review by GP, dietitian, and falls clinics.

of gait and/or balance, should be offered multifactorial falls risk assessment and be considered for individualized multifactorial intervention.

Multifactorial assessment may include the following factors.

- **Identification of falls history**—This can establish emerging patterns in someone's suffering falls.
- **Assessment of gait, balance, mobility, and muscle weakness**—Weakness can arise when a lack of mobility and activity reduces muscle strength, or be due to a medical condition that needs further assessment, diagnosis, and treatment.
- **Assessment of osteoporosis risk**—See 'Osteoporosis' below.
- **Assessment of the older person's perceived functional ability and fear related to falling**—If someone has a fear of falling, then they are five times more likely to have a fall and a referral to a falls service is required (see 'Fear of falling' below).
- **Assessment of visual impairment**—See Table 6.1 above on the intrinsic causes of falls.
- **Assessment of cognitive impairment and neurological examination**—If identified, then a referral to a specialist

Table 6.2 Extrinsic factors play an important role in the cause of falls for older people

Extrinsic factors	Assessment and management
Physical environment and hazards **Indoors:** Cot sides can increase the force of a fall; low staffing levels; slippery floors; loose rugs; obstructions; low or high cupboards; step ladders; spilt liquids; pets; low chairs and toilets; unstable furniture; high beds; no rails for baths/showers or stairs; steep stairs; poor lighting. **Outdoors:** Weather conditions, including ice, snow, strong winds and rain; uneven pathways; leaves on paths; lack of places to rest.	Environmental assessment/review. Non-glare and non-slip floors. Any spillages cleaned immediately. Make all staff aware of the need to avoid obstructions and clutter, including domestic and medical staff. Clear signs. Referral to occupational therapy. Staff need to be aware of bed-rail policies.
New environments/ relocation: Disorientation and confusion can occur when an older adult is relocated, particularly to a healthcare setting or institution; falls maybe attributable to lack of familiarity or changes in mobility and functional state.	Allow time for reorientation, including explanations and guided tours if appropriate, and repeated messages. Accessible call bells.
Footwear: Improper footwear, including poorly fitting and worn-down footwear that has lost its grip can affect gait and balance leading to a fall; high heels, slippery soles, and loose slippers/footwear are particularly hazardous.	Encourage and advise use of well-fitting and safe footwear, including low, broad heels and firm-fitting shoes/trainers that are laced or fasten with Velcro.
Nocturnal falls: Older people, particularly in care environments, who wake during the night (often to go to the toilet) are at risk of falling due to factors such as night sedation, poor illumination, inability to transfer safely out of bed and unfamiliar surroundings; it may be further exacerbated by low staffing levels.	Increased observation and use of movement sensors may help to monitor at risk patients at night. Additional review of allocation of staff to monitor patients at risk. Minimal distances to toilets. Height-adjustable beds. Awareness that some agency staff may not be as familiar with patients and residents under their care and with the relevant safety aspects.

is required. When there is a high level of cognitive impairment, there is less ability to retain information on falls prevention.

- Assessment of urinary incontinence—For example, urgency can result in falls when the person hurries to get to the toilet. Thus assessment and treatment of incontinence is required.
- Assessment of home hazards—See Table 6.2 above on the extrinsic causes of falls.
- Cardiovascular examination and medication review—See 'Medicines and falls' below.

Falls risk assessment and the management care plan

A&E admission

There is evidence that falls prevention initiated in A&E can be effective (Close et al., 1999; Davison et al., 2005). The best practice guidance from the Department of Health (2007) emphasizes that A&E professionals should routinely ask all older people if their emergency is due to a fall or a blackout, and assess gait and balance by observing the patient standing and walking (using usual walking aids). The guidance also highlights the importance of case identification in a falls care pathway in which the person is asked whether they have fallen in the past year, and about the frequency, context, and characteristic of the falls.

Risk assessment

Each patient admitted because of a fall and/or who has a history of falls should have a falls risk assessment completed within 24 hours of admission. Reassessment should occur weekly, or if the patient falls, or if their clinical condition changes. It is the responsibility of the clinician coordinating the patients care to ensure that it is completed.

The falls and injury risk screening and management plan (see Figure 6.2) was developed following the advice from the National Patient Safety Agency report on *Falls, Slips and Trips in Hospital* (2007). This radically changed falls management in institutional care compared to the previous

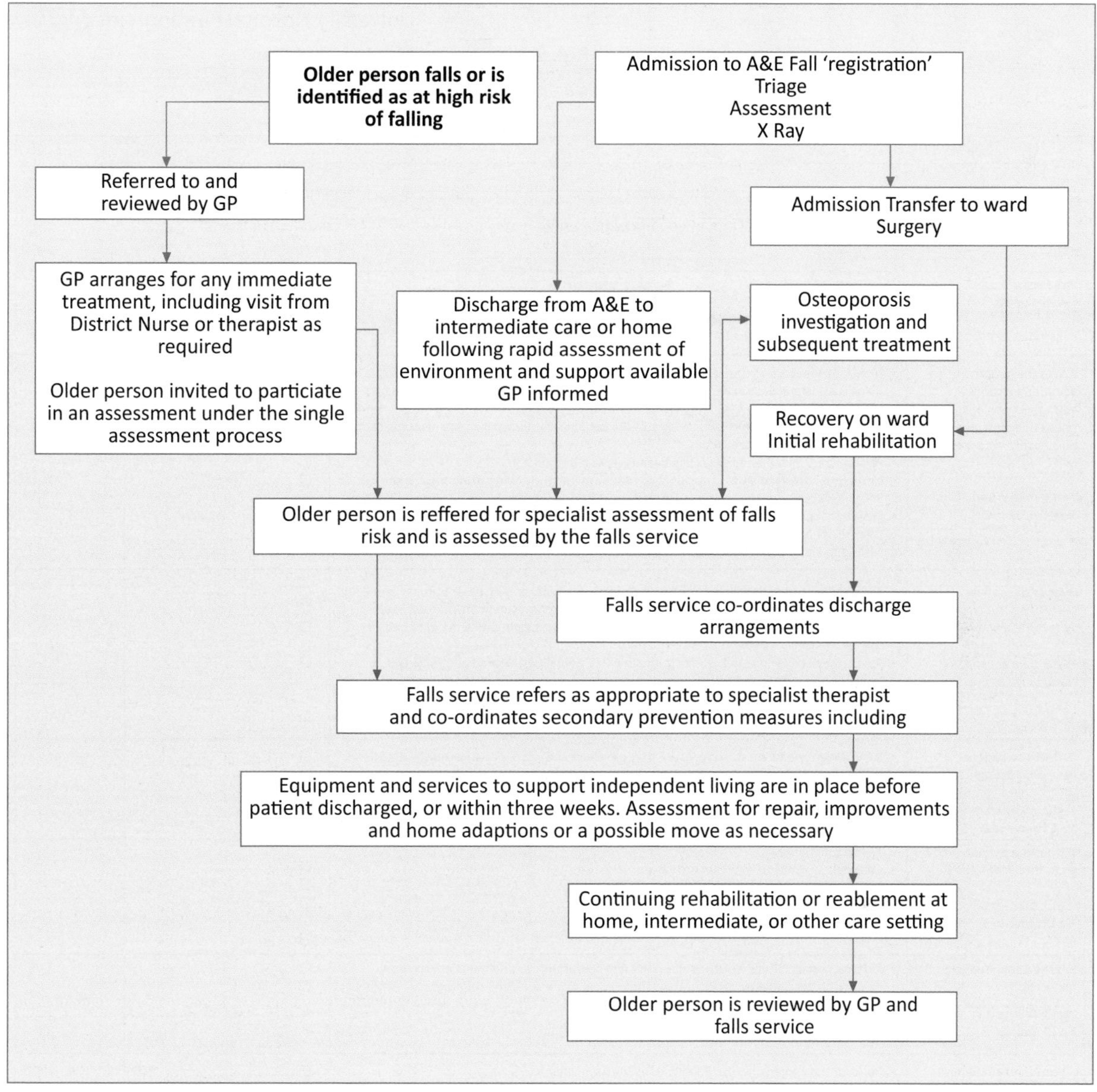

Figure 6.1 Falls care pathway
Source: DH, 2001 © Crown Copyright.

guidelines issued by NICE in 2004, in that there were a wide range of policies and interventions that were offered to reduce the number of falls and injuries.

A large randomized controlled trial (RCT) of implementing multifaceted interventions took place over two community hospitals and six elderly medicine wards, and achieved a statistically significant reduction in the number of falls by staff routinely looking for reversible risk factors for falls structured through a core care plan (Healey et al., 2004). Interventions include straightforward assessments, highlighting medications that might cause falls, urine, and lying and standing blood pressure checks, and alerting medical colleagues via a yellow sticker if a patient had fallen.

Further evidence of the importance of undertaking falls assessments for each patient has come from NHS North West, which has seen a significant drop in the number of falls in its hospital trusts since it introduced a falls assessment quality indicator or metric (Mooney, 2009). Each hospital in the north-west is assessed for its falls risk and controls that are in place, and falls that occur are reported and analyzed.

NICE Guidelines (2004) state that all older people with recurrent falls or assessed as being at increased risk of falling should be considered for an individualized, multifactorial intervention. The following areas consider the components of successful multifactorial interventions.

Patient Label	University Hospital Birmingham NHS NHS Foundation Trust **Falls and Injury Risk Screening and Management Plan** The Falls Screening Tool Section must be completed on admission or transfer for all patients aged over 65 and younger patients with multiple or complex needs or who are thought to be at risk of falling. **Appendix 2**

FALLS RISK SCREENING TOOL			
History of falls before or on admission?	**Yes/No**	Tries to walk alone but unsteady/unsafe with/without walking aid/s?	**Yes/No**
Falls since admission?	**Yes/No**	Patient or relatives anxious about patient at risk of falling?	**Yes/No**

If YES to any of the questions above, complete the Falls Management Plan below

Name..Signature ....Designation................................ Date................. Time.............

Risk Factor *Tick Yes or No*	**Action suggested** **A plan of care will be required for all actions identified and implemented below**	**Tick box when completed** **State Action Taken**	**Date / time/ sign** **Print Name** **Designation**
A.Was the patient admitted following a fall? Have they fallen since admission or do they have a history of falls? *Yes☐ take action* *No ☐ move to **B***	• Monitor and record lying and standing BP, if systolic BP drops > 20 mmHg inform doctor. If there is a postural drop in BP, or the systolic BP is <90 mmHg, consider compression stockings. • Refer to doctor to consider examination of the patient's cardiovascular and neurological systems to look for causes of falls. • Perform an ECG and ensure ECG has been reviewed by a doctor. • Liaise with doctors to assess osteoporosis risk. Consider prescribing a bisphosphonate in line with NICE. • Ensure that physiotherapist and occupational therapist are aware that patient has fallen. • Offer the patient, and their family or carers, a copy of the University Hospital Birmingham NHS Foundation Trust (UHB) Falls Advice leaflet.	☐ ☐ ☐ ☐ ☐ ☐	
B. Does the patient seem to be confused or agitated at any time? *Yes☐ take action* *No ☐ move to **C***	• Refer to the UHB Agitation and Confusion Guidelines, Poster and Acute or Chronic Care Plan. • Ensure an abbreviated Mental Test is completed and record result in the medical notes. • Establish the appropriate level of observation required. Is the patient in the right bed, in the right bay? • Assess the need for bed rails (Refer to the Bed Rail Guidelines). Use a low-profile bed, if available. If not, keep the bed at its lowest level. Seek advice from psychiatric services if appropriate. • Refer to occupational therapy if acute in onset.	☐ ☐ ☐ ☐ ☐	
C. Does the patient have poor eyesight? *Yes☐ take action* *No ☐ move to **D***	• If the patient wears spectacles, ensure they are clean and worn, or within reach, at all times. • If eyesight is poor with spectacles, advise patient to arrange to see an optician after discharge from hospital. • Ensure lighting is adequate where possible.	☐ ☐ ☐	
D.Does the patient need to go to the toilet frequently? *Yes☐ take action* *No ☐ move to **E***	• Assess continence. • Consider proximity to the toilet on ward. • Ensure call bell is in reach. • Offer a routine of frequent toilet visits (if appropriate). • Refer to occupational therapist.	☐ ☐ ☐ ☐ ☐	
E.Is the patient **on** any medication? *Yes☐ take action* *No ☐ move to **F***	• Refer to poster: "Drugs which increase falls and confusion" for additional information. • Refer to doctor and pharmacist, if the patient takes 4 or more different drugs.	☐ ☐	
F. Does the patient have any mobility or transfer problems with or without walking aids? *Yes☐ take action* *No ☐ move to **H***	• Perform and implement UHB Patient Handling Assessment. • Refer to physiotherapist. • Ensure walking aids (specify...........................) are within easy reach. • Ensure patient wears own shoes or sturdy slippers that fit. Patients who have fallen must **not** wear foam slippers. • Ask relatives or carers to bring in the patient's usual indoor footwear. • Cut, or file, the patient's toenails in line with UHB Nail care guidelines.	☐ ☐ ☐ ☐ ☐ ☐	
G. Does the patient have any problems at home which may need community services on discharge? *Yes☐ take action* *No*	• Liaise with therapists and community care team for therapy needs and community follow up on discharge. • Consider alarm raising.	☐ ☐	
	Completion of Section H below is compulsory for all patients requiring the implementation of this management plan		
H.Are there any environmental hazards that could contribute to a fall?	• Minimise any trip/slip hazards such as wet floors, trailing flexes, leads, drips and catheters. Ensure patient can reach his/her possessions (e.g. water and tissues) safely. Minimise bedside clutter. Ensure use of call bell is explained and it is within reach. • Ensure the bed and chair are of a height and size that allow safe transfers. If not available – liaise with occupational therapy, where required. • Consider use of a one-way glide sheet to prevent patient from slipping from chair.	☐ ☐ ☐	

Figure 6.2 Example of a falls and injury risk screening and management plan
Source: Reproduced with kind permission from the University Hospital Birmingham NHS Foundation Trust.

Home environment and community: Falls prevention and strategies, and falls health promotion

The following areas are all important elements for the nurse to consider when supporting the older person who has had a fall or when aiming for the prevention of falls.

Foot care

Older people need to take particular care of their feet, including washing them regularly and carefully drying them—particularly between the toes. The application of moisturizing cream can keep the skin supple.

For toenails that are difficult to cut, or if nails and corns are causing discomfort, then a referral to a podiatrist is required for assessment. Further information on care and advice for feet is supplied by the Society of Chiropodists and Podiatrists online at http://www.feetforlife.org/

Because unsafe footwear can be a cause of falls, shoes need to be supportive, low-heeled, feature a non-slip sole, and allow the wearer the ability to wriggle their toes, but fit snugly around the heel and not rub anywhere. Slippers particularly need to be supportive. Feet change in shape with age, so it is advisable to get feet measured.

NURSING PRACTICE INSIGHT: SIMPLE FEET EXERCISES

The nurse can encourage the older person to do simple feet exercises, which help the blood supply to the feet. The exercises can include raising the heels, stretching, ankle rotating, moving, squeezing, and opening and curling toes. Ideally, the older person will do these exercises at least daily as part of a general exercise routine, and without shoes and socks on to allow more flexibility. They can also be done while sitting down.

Looking after eyesight

An eye test does not only check vision, but also eye health. It can identify a condition in the early stages, enabling early treatment. NHS eye tests are free to the over 60s and it advisable that the over 70s have a test every year. (See also the intrinsic factors in Table 6.1 above.)

If bifocals or varifocals are prescribed for the older person, these can take some getting used to and are often a cause of falls.

With age, eyes need more light to function well, so it is important that homes or care environments are well lit, with good-quality lighting that does not throw shadows.

Dietary factors

A poor diet—and particularly a lack of adequate fluids—can put an older person at risk of falls, because this can lead to dehydration, and light-headedness and confusion.

Vitamin deficiencies—particularly vitamin B1 and vitamin B12—can also contribute to falls.

See Chapter 13 for more on maintaining an adequate diet and fluid intake.

Home and personal safety

The nurse needs to be aware that a large proportion of falls can occur in the home environment and that many of these are preventable. The following are simple measures that can be put in place to prevent falls from occurring.

- **Lighting**—Good lighting levels are important, particularly on stairs and steps. Use 100 watt bulbs (with compatible light shades for fire safety) and utilize natural light, avoiding curtains that are drawn in the daytime. Use night lights at night-time if required.
- **Obstacles**—Check for trailing flexes, loose rugs, frayed or loose carpets, or other uneven or slippery flooring, clutter, or pets and their toys, all of which could cause a fall.
- **Spillages**—These need to be wiped promptly. Trailing bed covers or soft furnishings should be avoided, because these can easily be tripped over.
- **Easy to reach**—Cupboard space needs to be at a level that avoids the older person reaching or bending too low. Electric sockets need to be at an easy-to-reach level and may need to be moved higher. Beds and chairs need to be at the right height, and not too low or high.

Box 6.1 Advice on looking after spectacles

- Keep spectacles clean and preferably in their case when not in use.
- Clean them with the special soft cloth supplied, not use tissues or clothing, because these could scratch the lenses.
- Do not rest lenses down on a hard surface.
- If the frame becomes loose or is uncomfortable, or the lenses are badly scratched, see your optician.

- **Bathing**—Use non-slip bath mats. Grab rails can be fitted (via occupational therapy referrals) to enable an older person to get in and out of the bath more easily. Raised toilet seats can also be ordered.
- **Warmth**—Older people feel the cold more as they get older use they are not as active and their bodies are generally not as efficient at keeping warm. This can lead to a lowering of body temperature (hypothermia). Extra layers of clothing assist in holding in the heat. Warm drinks and food, and gentle exercise, also help in keeping the body warm. The older person should avoid sitting for long periods. There are many agencies available that can assist older people to keep their homes warm and a local Age UK organization can provide further information on these.
- **Technology (tele-care)**—Nearly all local authorities offer a call alarm service within which individuals wear an alarm that can be activated as needed. These can provide reassurance and confidence for the older person. There are also now sensors that can be used in the home to detect if a person may have fallen. These can be designed to alert a response service automatically should an older person have a fall.

Medicines and falls

As noted in the intrinsic factors listed in Table 6.1 above, many medicines can change the way in which the body's natural balance works and can cause falls—particularly as a consequence of hypotension and side effects, including drowsiness and dizziness. A medication review should be carried out at a minimum of annually in older people; for those who are taking more than four medicines, a biannual medication review is recommended (DH, 2001).

Although the following list is not exhaustive, groups of medications that may cause an older person to fall due to the side effects include:

- tricyclic antidepressants (see Figure 6.3 below);
- phenothiazine antipsychotics;
- cardiovascular drugs, such as beta blockers and ace inhibitors, and diuretics, reduce blood pressure, may cause postural hypotension, and may precipitate urgency, which may in turn precipitate a fall; and
- sedatives, including benzodiazepines and barbiturates. (Due to reduced renal clearance in older people, the half-lives of benzodiazepines may often be quadrupled, resulting in an accumulation of the sedative effects of these drugs.)

The British National Formulary (BNF) offers further medication information online at http://www.bnf.org/

Osteoporosis

Osteoporosis is defined as a progressive, systematic skeletal disorder characterized by low bone mass and micro-architectural deterioration of bone tissue, with a consequent increase in bone fragility and susceptibility to fracture (National Institute of Health Consensus Development Panel, 2001).

Osteoporosis is a silent condition. In most patients, the condition is diagnosed following a low-trauma fracture.

Falls and osteoporosis are common in older people: if a person with osteoporosis falls, it is likely to result in a worse outcome due to the increased risk of fracture. However, osteoporotic fractures do occasionally occur in the absence of a fall.

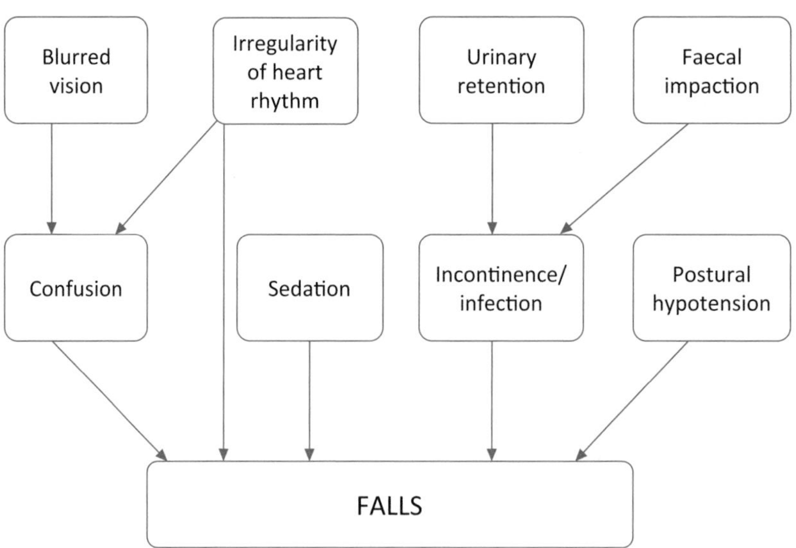

Figure 6.3 Tricyclic antidepressant side effects

Osteoporosis prevalence increases exponentially with age. The risk of fracture is 24.8-fold higher in a woman in her early 60s with osteoporosis and a fall in the previous 12 months than it is in a woman without either of those risk factors (Geusens et al, 2002).

Bone consists of cortical bone tissue, which is solid (80 per cent), and cancellous, which is a spongy bone tissue and has a honeycomb structure (20 per cent). Changes in the bone cause osteoporosis. The cortical bone is a compact layer that is dominant in the shafts of long bones. The cancellous bone forms the interior meshwork of bones—particularly the vertebrae, pelvis, and ends of long bones. In cancellous bone, the trabecullar tissue forms an interconnecting lattice (see Figure 6.4). The effect of a decrease in bone mineral density on bone strength is more marked in cancellous bone, because trabecular tissue may become discontinuous or even disappear, destroying the bone architecture and markedly impairing the ability to withstand stress, so that the risk of fracture increases disproportionately to the amount of bone lost.

Any osteoporotic condition makes any fall much more serious because of the increased risk of fracture, and thus identification of osteoporosis is important, so that prevention and risk factors can be addressed.

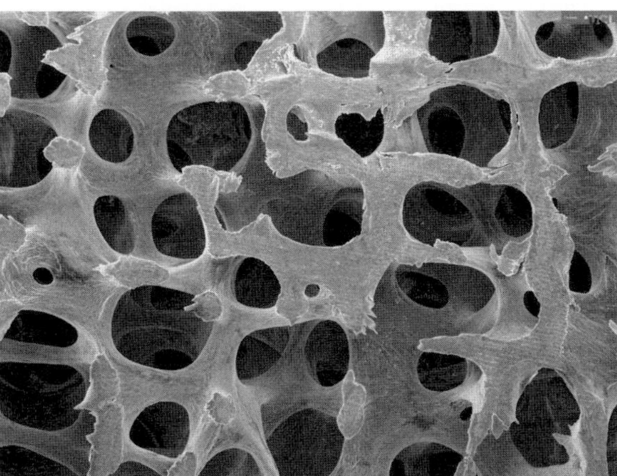

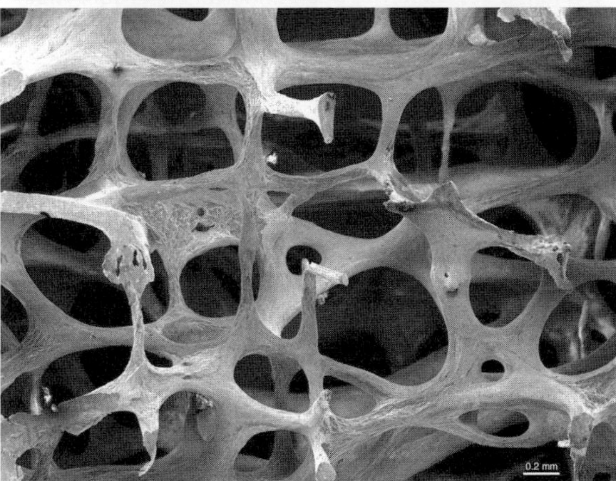

Figure 6.4 Comparison of fragile osteoporotic bone with strong dense bone
Source: Reproduced with permission from Professor Tim Arnett, UCL.

Clinical risk factors

The clinical risk factors for osteoporosis include:

- a low body mass index (BMI) of less than 19kg/m2;
- family history;
- a history of fractures;
- menopause;
- inflammatory bowel disease;
- rheumatoid arthritis;
- hypothyroidism;
- coeliac disease; and
- immobility.

Diagnosis

Bone mineral density (BMD) measurement of the hip is the standard for diagnosing osteoporosis. This is performed using a dual energy X-ray absorptiometry (DEXA) scan.

Management and prevention

Osteoporosis can be managed and, in some cases, prevented in the following ways.

- Primary prevention includes exercise programmes that increase bone density. Evidence has shown that post-menopausal women who do weight-bearing exercises regularly have higher bone density than those that do not exercise (Bonaiutu et al., 2003).
- Hormone replacement therapy (oestrogen) can help post-menopausal women.
- Vitamin D and calcium supplementation can also be helpful. This should involve doctor and dietician review.
- Osteoporosis risk assessment should be carried out to identify the possible need for soft shell hip protectors in specific cases and treatment options.

➲ Other consequences of falls (negative connotations)

Prolonged bed rest produces profound changes in muscle and bone, and muscle strength can be decreased by up to 40 per cent within four to six weeks (Bloomfield, 1997).

Because nursing home residents and hospital in-patients spend considerable periods of their time seated or lying down, they are thus at great risk, and mobility regimes or exercise/activity programmes should be in place to meet individual needs and capabilities.

Fear of falling and the psychological impact

Fear of falling is a significant issue and prevalent in older people. It is associated with previous falls, poor health status, functional decline, and frailty (Lord et al., 2007). Research has also established a relation between the fear of falling, and social and physical activity restrictions, anxiety, depression, and social isolation (Lord et al., 2007). As part of a holistic assessment, the nurse should ascertain if an older person is affected by the aforementioned factors and take or suggest remedial actions, such as a referral to a day centre.

In the community, the aim is to avoid admission by assessing the individual and facilitating multifactorial interventions to reduce the risk of further falls.

See Chapter 11 on mental health.

Further nursing aspects of falls and falling, and home environment prevention and advice

The nurse has a pivotal role in the assessment of an older person who has presented with a fall. Very often, it is the nurse who can relate to the older person's home setting and their normal environment. They will thus have the knowledge of the older person's usual lifestyle and needs, and can view the person holistically and propose appropriate interventions. This is all the more important in adopting a compassionate, yet positive, approach to supporting the older person in a difficult time for them and avoiding the often negative association of a fall with a decremental decline in older age (Kingston, 2000).

Interventions following a fall

Interventions following a fall should include the following.

- The nurse should always have a sympathetic approach, given that the older person may have been scared or traumatized following the fall. To differing degrees, their independence can be affected, and, as such, the nurse has a role both in ensuring confidence in the older person and alleviating the reasons why the person may have fallen.
- All incidents and accidents, including falls, should be recorded in an appropriate accident/incident book.
- Good practice includes keeping a falls register, so that any multiple falls and patterns can be identified.
- Periodic review will help to identify trends: for example, a person who has had a fall may demonstrate unsteadiness at particular times of the day that may be associated with medication, mealtimes, or certain activities.
- Ensure that the older person who has had a fall has the opportunity to recount what happened. This should entail how the person managed and what they would do should they have a fall again. This is particularly important for working out strategies for summoning help and to avoid the complications that can arise when spending a long time on the floor.
- Document the circumstances in the patient's records.
- Physical examination must take place and results must be documented.
- If no extrinsic factors can be associated with the fall, medical advice should be sought in order to rule out patho-physiological factors.

It must be noted that it is impossible to prevent all falls and accidents, and that interventions to minimize falls can result in restriction of activity and autonomy to an unacceptable degree, and may adversely affect rehabilitation.

NURSING PRACTICE INSIGHT: FALLS

- **Nurses need to have an understanding and awareness about falls.**
- **Wherever possible, keep people mobilizing.**
- **If a falls assessment has been undertaken, ensure that all colleagues are informed of the outcomes.**
- **If a fall has taken place, ensure that action is taken—that is, incident forms are completed, environments are clutter-free, a call bell is within reach, or, if in the community, a pendant call alarm has been considered.**

Physical activity and exercise programmes

Exercise is an important intervention for preventing falls in older people. Low levels of activity can make a person more at risk of falls. Exercise that helps to strengthen muscles, improve balance and coordination, and improve functional ability can help in preventing falls. The Cochrane Review of

Interventions for Preventing Falls in Older People Living in the Community (2009) concluded that multiple-component group exercise reduced rates of falls and risk of falling, as did t'ai chi and individually prescribed, multiple-component, home-based exercise. Figure 6.5 illustrates some postural stability exercise programmes based on NICE Guidelines.

RCTs of an individually tailored home exercise programme consisting of strength and balance retraining exercises, such as postural stability, concluded that they are effective in improving physical function, and reducing falls and injuries in women aged 80 years and over (Campbell at al., 1997; Campbell et al., 1999).

A detailed analysis of the specific components of exercise from 44 RCTs of exercise interventions for falls prevention was undertaken by Lord et al. (2007). They concluded that effective exercise programmes for preventing falls comprise a combination of challenging and progressive weight-bearing balance exercises, and particularly those that minimize the use of the upper limb for support.

Elements of a successful falls prevention programme

In order to be successful, the falls prevention programme will include the following elements.

- Exercise must be targeted, concentrating on strength, balance, and stability, and focused on the muscle groups that enable improvements in daily living tasks—for example, an hour of progressive exercises and endurance.
- Exercise is specifically tailored to meet the needs of each individual and progressed over time. This includes targeting it to a person's ability and lifestyle.
- The instructor should have the appropriate training in exercise for the prevention of falls and injuries.
- Exercise should be supplemented by education, such as talks on relevant topics that can prevent or cause falls, including foot care, medical conditions, nutrition, and safety.
- Follow-up telephone support is very helpful, both during the programme and after completion.
- Clients should be able to return to an earlier phase of the falls exercise programme if their condition worsens.
- Medical assessment is mandatory before the client embarks on a falls exercise programme.
- All clients should be encouraged to perform and record home exercise to nurture their ability to take regular exercise alone.
- Clients should be able to graduate to appropriate, safe, and effective community-based exercise programmes.

The nurse can encourage and help the older person to keep as active as possible. This can include referring them to an appropriate exercise programme, encouraging simple repeat exercises such as for the feet (previously discussed), or, if they are in hospital, walking with them rather than, for example, providing a wheelchair to go to the toilet. The nurse should also take the opportunity to talk with the physiotherapist for advice and to find out what can be achieved.

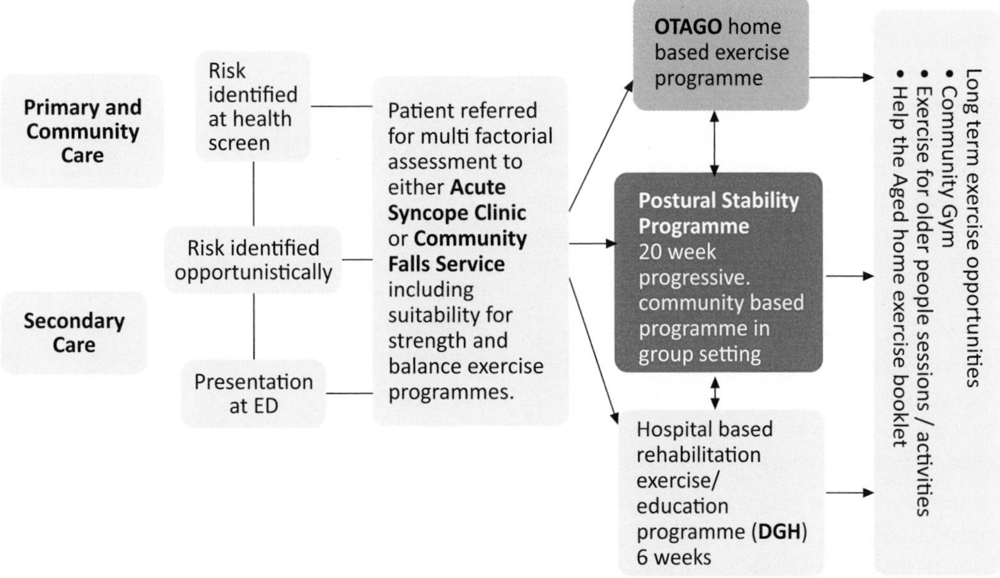

Figure 6.5 The Dudley Postural Stability Programme
Source: Reproduced with kind permission by the Dudley Community Falls Service.

Case study

Clare Brown is a 74-year-old lady who is to be discharged from A&E after falling in her house. She has not fractured any bones, but has arthritis and hypertension, and has been advised to go to an intermediate care centre for further assessment and observation. Mrs Brown is adamant that she return home, where she lives alone.

- Explain the potential impact of a fall on Mrs Brown.
- Consider where Mrs Brown would be in the falls care pathway and the referrals that could be made.
- What immediate elements of management and care will be required?

The district nurse who assessed Mrs Brown the following day noted several extrinsic and environmental factors, including clutter, a very cold house, poor lighting, and ill-fitting footwear.

- Describe the management that you would put in place to address these issues.
- What advice would you give Mrs Brown on falls prevention?

The perspective of an occupational therapist

Carol Portik is an occupational therapist specializing in risk and independence of older people. The following summarizes her perspective:

- Although falling can and does have a devastating effect on older people, it is crucial to instill a rehabilitation ethos from the beginning of any intervention. Falls and fractures, even with older people, should be considered a temporary disability, and it is imperative that all members of the multidisciplinary team work towards this goal and focus on giving positive reinforcements, rather than dwelling on negatives. Previous levels of ability should be a guide to the expected outcomes following a period of rehabilitation.
- From the onset of any fall or resulting injury, it is important that people are encouraged to take up and maintain their usual roles and functions. These normal activities encourage appropriate balance and gait, which are important components of functional mobility and are required in all aspects of independence.
- Families, especially of older people, can become overcautious and fearful on behalf of their relative. Therefore families and carers should be included in the goal-planning process, whilst encouraging the older person in working towards independence both in mobility and in the activities of daily living.
- Occupational therapists play a key role within the multidisciplinary team, providing a comprehensive and holistic assessment of patient need. Early intervention is essential, because all fallers should have a home assessment to identify potential hazards and possible causes of falls. Occupational therapists provide a variety of equipment to enhance independence in the home. However, consideration of need versus risk is imperative, because equipment can clutter up the environment, creating a greater falls risk. The occupational therapist will utilize the assessment process to identify alternative methods of conducting everyday activities prior to providing equipment. This approach reduces dependence and promotes independence in a more appropriate way.
- Equipment, such as chair raisers, toilet raisers, perching stools, and long-handled equipment such as shoe horns, easy reaches, and sponges, etc., help to maintain these precautions and promote independence in most activities, but individual assessment is necessary, because not all equipment will be necessary or environmentally suitable.
- Earlier discharges from hospital have meant the creation of community rehabilitation teams. Focusing on rehabilitation in a person's home is far more appropriate than doing so in hospital, because difficulties experienced will be specific to that individual and can be addressed appropriately. Good handovers of goals, and seamless transfer of information and supportive community staff, are imperative to ensure that rehabilitation continues within the person's home on hospital discharge.
- Competencies specific for clients post-hip fracture in the community include understanding the impact of cognitive deficit on rehabilitation and skills in managing people with cognitive deficits, dementia-specific skills for clients with dementia and hip fracture, as well as skills in prevention of falls.

Conclusion

Evidence suggests that:

all healthcare professionals dealing with patients known to be at risk of falling should develop and maintain basic professional competence in falls assessment and prevention.

(NICE, 2004)

- Fractures, falls, and osteoporosis are major public health problems.
- Fractures occur because people fall and/or their bones are fragile.
- High-risk people need to be identified and treated.
- Person-specific and environmental factors must be considered.

- A mulitfactorial falls risk assessment and management programme is the most effective intervention.
- Effective exercise programmes are individually tailored and comprise a combination of challenging and progressive weight-bearing balance exercises.

Questions and self-assessment

Now that you have worked through the chapter, answer the following questions:

- Why are falls are so debilitating to health?
- What are the main causes of falls and how might they be prevented?
- What are the key elements of a risk assessment used to identify a person who is vulnerable to falls?
- What are the key elements of a management programme for someone vulnerable to falls?

Self-assessment

- Having read the chapter, how will you change your practice?
- Identify up to three areas relating to falls in which you need to develop your knowledge and understanding further.
- Identify how you are going to develop this knowledge and understanding, and set deadlines for achieving this.

Podcast

Visit the Online Resource Centre for a podcast of someone who has suffered from a fall and questions to aid reflection.

References

American Geriatrics Society/British Geriatrics Society/American Academy of Orthopaedic Surgeons Panel on Falls Prevention (2001) 'Consensus of evidence-based guidelines for the prevention of falls in older persons', *Journal of the American Geriatrics Society*, 49: 664–72.

Bloomfield, S. (1997) 'Changes in musculoskeletal structure and function with prolonged bed rest', *Medicine & Science in Sports & Exercise*, 29(2): 197–206.

Bonaiutu, D., Shea, B., Levine, R., Negrini, S., Robinson, V., Kemper, H.C., Wells, G., Tugwell, D., and Cranney, A. (2003) 'Evidence for preventing and treating osteoporosis in postmenopausal women', *Evidence Based Nursing*, 6(2): 50–1.

Campbell, A.J., Robertson, M.C., Gardner, M.M., Norton, R.M., Tilyard, M.W., and Buchner, D.M. (1997) 'Randomized controlled trial of a general practice programme of home based exercise to prevent falls in elderly women', *British Medical Journal*, 315: 1065–9.

Campbell, A.J., Robertson, M.C., Gardner, M.M., Norton, R.M., Tilyard, M.W., and Buchner, D.M. (1999) 'Falls prevention over two years: A randomized controlled trial in women 80 years and older', *British Geriatrics Society*, 28: 513–18.

Chang, J.T., Morton, S.C., Rubenstein, L.Z., Mojica, W.A., Maglione, M., Suttorp, M.J., Roth, E.A., and Shekelle, P.G. (2004) 'Interventions for the prevention of falls in older adults: Systematic review and meta-analysis of randomized clinical trials', *British Medical Journal*, 328: 680.

Close, J., Ellis, M., Hooper, R., Glucksman, E., Jackson, S., and Swift, C. (1999) 'Prevention of falls in the elderly trial (PROFET): A randomized control trial', *Lancet*, 353: 93–7.

Cooper, C., Atkinson, E.J., Jacobsen, S.J., O'Fallon, W.M., and Melton, J.L. (1993) 'Population based study of survival after osteoporotic fractures', *American Journal of Epidemiology*, 137(9): 1001–5.

Davison, J., Bond, J., Dawson, P., Steen, N., and Kenny, R.A. (2005) 'Patients with recurrent falls attending A&E benefit from multi-factorial intervention: A randomized control trial', *Age and Ageing*, 34: 162–8.

Department of Health (2001) *National Service Framework for Older People*, London: DH.

Department of Health (2007) *Care Pathways for Older People with Complex Needs: Best Practice Guidance*, London: DH.

Department of Health (2009) *Falls and Fractures: Effective Interventions in Health and Social Care*, London: DH.

Eddy, D.M., Johnson, C.C., Cummings, S.R., Dawson-Hughes, B., Lindsay, R., Melton, L.J., and Slemenda, C.W. (1998) 'Osteoporosis: Review of the evidence for prevention, diagnosis, treatment and cost-effectiveness analysis', *Osteoporosis International*, 8(Suppl 4):S7–80.

Fonda, D., Cook, J., Sandler, V., and Bailey, M. (2006) 'Sustained reduction in serious fall-related injuries in older people in hospital', *Medical Journal Australia*, 184(8): 372–3.

Geusens, P., Boonen, P., Johan, S., Vanhoof, J., Declerck, K., and Raus, J. (2002) 'The relationship among history of falls, osteoporosis, and fractures in postmenopausal women', *Archives of Physical Medicine & Rehabilitation*, 83: 903–6.

Gillespie, L.D., Robertson, M.C., Gillespie, W.J., Lamb, S.E., Gates, S., Cumming, R.G., and Rowe, B.H. (2009) 'Interventions for preventing falls in older people living in the community', *Cochrane Database of Systematic Reviews*, available online at http://www.cochranejournalclub.com/preventing-falls-in-nursing-care-facilities-and-hospitals/pdf/CD007146_standard.pdf.

Healey, F., Monro, A., Cockram, A., Adams, V., and Heseltine, D. (2004) 'Using targeted risk factor reduction to prevent falls in older hospital inpatients: A randomized control trial', *Age and Ageing*, 33: 390–95.

Help the Aged (2005) *Preventing Falls: Don't Mention the F-Word*, available online at http://www.slips-online.co.uk/downloads/dont-mention-the-f-word.pdf.

Kingston, P. (2000) 'Falls in later life: status passage and preferred identities as a new orientation', *Health: An Interdisciplinary Journal for the Social Study of Health, Ilness and Medicine*, 4(2): 216–33.

Lord, S., Sherrington, C., Menz, H., and Close, J. (eds) (2007) *Falls in Older People: Risk Factors and Strategies for Prevention*, 2nd edn, Cambridge: Cambridge University Press.

Mooney, H. (2009) 'Assessment metric cuts falls by a quarter in pilot programme', *Nursing Times*, 105: 1–2.

National Institute for Health and Clinical Excellence (2004) *Falls: The Assessment and Prevention of Falls in Older People*, Clinical Guidance No. 21, London: NICE.

National Institute of Health Consensus Development Panel (2001) 'Osteoporosis prevention, diagnosis, and therapy', *Journal of the American Medical Association*; 285(6): 785–95.

National Patient Safety Agency (2007) *The Third Report from the Patient Safety Observatory: Slips, Trips and Falls in Hospital*, London: NPSA.

Royal College of Physicians Clinical Effectiveness and Evaluation Unit (2007) *National Clinical Audit of Falls and Bone Health in Older People*, London: RCP.

Salkeld, G., Cameron, I.D., Cumming, R.G., Easter, S., Seymour, J., Kurrle, S.E., and Quine, S. (2000) 'Quality of life related to fear of falling and hip fracture in older women: A time trade-off study', *British Medical Journal*, 320: 341–6.

For further reading and information

College of Occupational Therapists (2006) *Falls Management*, London: COT.

Downton, J.H. (1993) *Falls in the Elderly*, London: Edward Arnold.

Lord, S.R., Sherrington, C., and Menz, H.B. (2007) *Falls in Older People*, Cambridge: Cambridge University Press.

Tideiksaar, R. (2002) *Falls in Older People: Prevention and Management*, Baltimore, MD: Health Professions Press.

http://www.ageuk.org.uk/

http://www.bbc.co.uk/health/physical_health/conditions/osteoporosis1.shtml

Later Life Training Ltd—http://www.laterlifetraining.co.uk/

(includes physical activity programmes for falls).

National Osteoporosis Society—http://www.nos.org.uk/

National Strategy Framework for Older People and Standard 6 on Falls—http://www.dh.gov.uk/olderpeople

NICE Guidelines on Falls—http://www.nice.org.uk/CG021

Prevention of Falls Network Europe—http://www.profane.eu.org/

Royal Society for the Prevention of Accidents—http://www.rospa.com/homesafety/adviceandinformation/olderpeople/accidents.aspx#falls

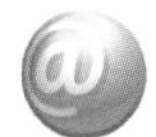

Online Resource Centre

You can learn more about falls and older people at the Online Resource Centre that accompanies this book: **http://www.oxfordtextbooks.co.uk/orc/hindle/**

Medicines management

Maggi Banning

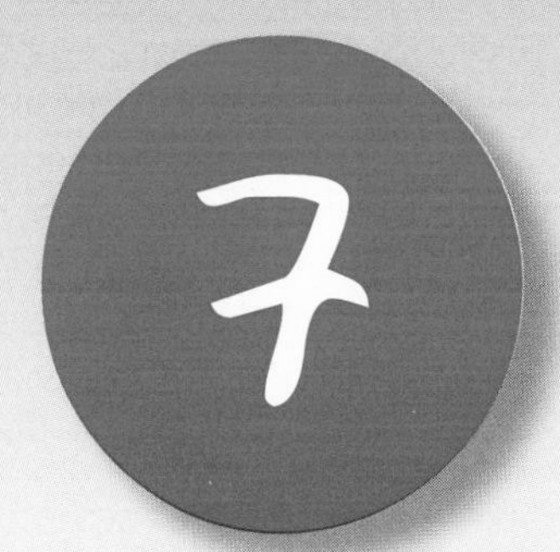

Learning outcomes

By the end of the chapter, you will be able to:

- understand the term 'medication management';
- appreciate the components of medication management;
- discuss the importance of medication management and its relevance to older people;
- assess the relevance and patterns of adherence to medication in older people;
- acknowledge the importance of the medication review process;
- review the concept of medication errors, their aetiology, frequency, and types, and preventative measures;
- appraise the importance of medication education as a component of the discharge planning of older people from acute NHS trusts; and
- identify the key nursing roles and responsibilities, and educational needs of nurses, specific to medicines management and older people, and how to improve medication self-management in older people.

Introduction

The aim of this chapter is to explore the issues related to medication management in older people, and to explore how nurses can support patients to take medication in a safe and effective way. In the UK, older people comprise more than 18 per cent of the population and receive 45 per cent of the total medicines prescribed (DH, 2002b). It is not uncommon for an older person to take several medications at once (polypharmacy) usually due to the higher likelihood of having one or more long-term conditions and multiple health needs.

See Chapter 12 on key health conditions in older age.

Polypharmacy increases the risk of adverse drug reactions, partly due to increased incidence of drug interactions. Older people may not always be aware of the occurrence of adverse drug reactions, and need support to reduce any unwanted side effects and to manage medications safely. In this regard, nurses are in an excellent position to educate patients on the safe, therapeutic use of medicines and the timely recognition of adverse side effects (NMC, 2010).

Improving medication management amongst older patients and service users overall is important for several reasons, including:

- increasing awareness of the need to reduce adverse drug reactions and iatrogenic disease amongst older people;
- poor management of long-term conditions in older people;
- the long-term effects on resources, including:
  - the costs of caring for older people in acute NHS trusts in terms of nursing and medical care, bed allocation costs, and costs of medical interventions;
  - the increasing costs of the drug budget for older people; and
  - that costs of iatrogenic (that is, inadvertently caused by treatment) disease management.

The UK government has been proactive in its provision of education and training of healthcare professionals in medication management, and the development and implementation of medication review processes and procedures, which aim to improve medicines management specifically targeting older people. The development of healthcare policy has also raised awareness of the issue of medication management in this group of patients by specifically targeting the need to improve current services, and to reduce the financial costs of unplanned and unscheduled care, and the ever-increasing drug budget. These policies and the resulting implications for nursing practice will be discussed later in this chapter.

What is medicines management?

The Medicines and Healthcare Products Regulatory Agency (MHRA) (2004) defines medicines management as '*the clinical, cost effective and safe use to ensure patients get the maximum benefit from the medicines they need, while at the same time minimizing potential harm.*'

Medication management is not only specific to pharmaceutical care; it is also an important concern for all healthcare professionals who are involved in the care of older people. Medication management is a broad term, which includes the following factors.

- **Patient-centred medication review**—This is a structured approach to identifying medication issue, assessing for adverse effects, and ensuring concordance with medication. Adherence to medication can be affected by cognitive impairment, memory lapses, and also dexterity problems secondary to arthritis.
- **Rational prescribing and prescribing support**—This refers to prescribing the correct medication for long-term conditions, and assessing the efficacy of treatment and the correct medication dose on its ability to manage the symptoms of patho-physiological conditions.
- **Repeat prescribing**—Older people should have regular reviews of their medicines at least every six months. It is essential that, before a repeat prescription is issued, the prescriber considers any essential drug monitoring that needs to be undertaken, and monitors patients for any adverse drug effects on hepatic or renal function and other bodily functions.
- **Patient education**—Older people need to be informed about their medicines in order to recognize side effects or adverse drug effects and to reduce the incidence of medication errors. Drug-related information needs to be provided in a logical and comprehensible manner, in order to improve patient knowledge of their medicines and to assist the recollection of drug regimens. Among hospital in-patients, medication education should be a component of discharge planning.
- **Access to medicines**—This aspect of medication management refers to the need for older people to be able to access their medicines in order to administer them at the correct time and correct dose. Many older people either live alone or may have limited mobility, which can render them housebound and can result in impaired access to medicines.
- **Improvements at the primary and secondary care interface (RPSGB, 2003)**—When care is shared between the primary and secondary care interface, and when patients are discharged from hospital into the community, the community healthcare team, general practitioners (GPs), and prescribers require accurate, effective communication about the older person's medication regimen and treatment. The sharing of information and good communication is needed to ensure that the care provided to the older person is safe and seamless.

Why older people?

Both the *National Service Framework for Older People* (NSFOP) (DH, 2001a) and the *National Service Framework for Older People: Medicines and Older People* (DH, 2001b) emphasize the importance of medication management in older people and their long-term conditions. In a survey of older people, the London Older People Services Development Programme (2003) found that 90 per cent of older people administer more than six medicines per day. In older people, polypharmacy (that is, the concurrent administration of four or more medicines) and not adhering to medication instructions can lead to medication-related adverse effects (DH, 2001b; Ellenbecker, 2004), but can also lead to medication mismanagement (Lindley and Tulley, 1992; Woodhouse and Wynne, 1992).

Medication mismanagement can take several forms, including inaccuracies with respect to the medication regimen, and memory lapses and forgetfulness regarding the timing and dose of drug administered. Medication-related side effects, or adverse drug effects, can be the result of a drug interaction. There are numerous drug interactions, including:

- drugs that have opposing actions on the same receptor sites, such as the use of dopamine agonists (levodopa) and dopamine antagonists (domperidone) in a patient with Parkinson's disease in which case the prescribing of the dopamine antagonist renders the dopamine agonist ineffective;
- drug interactions can occur when two drugs are prescribed concurrently, such as the use of warfarin and aspirin where the interaction is related to aggravated clotting and an increased risk of bleeding; and
- drugs interacting in the way in which they metabolize, such as diclofenac and phenytoin, which can interact with the drug-metabolizing enzyme cytochrome P450.

In addition, the frequency and severity of medication-related side effects can augment non-adherence with medication.

For example, it is established that the concurrent use of more than one oral non-steroidal anti-inflammatory (NSAID) drug increases the risk of dyspepsia, gastrointestinal bleeding, and abdominal pain (Vaile and Davis, 1998). It is now accepted that only one NSAID should be used. Commonly used NSAIDs include ibruprofen, diclofenac, indomethacin, or proxicam.

Such effects can result in unplanned hospital admission. Pearson (2000) supports the view that 10 per cent of unplanned admissions to hospital are due to a drug-related cause. These figures may even be as high as one in six unplanned admissions and may relate to the adverse effects of drugs (Mannesse, 1997). The impact of high unplanned admission rates among older people and the associated spiralling financial costs led to the implementation of policy on the management of long-term conditions (DH, 2005), and also to healthcare practitioner education and training.

The nursing role

There is currently a paucity of specialists who can manage older people and their medication needs (Fletcher, 2002). In this respect, the government has been keen to educate and prepare nurses to take on roles as community matrons (DH, 2006). Community matrons are senior nurses who possess extensive experience in patient management either as district nurses with both independent and/or extensive or non-medical prescribing qualifications, a nurse practitioner, or may hold additional organ-based specialist knowledge and qualifications, such as cardiac, haematology, or respiratory nurse specialisms. The education and training that is provided is based at the Master's degree level, and is focused on educating practitioners for case management responsibilities and risk prediction tools to assess risk of rehospitalization. Each community matron can manage a caseload of up to 50 patients, with patients being treated for one or several concurrent long-term conditions (Banning, 2009).

The *National Service Framework for Older People: Medicines and Older People* (DH, 2001b) identified several medication issues as problem areas, including:

- adverse drug reactions due to increased sensitivity to the pharmacokinetic and pharmacodynamic effects of medicines (Shelton, 2000; Swift, 2003). This is an important aspect of drug management of which nurses should be aware (NMC, 2010);
- non-adherence with the drug regimen;
- inappropriate prescribing of long-term drugs (Shelton, 2000);
- incidence of side effects, such as falls and gastrointestinal bleeding (Feder et al., 2000), meaning that nurses should be familiar with the common side effects of drugs (NMC, 2010); and
- inadequate therapeutic drug monitoring, especially of drugs that have a narrow therapeutic index and require regular monitoring, such as digoxin, theophylline, and gentamicin (Sheehan and Feely, 1999).

Older people and concordance/adherence with medication

The concept of medication-taking behaviour has been studied extensively (Allard et al., 2001; Barat et al., 2001). Medication-taking behaviour is a complex issue that is underpinned by the complexity of drug regimes. Any change to drug regimens—for example, the timing or dosage of a drug—can alter the medication-taking process. Muir et al. (2001) suggest that if the complexity of the regimen is reduced, this can have positive impact on medication-taking behaviour, or if the regimen is reduced by preferentially including medicines with a longer mode of action. Medication-taking behaviour can also be improved if the medications that are prescribed include those that have a licence to be used as drug treatment for that particular condition. Using only licensed drugs provides patients with the best chance of success with a drug regimen (Hames and Wynne, 2001).

So why is concordance and adherence to medication so important in older people?

A key issue that underpins medication-taking behaviour is to what extent the patient adheres to their medication. In older people, adherence to medication is a complex issue Non-adherence to medication involves several factors (Banning, 2008), some of which are illustrated in Figure 7.1.

Additional key factors include previous experience with the prescriber, medication history, illness, physical deterioration, lack of comprehension of the role of drugs in the management of the condition, dislike of taking medicines, lack of faith in the prescriber's diagnosis, disbelief or reluctance to accept diagnosis, possible confusion over conflicting advice provided by more than one prescriber, the severity and frequency of unpleasant medication-derived side effects (such as taste), and cognitive impairment (Salas et al., 2001).

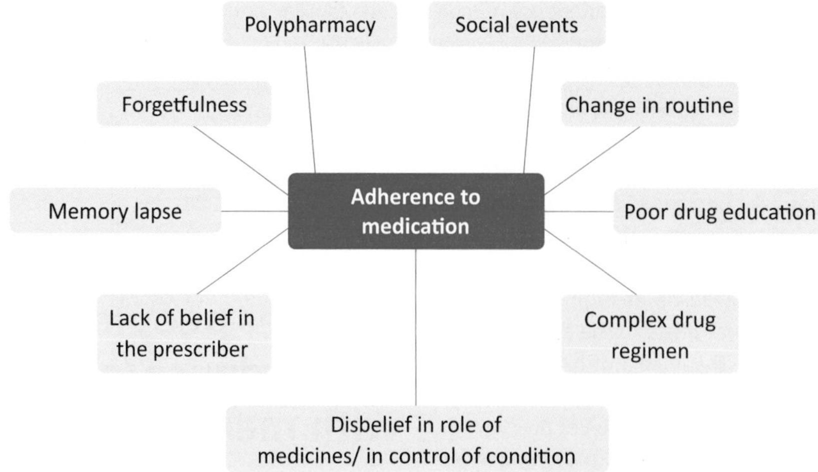

Figure 7.1 Factors affecting the development of adherence to medication

How many forms of non-concordance and non-adherence are known?

The current literature suggests that there are two forms of medication non-adherence: intentional non-adherence and non-intentional non-adherence (Johnson et al., 1999). Both types relate to the lack of an established pattern of medication-taking, which can lead to the incidental omission of medicines. Although these types of non-adherence are quite distinct and have different identifying distinguishing characteristics (as outlined in Table 7.1 below), they may occur concurrently (Banning, 2008).

In the older patient, non-adherence to medication is dependent on three phases of decision-making, as follows.

1. A patient's knowledge about their illness and treatment, medication-taking behaviour, and testing of medicines.
2. A patient having faith in the prescriber's ability to diagnose and manage their condition correctly. In many cases, patients will sample their medicines to explore drug-related side effects, and then omit or control the quantity of medicines that they administer according to their symptoms and the severity of side effects, and how these can be managed.
3. A patient's acceptance of their pathological condition. This acceptance ranges from passively accepting that they have a condition that requires treatment, to actively rejecting their diagnosis.

Table 7.1 Characteristics of non-adherence

Intentional non-adherence	Non-intentional non-adherence
Lack of faith in the prescriber	Change in lifestyle
Failure to accept diagnosis	Forgetfulness
Recognition or anticipation of side effects	Period of illness
Fears of prescribing errors	Having periods of feeling well and being asymptomatic
Fears of addiction	Altering dosing regimen
Dislike of taking medicines	Drug-related memory loss
Perception of health risk	Disruption to routine
Testing medicines against symptoms	

Improving medication concordance and adherence

Compliance aids

> ***Student activity***
> - Can you name three compliance aids that you have seen used in clinical settings?
> - What is the NMC Standard in relation to compliance aids? (See NMC, 2010.)

For adequate therapeutic control of long-term conditions, it is essential that older people adhere to their medicine regimen as prescribed by the prescriber. Adherence and concordance to medication can be improved through the use of compliance aids (Winland-Brown and Valiante, 2000), such as monitored dosage systems, heat-sealed blister packs, and plastic Dosette boxes. One example of heat-sealed blister packs, or a sealed cassette that contains seven days of medication, is the Nomad system. In this cassette, the drugs are clearly marked with the day and time of administration notified for each separate medicine. Packs are stored in a metal tray, with morning, afternoon, and evening clearly identified.

Plastic boxes, such as the Dosette boxes, have separate compartments corresponding to days of the week and times of administration. Each compartment is enclosed by a plastic seal and contains all of the medications to be administered at that particular time. In addition to this, informal carers and family members are a source of invaluable support, because they can help older people to manage their medicines effectively in a controlled manner. In order to promote adherence and concordance with medication, it is important to educate patients, informal carers, and family members in relation to types of medicines, frequency of administration, dose of medicines, possible side effects, and role of medicines in the management of the long-term conditions that are being managed. Medication education is essential as a preventative tool to stop older people from trivializing the role of medicines as essential components in the management of long-term illness.

Patient-centred medication review

Medication review is an enhanced service that is commissioned on a local basis by the primary care organization and is a prerequisite for people aged 75 years and older, and is particularly important for patients that concurrently administer four or more drugs.

'Medication review' is defined as:

a structured, critical examination of a patient's medicines with the objective of reaching an agreement with the patient about treatment, making best use of medicines. Minimising the number of medication related problems and reducing waste.

(LOPSDP, 2003: 9).

Patient-centred medication review involves a single assessment process (SAP) that identifies and addresses medication issues, assesses possible adverse effects, and addresses compliance concerns, as indicated in Standard 2 of the National Service Framework for Older People (DH, 2001a) and the SAP (DH, 2002a). The purpose of the SAP is to:

ensure that older people receive appropriate, effective and timely responses to their health and social care needs, and that professional resources are used effectively.

(LOPSDP, 2003: 1).

Health care professionals, such as nurses, community matrons, and pharmacists, received training in the SAP to become single assessment assessors. This includes working to identify the type of assessment that the patient requires. This can range from an initial contact assessment to identify needs, to a comprehensive assessment that requires the use and referral to the wider multidisciplinary team to explore the patient's specialist needs.

Single assessment process (SAP)

The components of the SAP include:

- individuals being central to the process;
- the needs of the individual being central to the undertaking of the SAP; and
- all planning processes involved in the SAP being recorded and updated as necessary.

A key component of the SAP is four trigger questions that are used by non-medical professionals to identify medication-related problems, as follows, see figure 7.2.

Following this assessment, the SAP assessor will develop a comprehensive care plan that addresses the patient's needs. The care plan will be developed in agreement with the patient, and will include a summary of the identified needs, objectives for the management of future care, a brief account of how services will impact on identified needs, what support the patient requires in terms of level and frequency of help, and a description of the monitoring processes to be used, along with the care assessor's name. See also SAP in chapter 8.

Medication errors

Medication errors are a significant source of morbidity and mortality for the hospitalized patient—especially older people (DH, 2001b). This is particularly important because older people comprise 18 per cent of the adult population and administer 45 per cent of the total medicines prescribed in England (DH, 2002b). Medication errors add to the spiralling costs of patient care due to prolonged periods in hospital. Annual costs are estimated to be in the region of £2 bn (DH, 2001b).

In the UK, the National Patient Safety Agency (2008) suggests that, of the 2,964 incidents that occurred in a six-month period involving one strategic health authority, 6.4 per cent of these related to medicines.

In *Building a Safer NHS for Patients*, the Department of Health (2004) outlined the causes, potential instigating factors, and the roots of errors caused through inappropriate prescribing, dispensing, and the administration of medicines. The paper also provided measures that can be used by nurses with regard to the care and management of drug administration and supply, and associated care for the patient.

Definition of 'medication error'

A 'medication error' can be defined as '*any preventable event that may cause or lead to inappropriate medication use or*

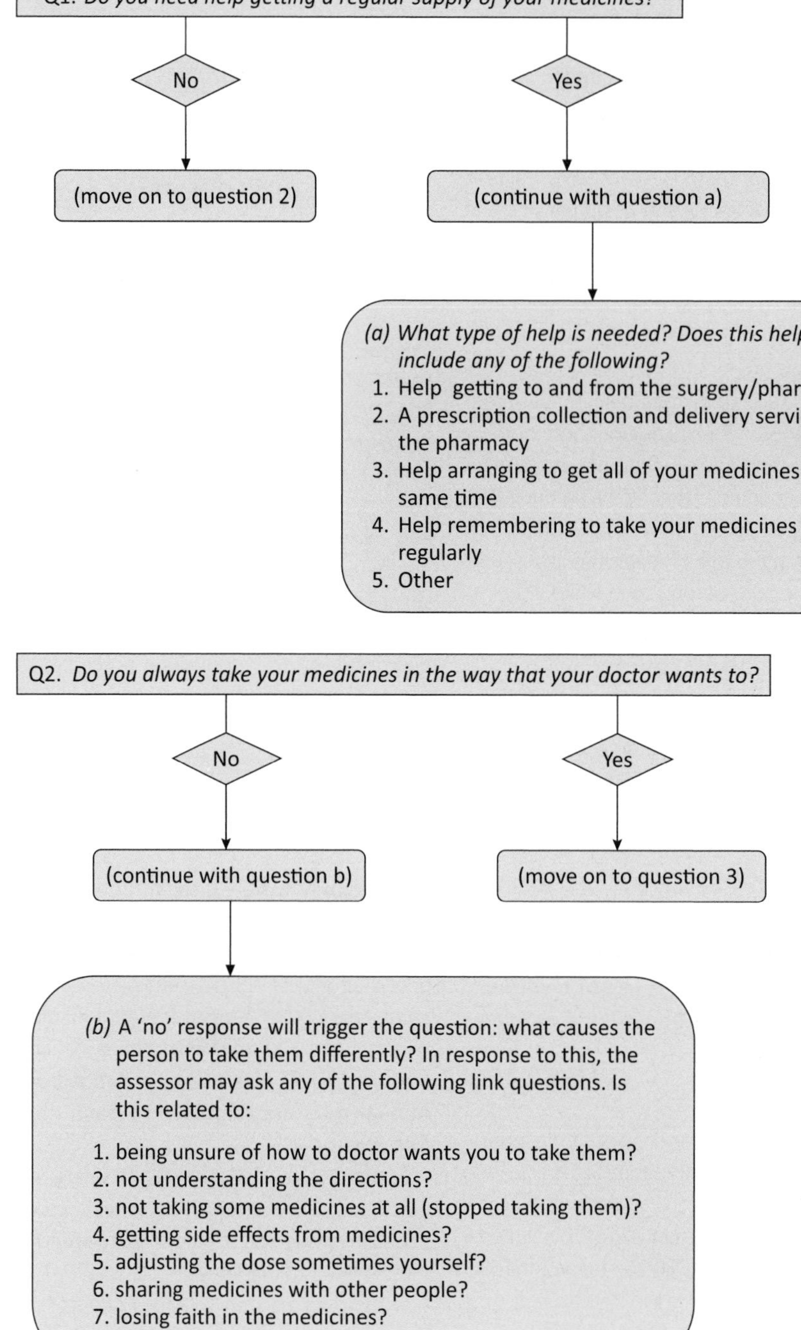

Figure 7.2 Single Assessment Process

patient harm while the medication is in the control of health professional, patient or consumer' (NCCMERP, 2002).

A typology of working definitions of medication errors includes the following.

- Omissions are errors that arise when a medication is not administered at the correct time. This excludes cases in which the patient refuses the medication or instances in which the patient is fasting in preparation for surgery.
- A wrong dosage medication error occurs when the nurse or medical practitioner administers an inaccurate dose of a medicine.
- An extra dose medication error occurs when the nurse or medical practitioner administers more doses of the prescribed medication than were prescribed on the patient's medication prescription chart by the prescriber.

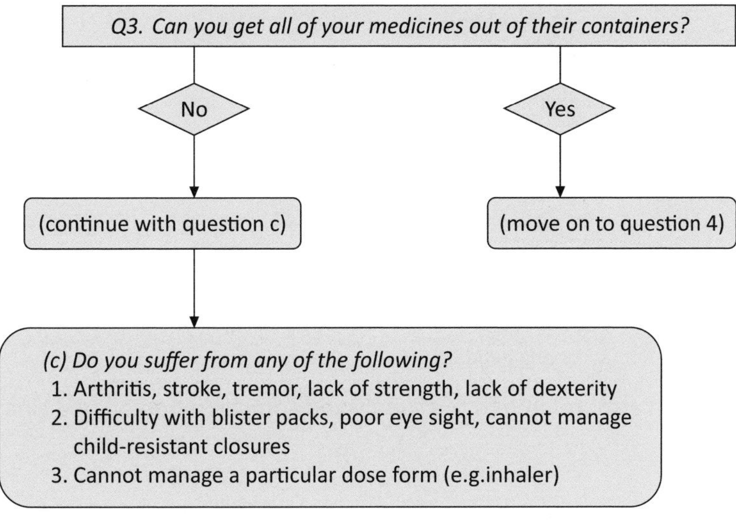

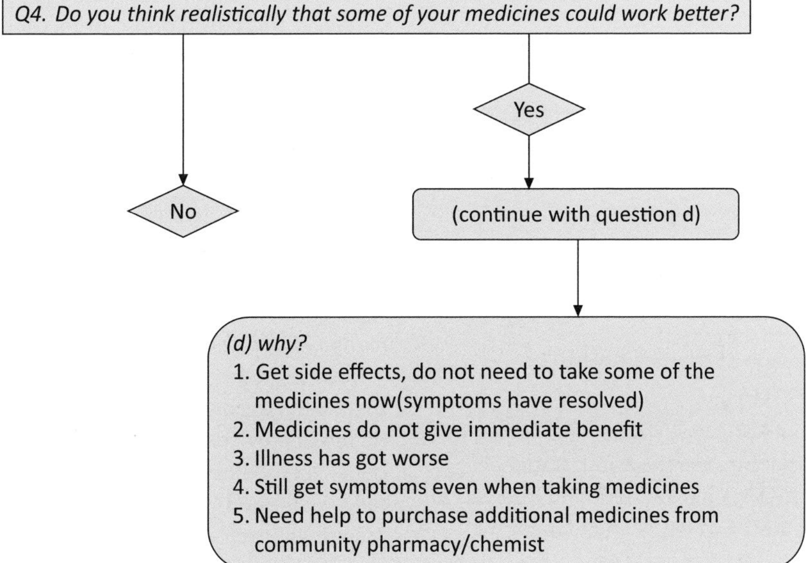

Figure 7.2 *(Continued)*

- An unordered medicine error occurs when the patient receives a medication that was not prescribed or authorized. In the older person, errors of this type can have serious consequences, due to the sensitivity of older people to the adverse effects of medicines.
- A wrong dosage form error occurs when a wrong dosage is administered—perhaps because the dosage has been incorrectly written in a prescription.
- A wrong route medicine error occurs when a dose is administered by the wrong route.

The wrong administration route, or the use of an inappropriate procedure or improper technique, in the administration of a drug can be detrimental to the rationale underpinning the pharmaceutical preparation—for example, splitting of medicines into two halves, in order to administer only half of the dose. Another common medication error amongst older people involves patients who have difficulties swallowing tablets whole. Many patients crush their tablets for easier administration, but this is problematic, particularly for slow-release drugs. It is important that nurses explain this to patients.

So medication errors can generally be caused by inappropriate prescribing, inaccurate administration, and the inaccurate supply of medicines (see Figure 7.2).

Nurses need to be vigilant when administering medicines to ensure that patients—in particular older people—receive the correct drug, at the correct time, and in the correct dose.

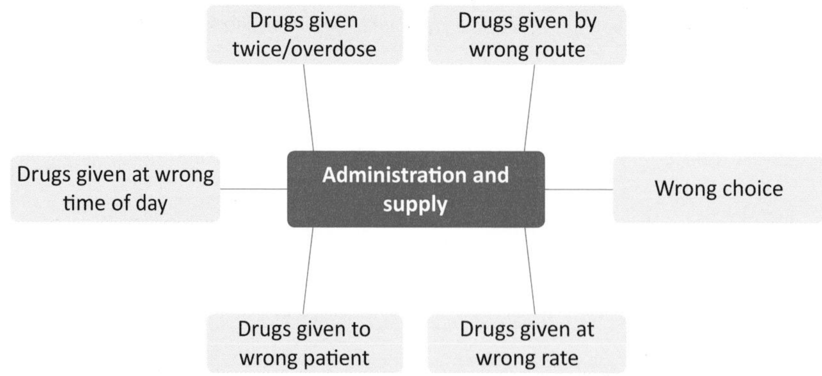

Figure 7.2 Types of medication error related to the supply and administration of medicines

Nursing practice on the administration of medicines is guided by the NMC *Standards for Medicines Management* (2010).

NURSING PRACTICE INSIGHT: ADMINISTRATING MEDICINES TO THE PATIENT

1. Check the patient's identity: ask the patient their name and their age.
2. Check that the prescription or the label on the medicine dispensed is clearly written and unambiguous.
3. Check the expiration date of the medicines to be administered.
4. Check that the dosage of the medicines to be administered is correct.
5. Check that the route of administration and timing of medicines is appropriate. Use the British National Formulary (BNF) to check individual dosing intervals for each medicine, if unsure of the timing of medicines.
6. If a patient refuses their medicines, this must be recorded in the patient's medicines administration chart.

Case study: Intentional non-adherence and non-concordance antihypertensive medication

Mr Davidson, a 75-year-old gentleman, lives alone and has a son who visits him every two days to check that he is okay. Mr Davidson is independent and he likes to socialize with his friends at his local pensioners' club. He plays cards on Tuesdays and goes old-time dancing on Fridays. He shops for food at the local supermarket and swims at least once a week at the local swimming pool. He was recently diagnosed with mild hypertension following a routine review of his lifestyle and health. Mr Davidson was prescribed a thiazide diuretic drug called bendroflumethiazide for treatment of his hypertension and was asked to attend a follow-up hypertension clinic managed by the nurse practitioner at his local GP surgery within the next two weeks. Mr Davidson has no other pre-existing health concerns.

During the following two weeks, Mr Davidson attended the hypertension clinic, where the nurse practitioner stressed the importance of adhering to his medication regimen. Advice was also given regarding the use of salt in his diet and the need for regular exercise.

However, during the next few weeks, Mr Davidson found that taking the diuretic interfered with his social activities. He felt depressed and unhappy taking the diuretic—especially when he had no physical symptoms and felt physically well—and questioned why he should take his prescribed medication. This resulted in Mr Davidson stopping his medication. Some time later, Mr Davidson collapsed at home and was admitted to hospital as an unplanned admission. Whilst in hospital, Mr Davidson's medication was reviewed and changed to a low-dose beta-adrenoceptor antagonist atenolol. Mr Davidson recovered and was discharged within a week.

A few days later, Mr Davidson was reviewed by his GP, who discussed the need to adhere to prescribed medication and to discuss any problems that he may have with his medication with the healthcare team at the GP surgery. The GP arranged an appointment for Mr Davidson to attend the hypertension clinic after one month, for blood pressure and medication monitoring.

As a result of the change in medication, Mr Davidson resumed his social activities and continued to take his medication as prescribed.

> **Reflection point**
>
> What can you learn from this case study?
>
> This case study raises concerns on how to persuade older people to adhere to antihypertensive medication when they are physically well and do not feel the effects of their illness—in this case, hypertension.

NURSING PRACTICE INSIGHT: IMPROVING ADHERENCE AND CONCORDANCE

Nurses can support older people through patient education initiatives. This is an important aspect of the continual management of long-term conditions. Ideally, patients in hospital should receive medication education as part of their discharge planning procedures. It is important to remember that medication education should be individualized and reinforced with written information, which may be in the form of educational leaflets. Older people need to receive information about new medicines in a staged manner to allow them to recall the information. In some cases, patient self-administration procedures are employed ,under which patients self-administer their medicines to adjust to new regimens prior to discharge from hospital.

Patients require information on:

- the timing of medicines;
- the mode of drugs and how they are used to manage their pathological condition;
- the importance of managing the drug regimen;
- the need to avoid certain foods when administering drugs;
- how to recognize side effects that arise from the medication and what to do if they experience side effects; and
- if there has been any change to their medication, for instance a new dose, brand or route.

(NMC, 2010).

For effective medication education, nurses require a working knowledge of applied pharmacology and therapeutics in order to explain proficiently how drugs work and what side effects may occur (Banning, 2003). Advice and support in relation to patient medication education can be provided by the ward pharmacist. By working in partnership with the pharmacist, the nurse can support the patient's needs and also learn basic pharmacological principles from teaching that the pharmacist offers the patient. In this way, working in partnership with other professionals can improve the medication management of older people.

Conclusion

Medication management is a continuing problem for older people. Many older people administer several medicines concurrently, which increases the risk of mismanagement, coupled with the problems of increased sensitivity to the actions of drugs, potential poor adherence and concordance to medication regimen, and possible medication errors. Medication mismanagement can be improved through medication review and patient-centred medication education. Nurses can be proactive, forming partnerships with pharmacists to teach patients about their medicines in order to reduce the incidence of medication-related problems.

Questions and self-assessment

Now that you have worked through the chapter, answer the following questions.

- What do you understand the term 'medication management' to mean?
- Identify why medication management is important and relevant to older people.
- What factors influence patterns of adherence and concordance with medication in older people?
- Why is the medication review process important?
- What preventative measures should nurses take to ensure that medication errors do not occur?
- Identify the key nursing roles and responsibilities in meeting the educational needs of patients and how to improve medication self management in older people.

Self-assessment

- Having read the chapter, how will you change your practice?
- Identify up to three areas relating to medication management and older people in which you need to develop your knowledge and understanding further.
- Identify how you are going to develop this knowledge and understanding, and set deadlines for achieving this.

References

Allard, A., Herbert, R., Rioux, M., Asselin, J. and Voyer, L. (2001) 'Efficacy of a clinical medication review on the number of potentially inappropriate prescriptions prescribed for community-dwelling elderly people', *Canadian Medical Association Journal*, 66: 1291–6.

Banning, M. (2003) 'Pharmacology education: A theoretical framework of applied pharmacology and therapeutics', *Nurse Education Today*, 23(6): 459–66.

Banning, M. (2008) 'Older people and adherence with medication: A review of the literature', *International Journal of Nursing Studies*, 45(10): 1550–61.

Banning, M. (2009) 'An evaluation of the impact of practice-based learning specific to the role of the Community Matron', *British Journal of Community Nursing*, 14(2): 76–80.

Barat, I., Andreason, F. and Damsgaard, E.M.S. (2001) 'Drug therapy in the elderly: what doctors believe and patients actually do', *British Journal of Clinical Pharmacology*, 51(6): 615–22.

Department of Health (2001a) National Service Framework for Older People, London: DH.

Department of Health (2001b) *National Service Framework for Older People, Medicines and Older People.* London: DH.

Department of Health (2002a) *Guidance on the Single Assessment Process for Older People*, Health Service Circular HSC 2002/001/ Local Authority Circular LAC 2002(1), London: DH.

Department of Health (2002b) *Statistics of Prescriptions Dispensed in the Family Health Services Authorities England 1989–1999*, Statistical Bulletin, London: DH.

Department of Health (2004) *Building a Safer NHS for Patients: Improving Medication Safety*, London: DH.

Department of Health (2005) *An NHS and Social Care Model for Improving the Care for People with Long-term Conditions*, London: DH.

Department of Health (2006) *Caring for People with Long-term Conditions: An Educational Framework for Community Matrons and Case Managers*, London: DH.

Ellenbecker, C.H. (2004) 'Nurses' observations and experiences of problems and adverse effects of medication management in home care', *Geriatric Nursing*, 25(3): 164–70.

Feder, G., Cryer, C., Donovan, S. and Carter, S. (2000) 'Guidelines for the prevention of falls in over 65s', *British Medical Journal*, 321: 1007–11.

Fletcher, A.E. (2002) 'The MRC trial of assessment and management of older people in the community: Objectives, design and interventions', *BMC Health Services Research*, 2(1): 21–31.

Hames, A. and Wynne, H.A. (2001) 'Unlicensed and off-label drug use in elderly people', *Age and Ageing*, 30(6): 530–1.

Johnson, M.J., Williams, M., and Marshall, E.S. (1999) 'Adherent and non-adherent medication-taking in elderly hypertensive patients', *Clinical Nursing Research*, 8: 318–35.

Lindley, C.M. and Tulley, M.P. (1992) 'Inappropriate medication is a major cause of adverse drug reactions in elderly people', *Age and Ageing*, 21(4): 294–300.

London Older People Services Development Programme (2003) *Medicines Management Pilot: Executive Summary*, available online at http://www.london.nhs.uk/olderpeople/contents.htm.

Mannesse, C.K. (1997) 'Adverse drug reactions in elderly patients as a contributing factor for hospital admission: Cross-sectional study', *British Medical Journal*, 315: 1057–8.

Medicines and Healthcare Products Regulatory Agency (2004) available online at http://www.mhra.gov.uk/home/idepg?Idosesewes=SS_GET_pageCnodeld=S.

Muir A., Sanders. L.L., Williams, M.S., Wilkinson, E. and Schamader, K. (2001) 'Reducing medication regimen complexity: A controlled trial', *Journal of General Internal Medicine*, 16(2): 77–82.

National Coordinating Council for Medication Error Reporting and Prevention (2002) *Consumer Information for Safe Medication Use*, available online at http://www.nccmerp.org/consumerinfo.html.

National Patient Safety Agency (2008) *Organization Patient Safety Incident Reports*, available online at http://www.nrls.npsa.nhs.uk/patient-safety-data/organisation-patient-safety-incident-reports/.

Nursing and Midwifery Council (2005) *Standards for Medicines Management*, available online at http://www.nmc-uk.org.uk/.

Pearson, B. (2000) 'Unplanned readmission to hospital: A comparison of the views of general practitioners and hospital staff', *Age and Ageing*, 31(2): 141–3.

Royal Pharmaceutical Society of Great Britain (2003*) Pharmacy in the Future: Medicines Management*, London: RPSBG, available online at http://www.rpsbg.org.uk/.

Salas, M., Int' Veld, B.A., Van der Linden, P.D., Hofman, A., Breteler, M., and Stricken, B.H. (2001) 'Impaired cognitive function and compliance with antihypertensive drugs in elderly: The Rotterdam Study', *Clinical Pharmacology & Therapeutics*, 70: 505–17.

Sheehan, O. and Feely, J. (1999) 'Prescribing considerations in elderly patients', *Prescriber*, 10: 75–83.

Shelton, P.S. (2000) 'Assessing the medication appropriateness in the elderly : A review of available measures', *Drugs and Ageing*, 16(6): 437–50.

Swift, C.G. (2003) 'The clinical pharmacological of ageing', *British Journal of Clinical Pharmacology*, 56(3): 249–53.

Vaile, J.H. and Davis, P. (1998) 'Topical NSAIDs for musculoskeletal conditions: A review of the literature', *Drugs*, 56(5): 783–99.

Wiland-Brown, J.E. and Valainte, J. (2000) 'Effectiveness of different medication management approaches on elders' medication adherence', *Outcomes Management for Nursing Practice*, 4(4):172–6.

Woodhouse, K.W. and Wynne, H.A. (1992) 'The Pharmacology of Ageing', in J.C. Brocklehurst, R.C. Tallis, and H.M. Fillit (eds) *Textbook of Medicine and Gerontology*, 4th edn, London: Churchill Livingstone.

For further reading and information

Mental Health Foundation (2004) *Medicines and Drugs: Pharmaceutical Care Services for Older People with Mental Health Problems Living in the Community*, available online at http://www.mhilli.org/medicines/rptpharmsum.htm.

Royal Pharmaceutical Society of Great Britain (1997) *From Compliance to Concordance: Achieving Shared Goals in Medicine Taking*, London: RPSGB.

Winterstein, A.G., Sauer, B.C., Helper, C.D., and Poole, C. (2001) *Implementing Medicine-related Aspects of the NSF for Older People*, London: HMSO.

Online Resource Centre

You can learn more about medication management and older people at the Online Resource Centre that accompanies this book: **http://www.oxfordtextbooks.co.uk/orc/hindle/.**

Part 3

Care settings

Primary and community care

Kay Norman

Learning outcomes

By the end of the chapter, you will be able to:

- recognize the importance of self-care and promotion of independence for the older person;
- identify the variety of care settings within the community in which the older person may access health services; and
- understand the role of the multidisciplinary team, and its importance in assessing and meeting the needs of the older person.

Introduction

Ninety per cent of people in the UK accessing health care will do so through a primary care or community care service (DH, 2004), and, for many, this is the only setting in which they will receive healthcare advice and treatment. The ultimate aim for many older people when accessing health care is to maintain independence; they want to feel secure and safe in knowing that any necessary support and resources will be effectively utilized to achieve this (Kane, 2001). This, alongside the older person's quality of life, must also be seen as the aim for health professionals when involved in healthcare planning and delivery.

It can be confusing when various terms are used to describe services delivered outside of the hospital care setting. 'Primary care' is an umbrella term for health services in the community, such as general practitioners (GPs), practice nursing, optometrists, and pharmacists (DH, 2004), and may be used interchangeably with 'community care'. The strategic direction identified within current Department of Health reports refer to 'community services', which incorporate primary care, social care, and all other community services, such as chiropodists, community nursing, physiotherapists, walk-in centres, etc., to ensure a holistic approach to care delivery (DH, 2008b). Therefore, throughout this chapter, all settings outside hospital care will be referred to as 'community care services'.

The scope of community care services for older people continues to expand, with more and more services seen traditionally as 'hospital-based care' now being shifted to community settings. For example, previously, an older person with one or more long-term conditions, such as asthma and diabetes, would be monitored and regularly reviewed within the relevant hospital clinics by a specialist consultant in that field. Now, the patient is reviewed either within a specialist clinic led by a GP or specialist practice nurse, or at home by a district nurse, community matron, or diabetes specialist nurse.

Various government documents have identified the need to ensure that the care of the older person is planned to consider the benefits of delivering treatment within the home environment, with the support to promote and enable them to make the most of their lives. *Our Health, Our Care, Our Say: A New Direction for Community Services* (DH, 2008b) states a vision for community-based services within three identified themes:

- putting people more in control of their own health;
- enabling and supporting health, independence, and well-being; and
- offering rapid and convenient access to high-quality, cost-effective care.

The *National Service Framework for Older People* (NSFOP) also highlights the need to strengthen community services for older people—in particular, within Standards 3 and 8, which address the importance of intermediate care and health promotion (discussed later in this chapter) (DH, 2001). National Service Frameworks (NSFs) were established to improve services by setting national standards, to improve quality and reduce variations in care across regions. It is important that these are read in conjunction with the NSPOP, because they will inform your knowledge about certain conditions that relate to the care of the older person. These NSFs can be accessed online at http://www.dh.gov.uk/ and include:

- cancer;
- coronary heart disease;
- diabetes;
- long-term conditions (neurological);
- mental health;
- renal;
- chronic obstructive pulmonary disease (COPD); and
- the national stroke strategy.

There is, at the time of writing, a process of transformational change to community care under way. *Transforming Community Services* is a change programme relating to the delivery of primary health care services in England and aiming to promote high-quality standards of care via modern, responsive community services (DH, 2009).

For more on Transforming Community Services, see the Online Resource Centre that accompanies this book.

The aim of this chapter is to explore the healthcare services available to older persons in the community, and the related nursing knowledge, attitudes, and skills required in order to deliver effective, high-quality care.

Self-care

Within the UK, an increased emphasis on the concept of 'self-care' has arisen within recent Department of Health reports, promoting the empowerment of individuals to actively self-care in improving and maintaining their health (DH, 2004; 2005a; 2006). The vision for reform within the National Health Service (NHS) is seen to be based on increasing self-care of patients to increase cost-effectiveness of resources, and to promote choice and independence for patients (DH, 2005a).

Many older people benefit and welcome the opportunity for support with self-care, including advice on long-term conditions, lifestyle, and minor illness, which helps to maintain their independence (Chambers et al., 2006). However, it is imperative that all health professionals collectively have up-to-date knowledge and skills in these particular areas so that they can give the most appropriate, evidenced-based advice. If conflicting advice is given, trust is diminished and any motivation to change may be lost. You may hear patients referring to an article in the local magazine, information received by a neighbour or friend, and Internet sources that may influence their decision on management of their particular condition. Therefore, it is important that all advice is given relating to the most current credible evidence available.

In the UK, it has been estimated that 80 per cent of all care episodes will be self-care (Chambers et al., 2006). The remaining percentage falls within shared-care and complex-care categories. Figure 8.1 demonstrates this as a healthcare pyramid. This concept originates from a US model—Kaiser Permanente—which aimed to organize levels of case management in relation to long-term conditions.

Any self-care strategy will not succeed unless all relevant multidisciplinary members of the community team are involved (see Figure 8.2). A whole-systems approach is needed to ensure that older people receive appropriate advice on how to self-care and manage their condition. Education and understanding is key, so adequate time must be taken in explaining the condition, how self-care will be monitored, discussing areas of concern, allaying any fears and anxieties, talking about what to do in an emergency, supplying relevant health professional contacts, offering understandable literature for future reading and reference, and detailing resource networks and support groups available.

Student activity

- Think of reasons why a self-care initiative may not be successful.
- How could these be overcome?

Example: The patient does not speak English as a first language, so is unable to understand. This problem could be overcome by enlisting the help of an interpreter and relatives (if non-confidential information is being discussed) to promote understanding. Use pictures, rather than wordy leaflets, to explain information, or access leaflets produced in the same language as that which the patient is able to read. Be culturally aware of differences relating to health perceptions and adjust information accordingly.

Self-management programmes

Self-management courses aim to empower patients to take more control of their health conditions, to be more active in the management of their conditions, and to take more responsibility for their health. Outcomes have included a reduction in doctors' and nurses' visits, a reduction in hospital in-patient bed days and emergency admissions, an improvement in

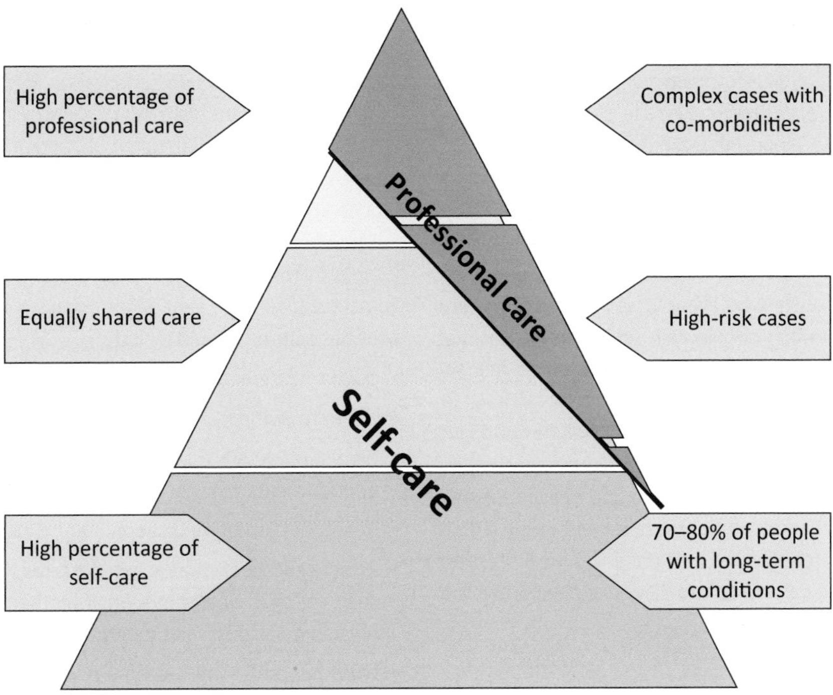

Figure 8.1 Self-care and long-term conditions pyramid
Source: Adapted from DH (2005a), © Crown Copyright.

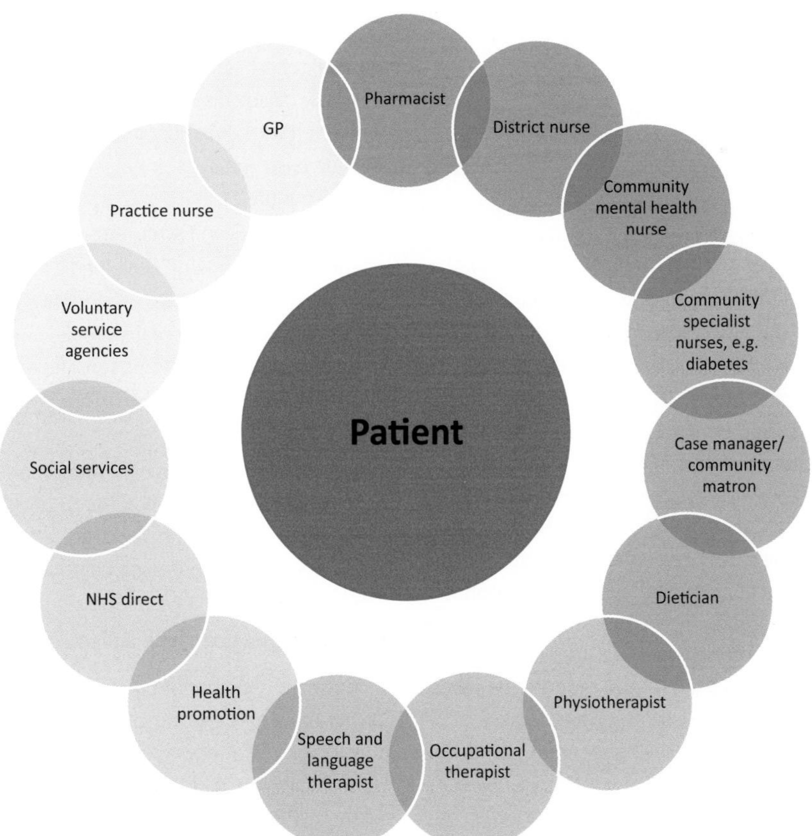

Figure 8.2 Self-care and the community team

medication compliance, and self-reported feelings of well-being. Across the UK, there are group training sessions for people living with long-term health conditions. Many programmes consist of 'chronic disease self-management courses', such as the Expert Patient Programme (EPP).

The EPP is a training programme that aims to improve quality of life by developing the confidence and motivation of people to use their own skills and knowledge to take effective control over life with a long-term health condition. It provides opportunities for people who live with long-term illness and their carers to meet other people with similar conditions, and to develop new skills and support networks to better manage their condition within the community.

The EPP is one among a range of new policies and programmes aiming to modernize the NHS that emphasizes the importance of the patient in the design and delivery of services. Fundamental changes are taking place within the NHS to empower patients, recognizing that patients and professionals each have their own area of knowledge and expertise, and need to work together.

Long-term conditions and self-care

Much of the current self-care initiatives within the community are concentrated on older people with long-term conditions aiming to reduce the risk of admission to hospital and to maintain independence. The Working in Partnership Programme (WiPP) was initially set up to address management of patient demand within general practice, with self-care being a key issue for promotion within the programme. Further useful information and case examples relating to self-care within general practice—and in particular for nurses and health care assistants—is available online at http://www.wipp.nhs.uk/

Your Health, Your Way: A Guide to Long-term Conditions and Self-care can also be found online at http://www.nhs.uk/

One of the roles of the practice nurse is to review individuals who have one or more long-term conditions. This may be through individual clinics with a GP, or a nurse-led clinic. All practices use a computer template to record information gained at the consultation review. A patient record card will also be completed at the first appointment and this may be continued by the patient at home to monitor their condition until the next review. The older person may need initial regular contact with the practice nurse until they feel more confident in managing their own health. It is important that they are given time and understanding, because intensive input at commencement of any self-care initiative reduces the risk of problems and lack of motivation later (Glasgow, 2002).

Any particular intervention or review needed within the home would be referred to a district nurse, and all relevant information disseminated following discussion with the patient. McDuff and Sinclair (2008) suggest that district nurses have an important role to play in promoting self-care, and that information concerning the district nurse's role should be highlighted in patient documentation and care plans.

Self-management planning of a long-term condition should always be formulated, understood, and agreed by the patient. Studies have suggested that self-management plans can reduce acute episodes and resulting hospital admissions (BTS/SIGN, 2008). There are a variety of self-management plan templates for different conditions available. As an example, an action plan or self-management plan for an older person who has asthma should include:

- doctor/nurse/health professional contact details;
- the date of the last review;
- discussion on any agreed goals that were set in the previous appointment;
- details of current medication and the date of diagnosis;
- asthma triggers—that is, what makes the asthma worse—such as cold weather, sunny weather, laughing, anxiety, pets/animals, dust, and damp;
- what happens when asthma is well controlled—for example, no coughing or wheezing, ability to continue with normal activities, normal peak expiratory flow (PEF) at 85 per cent of predicted value on PEF diary (advise usual treatment or inhalers);
- what are the symptoms to look for when asthma is getting worse, including reduced PEF (70–85 per cent of predicted value), chest tightness, wheezing, little effect from reliever inhaler, sleep disturbance—in which case, advise specific interventions dependent on current medication, such as:
  - increase reliever inhaler by X no. of puffs every 20 minutes;
  - monitor PEF and symptoms for improvement;
  - if no improvement, seek medical advice;
  - if improving, step up preventative treatment (again, give specific dosages), oral steroids, until PEF increases to 85 per cent and symptoms subside; and
  - book an appointment to see the GP or practice nurse within three days;
- how to recognize an emergency or acute episode—for example, difficulty in breathing, unable to talk, shortness of breath, reliever inhaler is not effective—in which case, contact practice nurse or GP immediately, or emergency services; and
- agree further goals with patient.

The self-management plan must be clear and readable, in a format that the patient can understand at a glance, with pictures/diagrams as appropriate. Following each review or episode of care, the plan must be updated accordingly.

For further information on asthma and care plans, see http://www.pcrs-uk.org/ and http://www.asthma.org.uk/

Tele-care and tele-health

'Tele-care' is an assistive technology service that enables people—especially older and more vulnerable individuals—to live independently in their own homes.

Equipment is provided to support the individual in their home and tailored to meet their needs. It can be as simple as the basic community alarm service, including pendant alarms, able to respond in an emergency and to provide regular contact by telephone. It can also include detectors or monitors, such as motion or falls, and fire and gas, which trigger a warning to a response centre.

As well as responding to an immediate need, tele-care can work in a preventative mode, with services programmed to monitor an individual's health or well-being. Often known as 'lifestyle monitoring', this can provide early warning of deterioration, prompting a response from family or professionals. The same technology can be used to provide safety and security through bogus-caller and burglar alarms.

Another technology development that is increasing in the community is the medication dispenser. Adults who risk deteriorating health by forgetting to take their medication can use a dispenser, which is preprogrammed to remind patients when and which pills to take. This could make the difference between a person staying in their own home and having to go into institutional care.

The concept of tele-health involves using assistive device technology in patients' homes to remotely monitor patients' vital signs—for example, blood pressure, blood glucose, weight, and oxygen saturation levels. The supporting clinician monitors readings to look for trends that could indicate deterioration in the condition. Readings that are out of range are flagged to the clinician via a traffic light system, or can be reviewed via a web-based database, and an appropriate response is made.

The purpose of tele-health monitoring is to:

- provide regular monitoring of a person's physical health and symptoms;
- ensure the early identification of an exacerbation with a view to an early intervention (including treatment regimes), thereby reducing the need for emergency admission to hospital; and
- promote the independence and confidence of individuals living at home who have long-term conditions.

In the UK, it has primarily been introduced for supporting people with complex conditions—particularly heart failure, COPD, and diabetes—although it can be utilized for other long-term conditions. The Department of Health is presently funding *Whole Systems Demonstrators*, a two-year research project to find out how technology can help people to manage their own health while maintaining their independence. It is believed to be the largest randomized control trial (RCT) of tele-care and tele-health in the world.

For updated information on *Whole Systems Demonstrators*, see http://www.dh.gov.uk/.

Personalized care plans

In the *National Operating Framework for the NHS in England* (DH, 2008c), one of the priorities was '*to ensure that those living with a long-term condition receive a high quality service and help to manage their condition, everyone with a long-term condition should be offered a personalized care plan*'. Personalized care plans are now central to taking forward care planning and integral to self-care.

A personalized care plan involves setting goals with the patient or carer, and should include questions such as:

- what would I like to change or improve?
- what do I feel I can change?
- what sort of things can be achieved?
- what one thing does the person want to achieve?
- how important is it for the person?
- what barriers to achieving the goal could occur?
- what can be done to overcome barriers?

The 'how', 'what', 'when', 'where', and 'how often' also need to be considered, along with timescales.

For an example of a personalized care plan, see the Online Resource Centre that accompanies this book.

To illustrate how many established services can support people with a long term condition see the stepped care model below for neurological conditions. The majority of people (high volume) will be cared for and access services in primary/community care.

Nursing in the older person's home

Community nursing involving older people within their own home environment can be an extremely rewarding experience. The vast array of nursing conditions, patient stories, and personalities that you will encounter will add a tremendous amount of understanding and skills to enhance your nursing career. It is important that you remember that you are a guest in the home, and do not make hasty judgements on lifestyle, living accommodation, or physical capabilities.

Research has shown that community nursing in the person's home consists of multiple agendas, such as long-term condition management (for example, of diabetes and COPD), acute

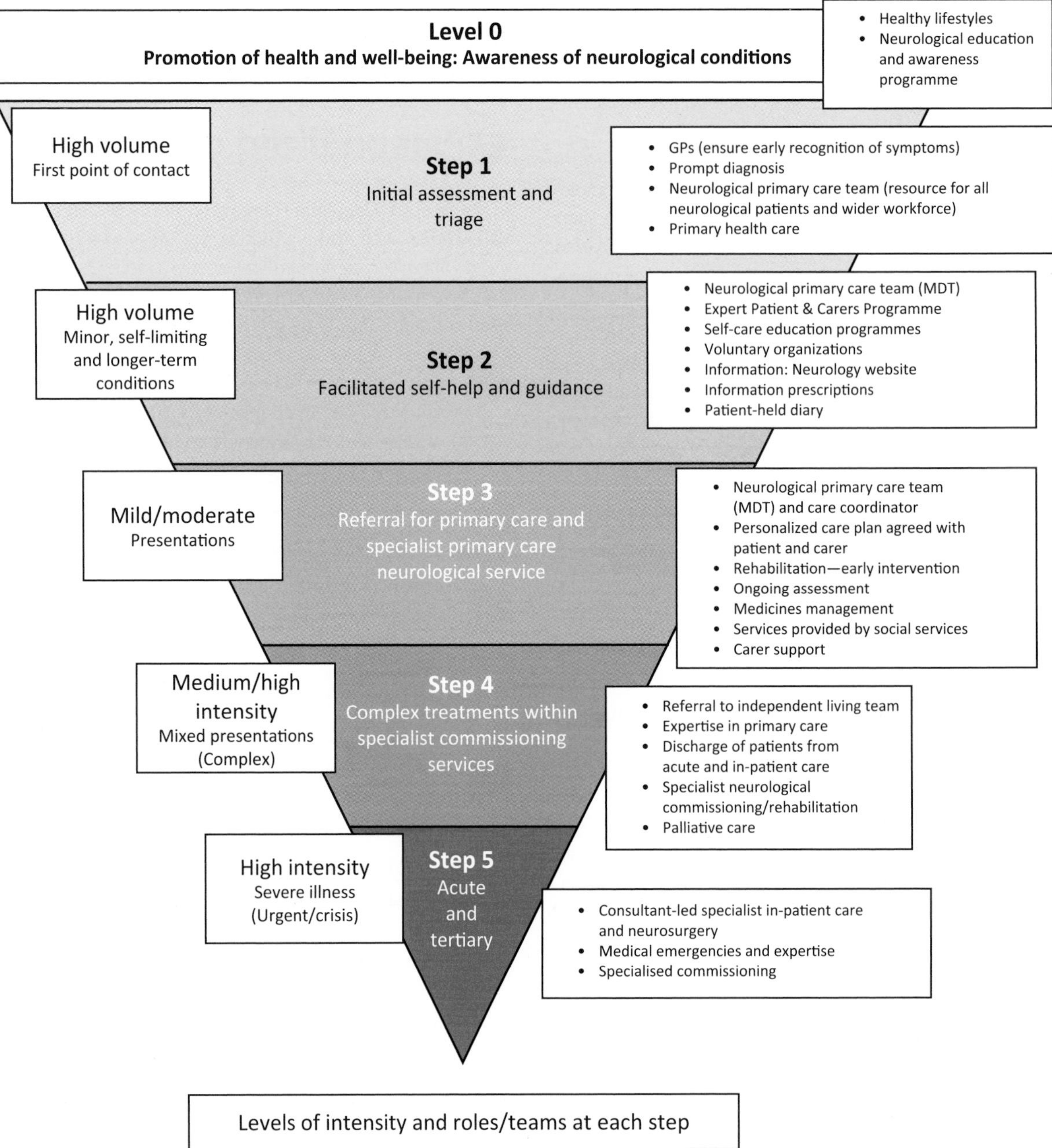

Figure 8.3 Neurological model of care: stepped care model

care (such as parental feeding and exacerbations of chronic diseases), end-of-life care, and post-surgical care (such as wound dressings) (Carr, 2001). However, many older people simply want someone to talk to if you may be the only person that they see each day. This interaction may be seen as their priority, rather than having their leg ulcer dressed, for example. Conflict between service needs and patient needs may arise, therefore it is important that a balance is achieved by appropriate assessment, care planning, and referral to appropriate health, social, and voluntary care services as needed (Dickenson, 2006).

There are no boundaries within the real-life home situation as there are within the constraints of a hospital setting. This is the patient's home and it does not conform to a specific set of standards, so the nurse needs to be adaptable and accepting of diverse situations and surroundings.

A holistic approach is required to ensure that physical, psychological, social, and spiritual needs are addressed in a non-judgemental manner, focusing on what the patient wants, even though it may be very different from your own standards and beliefs. The context of community nursing care in the home provides the very foundation for individualized care.

Although the reason listed for a visit may be 'leg ulcer dressing', you may be required to assess a change in the home environment, such as problems with an immersion heater causing no hot water to be available, or the patient's dog unable to be taken out for a walk, a risk of falling due to excess wires from electrical equipment not being secured, poor nutritional intake due to lack of mobility and inability to walk to the shops, signs of depression due to isolation, and poor compliance of medication. These are only a few issues that may be present; the list is endless.

It is of the utmost importance to respect the older person at all times, demonstrating an interest in them as a person, no matter what the person looks like, their physical and mental capabilities, their home environment, or how they communicate (Miller, 2002). The need for an older person to maintain their identity is especially important when faced with illness or the possibility of further long-term care, and this can be an anxious time for many. They are accepting you as a stranger into their homes, relying on your professional responsibility as a nurse to adopt the principles of non-maleficence and beneficence. They have the right to expect competent, reliable, compassionate nurses to deliver quality care, who will challenge poor practice to ensure the safeguarding of older people.

Within the recent Nursing and Midwifery Council (NMC) *Guidance for the Care of Older People* (2009), one of the fundamental principles is:

The essence of nursing care for older people is about getting to know and value people as individuals through effective assessment [...] providing care which ensures respect, dignity and fairness [...]

(NMC, 2009: 6).

NURSING PRACTICE INSIGHT: EFFECTIVE ASSESSMENT

- Be aware of changes and risks within the home.
- Take time to talk to the person whom you are visiting.
- Listen to their story and ask what they see as their problems/concerns.
- Ask how you can help.
- Suggest services available that may be appropriate to help with concerns (for example, voluntary services, dog-walking services, neighbour and family help, spiritual involvement from their local church/temple, etc., social services to help with meals and cleaning, etc.).
- Involve relatives or carers as appropriate.
- Document discussions in order that others are updated with appropriate information.
- Refer to a senior member of the team if there is anything that you feel needs to be addressed urgently.

Single assessment process

The NSFOP (DH, 2001) suggested that assessment should be person-centred, matched to individual circumstances, and that all relevant needs should be identified and should not be culturally biased. Older people should be invited to play a full part in the assessment. Previously, multiple and repetitive assessments were carried out by varying professional groups with little collaborative working or sharing of information. The single assessment process was to encourage cross-boundary working, with information obtained within the assessment given once and consent given to share this between all relevant personnel, involving decision-making by the patient in which their wishes and views are central.

This information gives a summary for planning and monitoring services.

The interpretation and documentation used for assessment varies across regions, with more than one assessment needed for complex case management and referral to intermediate care or residential care.

see also SAP in chapter 7

Student activity

- Discuss with your mentor the types of assessment used within your area.
- Look at the types of documentation that are currently used for assessment for varying types of care. Are they easy to complete and understand?
- How have the patients been involved with this process?

Examples of information required on the single assessment documentation may include:

- full name and preferred name, date of birth, address, NHS number, GP and care coordinator;
- main language spoken and whether a translator is needed;
- preferred medium of understanding, such as written information, verbal discussion, pictures, listening to tapes;
- medical conditions and impairment—for example, memory loss, visual and hearing impairment, hearing loss, mobility problems;
- needs being met by others—for example, friends, families, or carers;
- details of others involved (other than families or friends), such as voluntary service personnel, GP, occupational therapist, physiotherapist;
- timetable of care;
- telephone contact list for all nursing and social care services involved (normal and out of hours); and
- medication (prescribed and over-the-counter).

For an example of the single assessment process, see the Online Resource Centre that accompanies this book.

A full history would be required to ensure a holistic assessment and that an appropriate care plan is devised, and there are various nursing models of assessment available that can be utilized. It is not possible within this chapter to discuss the wide variety of assessment tools available, although you may have already used some nursing models, tools, or frameworks that can be applied.

One example is provided by the Royal College of Nursing (RCN) in its *Nursing Assessment in Older People: A Royal College of Nursing Toolkit* (2004). This was originally formulated for registered nurses to use as part of the single assessment process and for use within care homes. It offers templates that can be used to gain a holistic assessment of the older person and their environment, and to develop nursing care plans that are person-centred. It also helps to quantify hours of nursing interventions that may be required.

Case study

Mrs Patel is a 78-year-old lady who lives with her extended family in a four-bedroom terraced house in a busy urban location. She has recently been discharged from hospital following a stroke. She has limited mobility, but can walk short distances with a walking frame. She has a left-sided weakness, and needs help with drinking and eating. Her family has moved her bed into the lounge downstairs because she cannot walk upstairs. Her husband says that she cries a lot, but she will not talk about how she feels. He says that she was always the strong person in the family and made all of the decisions in the household.

Before the stroke, Mrs Patel was the main carer for her two young grandchildren (aged 2 and 3) while their parents went to work. She is not able to look after the children now and they attend a nursery. She was diagnosed with non-insulin-dependent diabetes mellitus (Type 2 diabetes) three years ago, which is poorly controlled by diet and medication. Her main wish is that she remains at home with her family.

- Reflect on what further information you would require and what questions you would need to ask in order to formulate a holistic assessment and robust care plan, including what other health or social care personnel may need to be involved.
- Discuss this with your mentor.

An example of an initial care plan for Mrs Patel has been given below for mobility and diabetes (Table 8.1). In reality, all goals and interventions would be agreed with the patient and family, as appropriate.

Table 8.1 Example of a nursing care plan

Nursing diagnosis	Agreed goals	Interventions	Evaluation / review date
Reduced mobility	To promote independence and increase mobility	Liaise with social services and occupational therapist to ensure appropriate equipment/aids and adaptations to home.	Initial request on discharge from hospital – review 1/52
	Respect dignity	Discuss with Mrs Patel and family the importance of increasing mobility and reducing the risk of pressure sores.	1/52
	Reduce isolation	Access to the bathroom and bedroom; stair lift request to occupational therapy.	1/52
		Agree that Mrs Patel's daughter-in-law will help with hygiene needs; care staff to demonstrate techniques	Ongoing
		Respect Mrs Patel's need for independence. Information given on local resource centres/day centres/ voluntary services; positive reinforcement of social networking to encourage independence.	Ongoing
Poorly controlled non-insulin-dependent diabetes mellitus	Maintain blood glucose levels within normal range	Discuss diet and nutrition with Mrs Patel and family, considering cultural and religious dietary requirements.	Ongoing
		Blood glucose machine given and explained; diary to be completed and reviewed fortnightly.	Ongoing

Table 8.1 *(Continued)* Example of a nursing care plan

Nursing diagnosis	Agreed goals	Interventions	Evaluation / review date
		Advice on minimum/maximum levels; contacts provided for further advice or issues. Ensure the reasons for and importance of prescribed medication are understood; give contact details of local support groups to both Mrs Patel and family.	Ongoing

Intermediate care

Within the NSFOP (DH, 2001), Standard 3 relates to intermediate care, with the aim of providing integrated services to promote independent living as soon as possible following discharge from a hospital setting. It also suggests that intermediate care will prevent unnecessary admissions to hospital and long-term residential care through a range of acute and rehabilitative services.

Therefore, intermediate care can be seen as the link between hospital care services and community care services, ensuring continuity of care for the patient.

Intermediate care services should focus on three points:

- responding to or averting a crisis;
- active rehabilitation following an acute hospital stay; and
- whether long-term care is being considered.

The Department of Health defines 'intermediate care' as those services that meet all five of the following conditions.

- **They must be targeted at people who would otherwise face unnecessarily long hospital stays or inpatient care or long-term residential care when this is not appropriate.**
- **The services provided must be based on a thorough assessment. This should result in a structured individual-care plan agreed with each user and if relevant, their carer. The plan should involve active therapy, treatment or the opportunity for recovery. Intermediate care will always include a programme of active rehabilitation involving one or more of occupational therapy, physiotherapy, speech and language therapy.**
- **The services should plan to make the person as independent as possible. This should usually mean that the person can stay living at home.**
- **The services should be limited to a certain time—normally for no longer than six weeks and frequently as little as one to two weeks or less. If this time is extended, there should be a full reassessment, authorised by a senior clinician and including a review date within the six-week period.**
- **The services should work together within a single assessment framework. There should be one set of professional records and shared ways of working.**

(DH, 2008).

Regions across the UK have adopted various methods of addressing the above service conditions, with a range of teams providing the necessary assessment and care delivery required. Examples include rapid-response nursing teams, hospital-at-home teams, rehabilitation community teams, identified residential or attached hospital units that are used specifically for intermediate care, home support teams, day care provision, accident and emergency discharge coordinators, hospital and community social care teams, and community matrons. These services are coordinated through referral from a GP, social worker, hospital unit, or other health professional. Patients themselves can also ask for a referral to this type of service.

Intermediate care provided in the patient's own home is free, but there may be a charge for care in some residential homes. This must be advised at the time of assessment.

Long-term care

In April 2007, 420,000 people in the UK lived in care homes (Age Concern, 2009). For many, the transition to long-term care may have been an upsetting and anxious experience, following decades of independence and living in their own home. For others, it may be a welcome relief to be in a safe, secure environment in which their physical, social, and psychological needs can be met.

NHS continuing health care is a package of care that is arranged and funded by the NHS to meet physical and or mental health needs. This can be received in any care setting, including a care home, where a person is eligible for continuing health care. The primary care trust (PCT) in which the individual's GP is located will make a contract with the care home to pay the fees for accommodation and care. This should be completed before any assessment to identify nursing needs of a person who is in, or is about to go into, a nursing home (under the NHS Continuing Healthcare (Responsibilities) Directions 2007).

See Chapter 4 for more on the law relating to continuing health care.

Making a decision on care homes

Sources of funding can be an important issue for the older person and their relatives when considering long-term care; therefore, it is important that nurses are aware of current legislation and appropriate resources for direction. The *National Framework for NHS Continuing Healthcare and NHS-funded Nursing Care* (DH, 2007) sets out the principles and processes of funding arrangements for continuing care.

Further information for patients and families from the Care Quality Commission (CQC) is available online at http://www.cqc.org.uk/. The CQC is the independent regulator of health and social care in England, which includes services within the NHS, local authorities, private companies, or voluntary organizations. Previous inspection reports from the various care home organizations are available online and can be useful in informing decisions.

Davies and Nolan (2003) argue that health and social care practitioners have enormous potential to influence whether or not helping a relative to move into a nursing home is perceived as a positive choice. Feelings of guilt, anger, and sadness are common amongst relatives visiting their loved ones if this has not been the case prior to admission. Negative portrayals of care in care homes via the media can add to these feelings, and although substantiated cases are reported, there are many examples of good care that are not (Kydd and Kearney, 2009). Any instances of poor nursing practice must be reported. The NMC Code (NMC, 2008) states: '*You must act without delay if you believe that you, a colleague or anyone else may be putting someone else at risk*'.

Making the transition to a care home

Many older people making the transition to a care home understand that they need help with some activities. However, it is important to remember that this care should help the individual to retain some independence wherever possible, to ensure that the older person is able to make choices and have control over their life (Raynes et al., 2001).

Some studies have shown that perceptions of care given by nurses and carers do not correlate with residents' views of care received (Milke et al., 2006). Residents within care homes are regarded as 'vulnerable', and it may be difficult to make joint care decisions with the resident if this could result in risk-taking behaviour—for example, a resident suffering injury from a fall if allowed to walk unaided. Conflicts invariably will arise within this setting when deciding between protection from harm and respecting freedom of choice. It is important that all options are discussed with individuals, staff, and relatives, as appropriate, and that necessary documentation of the discussions completed. The Mental Capacity Act 2005 must be considered in terms of consent. The final part of the Act came into force in April 2009. Everyone working with and/or caring for an adult who may lack capacity to make particular decisions must comply with this Act when they make decisions or act for that person.

The nurse must take the time to show empathy, respect, and understanding both to the resident and also the relatives, and to try to allay any fears and worries that they may have. The first day moving into their new home can be an anxious experience for all concerned.

Student activity

Below is an initial list of ways in which the nurse can ensure a smooth transition into a care home for a new resident.

- Undertake a full assessment in partnership with the family prior to arrival.
- Understand the older person's life history.
- Gather information of their likes and dislikes prior to arrival.
- Ensure that all staff are aware of the new arrival.
- By what name does the new resident like to be called?
- Ensure that the room is ready and that any personal items supplied by relatives have been put in place.
- Talk to other residents to let them know of the new arrival.
- Ensure that a member of staff is allocated to greet the new arrival, and has time to talk and discuss needs (holistic assessment) as appropriate.

Can you think of any others?

Nursing within a care home can be a varied and rewarding experience, within which you can really get to know the resident. Remember that this is their home, and that maintaining dignity and respect is paramount. It is a wonderful opportunity to talk with clients and listen to their stories, gaining continuing information for ongoing holistic assessment. A person's life history can be fascinating and influences how they see, and feel seen, in the world; these discussions help to build a therapeutic relationship between resident and nurse. Bayer et al. (2005) suggest that the characteristics that older persons value greatly are helpfulness, respect, and friendliness, which are considered essential nursing skills. Although it is important to assess activities of daily living to identify areas of inability such as poor mobility, it is also important to assess the resident's likes and dislikes, in order that individualized care is maintained. Building a good rapport with the resident may help to overcome any sensitive issues or embarrassment, ensuring empathy and compassion.

Conclusion

There are many challenges for the future of community nursing, and *Transforming Community Services* will drive the need to strengthen clinical skills and leadership, support quality and time to care, and to develop evidence-based practice. There will be more use of information management, including risk stratification tools and assistive technology—particularly telecare and tele-health. Self-care and personalized care plans will also have increasing prominence.

As discussed, there are many care settings within the community, but care can also take place in areas not discussed in this chapter, including sheltered housing, prisons, homeless shelters, and among travelling families. Multidisciplinary working is essential within the community, with collaborative decisions made with the patient. It is important to remember that, whatever the community setting, whether it is a care institution or a hostel, this is the older person's home. You are a guest in that home and must respect their privacy, help to maintain their dignity, and promote their independence. Nursing older people in the community is a positive, rewarding experience that will give you a deeper understanding of social, psychological, spiritual, and physical care issues from the patient's perspective.

Questions and self-assessment

Now that you have worked through the chapter, answer the following questions.

- What are the benefits of self-care and how does this help to maintain independence?
- Where do most older people receive health care?
- List the main advantages of the single assessment process.
- Take some time simply to talk to a resident within a care home. Do not concentrate on 'nursing' interventions, but use the time to find out about their life, such as what job they did previously. What hobbies or interests did they enjoy? Where did they grow up and what adventures have they had? Reflect on whether this has made you see the resident differently. If you find that it has, how?
- How will the information gained from your conversation influence your plan of care?

Self-assessment

- Having read the chapter, how will you change your practice?
- Identify up to three areas relating to community or primary care in which you need to develop your knowledge and understanding further.
- Identify how you are going to develop this knowledge and understanding, and set deadlines for achieving this.

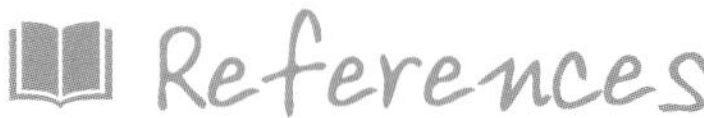

References

Age UK (2009) *Ageing Population*, available online at http://www.ageuk.org.uk/.

Bayer, T., Tadd, W. and Krajcik, S. (2005) 'The voice of older people', *Quality in Ageing*, 6(1): 22–9.

British Thoracic Society/Scottish Intercollegiate Guidelines Network (2008) *Guidelines on the Management of Asthma*, available online at http://www.brit-thoracic.org.uk/Portals/0/Clinical per cent20Information/Asthma/Guidelines/asthma_final2008.pdf.

Carr, S. (2001) 'Nursing in the community: Impact of context on the practice agenda', *Journal of Clinical Nursing*, 10(3): 330–6.

Chambers, R., Wakeley, G., and Bleckinsopp, A. (2006) *Supporting Self-care in Primary Care*, Oxford: Radcliffe Publishing.

Davies, S. and Nolan, M. (2003) 'Making the best of things: Relatives' experiences of decisions about care home entry', *Ageing and Society*, 23(4): 429–50.

Department of Health (2001) *National Service Framework for Older People*, London: DH.

Department of Health (2004) *NHS Improvement Plan: Putting People at the Heart of Public Services*, London, DH.

Department of Health (2005a) *Public Attitudes to Self-care: Baseline Survey*, London: DH.

Department of Health (2005b) *Self-care: A Real Choice—Self-care Support: A Practical Option*, London: DH.

Department of Health (2006) *Supporting People with Long-term Conditions to Self-care: A Guide to Developing Local Strategies and Good Practice*, London: DH.

Department of Health (2007)*The National Framework for NHS Continuing Healthcare and NHS-funded Nursing Care*, London: DH.

Department of Health (2008a) *NHS Next Stage Review: Our Vision for Primary and Community Care*, DOH London.

Department of Health (2008b) *Our Health, Our Care, Our Say: A New Direction for Community Services*, London: DH.

Department of Health (2008c) *The Operating Framework for the NHS in England: 2009–10*, London: DH.

Department of Health (2009) *Transforming Community Services*, London: DH.

Dickenson, A. (2006) 'Implementing the single assessment process: Opportunities and challenges', *Journal of Interprofessional Care*, 20(4): 365–79.

Glasgow, M. (2002) 'Self-management aspects of the improving chronic illness care breakthrough series: Implementation with diabetes and heart failure teams', *Annals of Behavioural Medicine*, 24(2): 80–7.

Kane, R. (2001) 'What older people want from long-term care', *Health Affairs*, 20(6): 114–27.

Kydd, A. and Kearney, E. (2009) 'Life in Care', in A. Kydd, T. Duffy, and R. Duffy (eds) *The Care and Well-being of Older People*, Devon: Reflect Press.

MacDuff C. and Sinclair J. (2008) 'Evidence on self-care support within community nursing', *Nursing Times*, 104(14): 32–3.

Milke, D.L., Beck, C., and Danes, S. (2006) 'Meeting the needs in continuing care of facility-based residents diagnosed with dementia: Comparison of ratings by families, direct care staff and other staff', *Journal of Gerontology*, 25: 103–19.

Miller, L. (2002) 'Effective communication with older people', *Nursing Times*, 17(9): 45–50.

Nursing and Midwifery Council (2008) *The Code*, London: NMC.

Nursing and Midwifery Council (2009) *Guidance for the Care of Older People*, London: NMC.

Raynes, N., Temple, B., Glenister, C., and Coulthard, L. (2001) *Quality at Home for Older People: Involving Service Users in Defining Home Care Specifications*, York: Policy Press.

Royal College of Nursing (2004) *Nursing Assessment in Older People: A Royal College of Nursing Toolkit*, London: RCN.

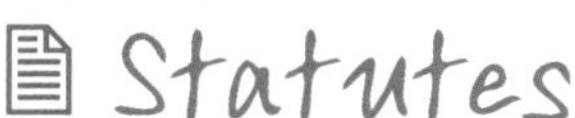

Mental Capacity Act 2005

Statutory instruments

NHS Continuing Healthcare (Responsibilities) Directions 2007

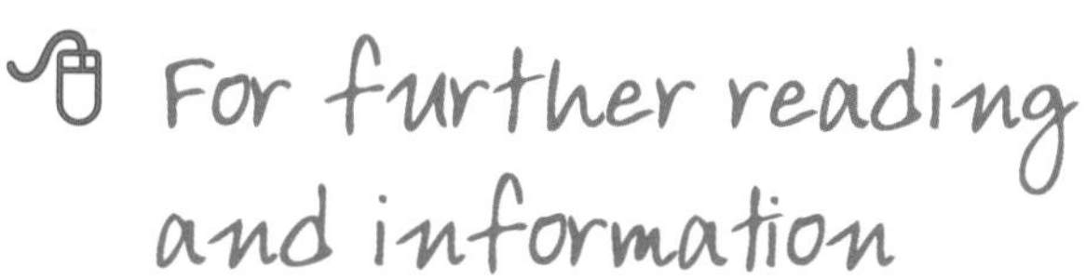

Department of Health (2007) *Supporting People with Long-term Conditions*, London: DH.

Drennan, V. and Goodman, C. (2007) *Oxford Handbook of Primary Care and Community Nursing*, Oxford: Oxford University Press.

Goodman, B. and Clemow, R. (2008) *Nursing and Working with Other People*, Exeter: Learning Matters Ltd.

http://www.cqc.org.uk/

http://www.dh.gov.uk/

http://www.nhs.uk/

http://www.nice.org.uk/

http://www.nmc-uk.org.uk/

http://www.rcn.org.uk/

http://www.wipp.nhs.uk/

Online Resource Centre

You can learn more about primary and community care for older people at the Online Resource Centre that accompanies this book:
http://www.oxfordtextbooks.co.uk/orc/hindle/

Hospital care

Professor Wilf McSherry and Judith Bennion

Learning outcomes

By the end of the chapter, you will be able to:

- consider the factors that impact the experiences of older people receiving hospital care;
- demonstrate an awareness of how care and services may be organized and delivered to older people while in hospital;
- be aware of the steps involved in discharging the older person from hospital; and
- transfer the knowledge and skills gained into caring for older people within the hospital environment.

Introduction

The National Health Service (NHS) has undergone significant changes in terms of policy and practice. These policies and practices have impacted either directly or indirectly upon older people services, with the aim of enhancing the older person's experience of receiving hospital care. Several healthcare reports have indicated that there have been many institutional failings in the delivery of care to older people, especially within hospitals (Age Concern, 2006; HCC, 2006). It must be stressed that many of the issues associated with the nursing of older people are not specific to the UK, but that these issues are also being debated across other regions of the world (Cheek and Gibson, 2003; Hweidi and Al-Hassan, 2005; Jones, 2005; Sand et al., 2006).

A landmark publication

The *National Service Framework for Older People* (NSFOP) (DH, 2001) was a landmark publication, setting a ten-year programme for improving health and social care for older people. The publication of this document was significant because it acknowledged that the care of older people within many sectors—and specifically within acute care—had fallen short of any minimum standard.

Standard 4 of the NSFOP focused specifically upon 'General Hospital Care', with the explicit aim of ensuring that '*older people's care in hospital is delivered through appropriate specialist care and by hospital staff who have the right set of skills to meet their needs*'. The aim of the NSFOP was not only to tinker with service delivery and organization, but also to revolutionize the entire care that older people receive specifically within a hospital environment.

In the several years since the launch of the NSFOP, considerable progress has been made in the implementation and achievements of the key standards (DH, 2008). Yet there is no room for complacency: publications are still emerging that stress that older people still face ageist attitudes, patronization, and care that does not respect the privacy and dignity of each person. Furthermore, in some hospital wards, older people are still receiving reduced standards of care and poorly managed discharges (HCC, 2006; 2007).

This chapter will therefore explore some of these important issues, offering strategies and skills that nurses can use to ensure that the care provided to older people is safe, holistic, and dignified. This chapter asks everyone involved in caring for older people within a hospital setting to evaluate traditional and contemporary practice.

In addition to the above learning outcomes, the authors will highlight the importance of ensuring that the nursing care of older people in hospital is underpinned by four key principles:

- communication (staff attitude);
- respecting the privacy and dignity of each older person;
- empowering the individual to maintain their autonomy and independence (choice and control); and
- nutritional support.

These are inherent themes within several publications targeted at improving care for older people (for example, Magee et al., 2008).

Consequence upon hospital care of living longer

National and global statistics indicate that the fastest growing age group in the UK is those aged 80 and over (National Statistics, 2010). The fact that people are living longer may have serious ramifications for all healthcare sectors. One of the biggest providers of health care are family 'carers'. With an ageing population and a subsequent decline in young people, there may well be a shortfall in this resource in the future. Despite individuals living longer, older people over the age of 65 are still the primary consumers of hospital care.

Chinn and Spink (2007: 17) reported that '*in 2005, in a three-month period, 25 per cent of those aged 75 and over had attended the casualty or out-patient department of a hospital, compared with 14 per cent of people of all ages*'. Referring to the General Household Survey data, they go on to point out that the average length of stay in hospital for those aged 75 and over was 13 nights.

NURSING PRACTICE INSIGHT

Where would you expect older people to be nursed within an acute hospital?

This question may seem a little simplistic—but it highlights an important point: *older people may be nursed anywhere within the acute care setting*.

Table 9.1 presents a snapshot of people in hospital over the age of 65 on a single day. This particular acute NHS trust has 723 beds across two hospital sites. The age range in Table 9.1 is from 65 years old to 97 years old. Approximately 68 per cent of the hospital beds are occupied by people over the age of 65, with the majority of these being cared for in the medical and surgical specialities.

Table 9.1 Number of people over the age of 65 in one hospital

Department	Number of people
Vascular	1
Urology	14
Thoracic medicine	28
Trauma and orthopaedics	59
Surgery	48
Rehabilitation	32
Radiology	2
OPH ophthalmic	1
Nephrology	14
Medicine	233
Haematology	4
Gynaecology	1
Geriatric	11
Gastroenterology	35
Ear, nose, and throat	4
Cardiology	7
TOTAL	494

The table supports the findings of the National Audit Office (2007: 8) indicating that '*older people occupy some 60 per cent of acute hospital beds and of these 40 per cent may have dementia*'. These figures reinforce the point that older people are not only cared for within elderly care units or departments.

Caring for older people in hospital is complex and often undervalued. There are still many myths, misconceptions, and prejudices surrounding the care of older people. Thankfully, the NSFOP (2001) has gone some way to challenging and eradicating age discrimination and ageist attitudes.

Older people are frequently admitted into hospital with more than one condition or illness (known as 'co-morbidity'). For example, an older person may be admitted into a ward with acute chest pain indicating a suspected heart attack (myocardial infarction) and this condition may be complicated because they also have diabetes (diabetes mellitus Type 1 or Type 2), which places them at greater risk of developing complications associated with admission to hospital, such loss of mobility and independence. The fact that some older people may present with co-morbidities requires those caring for them to be more informed about the impact of illness upon older people. Castledine (2005: 351) warns nursing staff that many of the institutional failings when caring for older people can be avoided by employing '*enlightened and motivated nursing staff*'.

Experience of older people within acute care

The Acute Coordination Centre for the NHS Patient Survey Programme reported:

Nearly 8 in 10 patients (79 per cent) rated the care they received in hospital as 'excellent' (43 per cent) or 'very good' (35 per cent) with those rating their overall care as 'excellent' increasing from 42 per cent in 2007 to 43 per cent in 2008.

(2008: 2)

These results indicate that the vast majority of adults are satisfied with the hospital care received. However, the results reveal that a small proportion of patients are dissatisfied with the care provided.

Two significant reports recently published (HCC, 2009; The Patients Association, 2009) suggest that some older people may be receiving care that is cause for concern.

For far too long now, the Patients Association has been receiving calls on our helpline from people wanting to talk about the dreadful, neglectful, demeaning, painful and sometimes downright cruel treatment their elderly relatives had experienced at the hands of NHS nurses.

(Rayner, 2009: 3)

Despite some major developments in both policy and practice, and high-profile political (DH, 2006a) and professional campaigns (RCN, 2008), the experience for some older people within hospitals remains disconcerting.

One of the key reasons for the launch of the NSFOP was to eradicate bad practice and ensure that the care older people receive in hospital is the same as that received by any other user group. The NSFOP was supposed to be revolutionary, tackling many of the negative stereotypical and discriminatory attitudes directed towards older people and health care. Despite all of the propaganda, policy, and development, some older people are still experiencing demeaning and neglectful care while in hospital.

A useful exercise to highlight these points is to explore how the media portray the care that older people receive in hospital.

What do the media say?

> ***Student activity***
>
> Undertake a general Internet search on 'older people, dignity and hospital care'. Review some of the cases presented, paying special attention to how the care of older people is perceived and presented by the mass media.

The following was reported by Narain (2009) in the *Daily Mail*:

An Alzheimer's patient lies in a grubby hospital bathroom because of a shortage of beds. Will the elderly EVER be treated with dignity in Britain?

This kind of headline might sell newspapers, but it paints a very negative and unrepresentative picture of health care in the UK. We are aware that such incidences are thankfully rare and that they can be sensationalized.

In contrast to this news story, there are many centres of excellence throughout the UK providing world-class care and services for older people.

Improvements to hospital care

There have been a number of very successful initiatives to improve the experience of older people receiving hospital care, including:

- the West Midlands Champions for Older People Programme (Hindle, 2008);
- nationally, the Department of Health has launched the ten-point Dignity Challenge (DH, 2006a), raising awareness of the importance of dignity in care for older people;
- the Nursing and Midwifery Council (NMC) (2009) published *Guidance for the Care of Older People*, offering a framework for enhancing the care provided to older people; and
- other initiatives, such as the creation of 'dignity maps' (DH, 2009b) to help healthcare professionals to evaluate and enhance the care provided to older people.

However, there is no room for complacency: the patient stories presented by the Patients Association (2009) reveal that some older people's dignity and self-respect are still violated in today's modern NHS. They also highlight that older people remain a vulnerable group, reinforcing the idea that staff must be vigilant and ready to safeguard the needs of older people at all times.

> ***Reflection point***
>
> Before proceeding with this section, reflect upon the skills and qualities that you, as a nurse, will need to develop and utilize when caring for older people.

Once you have done this, look at Box 9.1. You may have identified similar skills, qualities, and personal attributes. These are the 'core values', or 'essential skills', of nursing (NMC, 2007). These core skills are the foundations of all caring relationships and are fundamental to the delivery of nursing care.

Box 9.1 Skills and qualities associated with care and caring

- Caring with compassion.
- Dealing with older people with sensitivity and in a non-patronizing manner.
- Being prepared to spend time listening and attending to the needs of the individual.
- Using observation to assess the 'holistic' needs of the older person.
- Always treating older people with respect and courtesy.
- Striving for a non-judgemental approach to care.
- Challenging prejudice, poor practice, and discrimination where these are encountered.
- Preserving privacy and dignity in all interactions.

Care organization and delivery

This section will introduce you to the different models of organizing and delivering care to older people within the acute hospital environment. It will take you on a patient's journey, from admission through to discharge, highlighting the different steps and processes that nurses must consider in order to provide safe and competent nursing care for older people.

Communication is the key to preserving dignity and respect

The NSFOP suggests that, in order to deliver effective, dignified, and individualized care, staff must have the necessary skills and experience. These will be fundamental in achieving the key interventions, or key stages, in the journey of any older person admitted into hospital (DH, 2001)—that is, emergency response, early assessment, ongoing care, old age specialist care, and discharge planning. All of these require practitioners who are skilled, proficient, and excellent communicators, providing timely and appropriate—often life-saving—interventions in a dignified and respectful manner.

The nurse will need to integrate within their practice the fundamental principles of communication, which means respecting and empowering the older person, and offering reassurance and support so that they feel empowered and involved in decision-making and the caring relationship.

Reflection point

Before you proceed, we would like you to spend several minutes reflecting upon the following case study. As you undertake this activity, you may also want to reflect upon the skills and qualities that you identified earlier, establishing which ones you may use in this caring relationship.

You might want to consider the admission procedures that you use, or have observed, in practice. Ask these questions:

- Are the procedures welcoming and supportive?
- Could they make an older person feel vulnerable and isolated?

Case study: Representation of an acute admission into hospital

Charles, a gentleman aged 80, had been a little unwell for the past week, and had become increasingly confused, disorientated, and extremely agitated, which was totally out of character. Charles was normally a very active and physically well person, having enjoyed excellent health during the course of his life. Since his wife had died two years ago, he had lived alone, with the support of his daughter, who lived nearby. This daughter was very concerned by Charles' symptoms and contacted his general practitioner (GP), who visited.

Upon assessment, Charles was found to have pyrexia, with a temperature of 38.7. Physical examination revealed that his abdomen was distended and tender, and a provisional diagnosis was reached of urinary retention due to some underlying infection. The GP attempted to catheterize, but was unable to pass the catheter due to an enlarged prostrate.

Charles was admitted to the medical emergency centre, where he was assessed and transferred to a surgical ward, because no bed was available within the elderly care department. He was greeted by a nurse with the following term of endearment: 'Alright, lovey... We'll be with you in a minute'.

Charles remained on the ward for two days before being transferred. Upon admission to the surgical ward, Charles was placed in a four-bedded bay opposite two ladies.

This case study raises a number of questions relating to the admission of older people into hospital. The case study highlights that all of the skills, qualities, and attributes (see Box 9.1 above) are fundamental to the admission of any patient. In particular, it indicates that we must treat all patients with dignity and respect, and that we must give careful consideration to the way in which we communicate with older people. Furthermore, it asks us to pay specific attention to the environment in which we care for older people.

The nursing of any patient in mixed-sex bays should be avoided at all costs. The Rt Hon Alan Johnson MP, Secretary of State for Health, speaking on 28 January 2009 at the NHS Chairs Conference, *Care and Compassion in the 21st Century*, stated: '*I want to make clear today that mixed sex accommodation is no longer tolerable in the NHS, except when it is absolutely clinically necessary*'.

In the case study above, Charles should be offered a plan of care that is individualized and tailored to his own unique needs and circumstances. Despite considerable progress, some reports are still indicating that older people continue not to be involved in decision making and consulted in all aspects of their care (HCC, 2006).

Finally, we should also avoid, where possible, transferring older patients from pillar to post within our organizations in order to meet service demands.

The NMC's *Guidance for the Care of Older People* (2009) highlights three important elements that must be considered in our interaction with older people. Figure 9.1 illustrates how these three elements should inform Charles' care.

Multidisciplinary team approach

The case study above emphasizes the need for both excellent nursing and medical care. It reinforces a requirement for a coordinated and multidisciplinary model of care. This team should include all of the following: a consultant in old-age or geriatric medicine; specialist/consultant nurses; and allied healthcare professionals, including advanced practitioners, dieticians, social workers, and pharmacists. In addition, we would have added to our team old-age psychiatry and mental health liaison services.

The NSFOP suggests that this model of service delivery should be based around a specialist unit, or centre of excellence, so that specialist knowledge and skills can be cascaded and made available to the entire hospital. This model ensures that expertise can be used in the setting and monitoring of standards, outcomes, and practices that directly impact on the older person's experience of receiving hospital care.

A new development in many acute hospitals and social care sectors is the creation of 'older people champions', or 'dignity champions', to be proactive in promoting the needs and services of older people (DH, 2006a; 2006b; 2006c). These innovations suggest that there is a change in culture and attitude towards caring for older people; we are witnessing a renewed commitment to and valuing of, older people's health and well-being.

Models of service delivery

The NSFOP presents three mechanisms, or models, for delivering care to older people within acute hospital, each of which has its own strengths and limitations (see Box 9.2 below). Neither model is superior to the other. The adoption and utilization of these models is intended to make sure that the services provided to older people are coordinated and not

People

Nurses who are efficient and able to deliver safe, effective, quality care by being.

Competent: having the right knowledge skills and attitude to care for older people.

Assertive:
challenging poor practice, including attitude and behaviour and safeguarding older people.

Reliable and dependable.

Empathetic, compassionate, and kind.

Process

Delivering quality care which promotes dignity by nurturing and supporting the older person's self-respect and self-worth through:

- Communicating with older people by not only talking with them, but listening to what they say.
- Assessment of need.
- Respect for privacy and dignity.
- Engaging in partnership working with older people, their families, carers and your colleagues.

Places

Diverse environments in the community or hospital where care is provided for older people which is:

- Committed to equality and diversity.
- Appropriate.
- Resourced adequately.
- Effectively managed.

Figure 9.1 People, process, and place
Source: NMC (2009)

Box 9.2 Models of delivering hospital care to older people

- **Age-defined models**—Patients are admitted to specialist or general wards, with a locally agreed chronological age (usually 75+). The origin of these wards arose out of concern that older people's needs were being overlooked in more general wards. There was an assumption that such wards would provide a high level of specialist care for older people. However, this was not always the case, because some of these wards were isolated from the main services and facilities within the hospital, meaning that care was often under-resourced and fragmented.
- **Integrated models**—Physicians receive patients irrespective of age and there is collaboration with consultants in old-age medicine. This model operates around the principle of equality, suggesting that all people have the right to specialist acute care and services, irrespective of chronological age.
- **Needs-based models**—Patients are admitted to specialist areas or wards based on need, usually determined by locally based criteria.

fragmented, ensuring a seamless transition throughout the different stages of hospitalization and discharge. These models may help to reduce the 'hiccups' that older people experience when being transferred from one sector to the next—whether for intermediate or long-term care.

A systematic approach to care delivery

The term 'systematic' means that there are different steps that must be undertaken to provide care (see Figure 9.2 below). By adopting a 'systematic' and individualized approach to care delivery, the older person will feel empowered, having a sense of value and control. Importantly, they will report that they have been listened to and acknowledged as a unique individual.

Irrespective of which model of care (outlined above) is used to organize and deliver care to older people, there is still a fundamental requirement that the older person's needs be met within a holistic framework (that is, a framework that looks at the whole person), ensuring that their physical, psychological, social, and spiritual needs are addressed. Care must be culturally sensitive, respecting the older person's culture, race, and ethnicity, and adequate attention should be paid to religious beliefs and values.

Crucially, older people need to be involved in every stage of planning care whenever possible—but what we are advocating

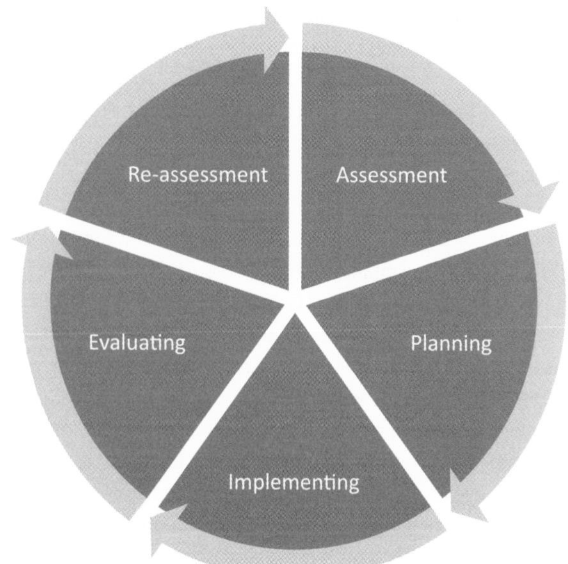

Figure 9.2 Stages involved in a 'systematic' approach to care
Source: Kratz (1979).

is not pioneering or innovative. The nursing profession seems to have lost sight of the power that the nursing process possesses. It is not about inventing new technologies and practices, but about refocusing and evaluating what we do well, and using this to enrich the older person's experience.

Benefits of simple strategies

These simple strategies will go a long way in promoting the older person's independence, self-worth, and autonomy. Nurses are familiar with the 'nursing process' (Kratz, 1979), or a 'systematic' approach to care and the stages involved in this cyclical process (see Figure 9.2 above). This process—assessing, planning, implementing, evaluating, and reassessing care—provides a framework and structure that involves the older person in the entire caring relationship, as an equal partner. It is a model that should ensure that the nursing care provided is individualized and person-centred.

There is nothing more frustrating than walking onto a ward and seeing registered nurses evaluating and writing care plans at the nurses' station or in the sister's office. This is a lost opportunity for interaction, enquiry, and observation—a lost opportunity for developing a rapport with the patient and a therapeutic relationship. Fundamentally, it is a lost opportunity to listen to the patient and their relatives, etc., demonstrating that nurses are present and care. Consequently, as a profession, we need to re-evaluate our practices: it is not about discarding our history, but about using some of the older rituals and traditional practices that we have at our disposal to enhance the patient experience. This humane and partnership approach to care is what all patients want (Maben and Griffiths, 2008).

Patient comfort rounds

There are many terms or phrases used to describe the practice of giving fundamental care to older people in the ward environment. During the era of task orientation, or ritualistic nursing, the most commonly used phrases would have been 'the back round', or 'pressure area care round'. As implied, it was often seen as a time to check on the patient's skin integrity and ensure that bed or pressure sores were not developing. These 'rounds' were much more than a cursory check, however, and would have involved the turning, washing, drying, powdering, or creaming of the patient's pressure areas, and then the repositioning of the patient. The care delivered would be documented—often on a turning chart and in the nursing notes, where any changes would be recorded. Other tasks undertaken at this time would include general observations of urinary catheters, toileting, and the offering of a drink.

In recent times, these ritualistic practices seem to have been frowned upon because of the lack of individualistic care and attention. Yet, while these 'rounds' served a specific function, they also enabled the nurse to enquire and engage in conversation with the older person, their relatives, and their visitors, perhaps about progress, level of satisfaction, or a general enquiry about comfort. Therefore, not everything about these rounds was 'bad', or detrimental to the care of older people.

A return to traditional nursing practices

In recent years, then, many traditional nursing practices have come under scrutiny; with the advent of evidence-based, individualized patient care and care planning, many would question the validity of the old-style 'back round', seeing it as defunct. But in defence of tradition, one could argue that these rounds were important in terms of patient contact and interaction—observation and interaction that allows the nurses to pick up on cues that are both verbal and non-verbal. The round helps to preserve the patient's independence, dignity, and privacy in relation to activities of daily living.

In some cases, these rounds have continued to be undertaken and referred to as a 'back round' by 'old-school' nurses who trained and practised through the 1960s, 1970s, and 1980s. It is reassuring also to see that these traditional nursing practices are experiencing a revival, being reintroduced under the more appropriate name 'patient comfort rounds' (PCRs) (Castledine, 2002)—a term that conveys a more individualized approach to the care delivered.

While the use of the term 'round' indicates a task-orientated model, rather than a patient-centred one, all of the care offered will be identified in the patient's care plans. The patient is asked about their needs at given periods of the day and these needs are then responded to by the nurses responsible for that patient's care. Much of the care being carried out is as it was in previous years. Patients are offered the opportunity to go to the toilet if they are able or to have catheters checked. The emphasis today is less on commodes and more on preserving the patient's dignity by taking them to the privacy of the toilet, because most wards today have better facilities. Bedbound patients are offered drinks as allowed in their care plans and are encouraged to change their position in bed to avoid developing pressure sores. Those patients unable to do this for themselves are repositioned by the nursing team and the opportunity to visualize pressure areas is taken.

Depending on the time of day, the care will vary as relevant (see Table 9.2 below). It must be stressed that this timetable for PCRs looks, at first glance, to be very mechanistic and ritualistic in nature. However, this is not the purpose behind the introduction of PCRs.

Castledine (2002) provides a list of at least 12 positive benefits for patients when these rounds are implemented with thought and regularity, such as opportunities for:

- discussions with patients or significant others about nursing or caring intervention;
- attention to cleanliness;
- updating records;
- enquiring about pain control and privacy;
- observing the patient's condition;
- environment checks; and
- encouraging and documenting fluid intake.

In today's busy climate, a lot of these practices have been fragmented and devolved within a team of practitioners. The net result is that older people may feel isolated because they feel that nursing staff are too busy to be bothered or approached. The introduction of PCRs may therefore reduce these feelings of isolation, and help to develop the sense of care and caring that has been eroded within the healthcare environment.

Key responsibilities/skills of the nurse

● *Reflection point*

Earlier, you were asked to reflect upon the skills and qualities required to provide compassionate and dignified care for older people. We would like now to develop this a little further and ask you to reflect upon the contents of Table 9.3.

Table 9.2 Organization of patient comfort rounds (PCRs)

Shift	Time	Example of care delivered
Night staff	06:00	Introduce self and enquire about how the older person is feeling and how they slept. Offer toileting and hand washing, and ask whether they would like to sit up in bed or chair. Give choice of morning drink.
Early	Mid-morning	Offer assistance or full support with personal hygiene needs—offer washes/shower or bath, again enquiring whether they would like to sit out of bed. Perhaps provide a drink, or ensure water jug and glass are at hand. Use of communication skills—providing the patient with time and presence, a feeling of being cared for.
Early	11:00	Toileting and hand washing Offer drink
Early	After lunch	Toileting and hand washing Offer a rest on bed and a drink
Late	Mid-afternoon 16:00	Toileting and hand washing Offer to sit out for meal/drink
Late	After supper 18:00–20:00	Toileting and hand washing Offer to wash and return to bed with a drink
Night staff	Pre-bedtime 22:00	Toileting and hand washing Offer drink
Night staff	Mid-night-time 01:00–04:00	Toileting and hand washing Offer drink and reposition as required

Table 9.3 Areas of responsibility

Communication	Listen to and facilitate positive communication with the older person. Avoid being patronizing and be courteous at all times.
Eating and drinking	Give the older person choice about food. Offer appropriate and sensitive assistance with eating and drinking if required.
Autonomy	Involve the older person in decisions about their care and treatment.
Pain	Ensure timely and appropriate intervention for pain or discomfort. Allow the older person to be responsible for their own pain relief, should this be desired. Avoid practices that may cause or contribute to discomfort or pain.
Personal hygiene	Offer and provide timely assistance as required. Maximize choice and independence. Ensure facilities are clean and suitable.
Privacy	Ensure that the older person's privacy is maintained at all times, especially when using wash or toilet facilities. Obtain consent for all care and examinations, and permission for students to be in attendance. Hospitals and wards should comply with all national directives regarding single-sexed accommodation.
Social inclusion	Older people should be able to practise and maintain their own personal, religious, and spiritual beliefs. Nurses should value the older person, ensuring that there is no age discrimination. Contact and access should be maintained with family, friends, and community, if requested.
Safety	Nurses must undertake a thorough individualized assessment of each older person, identifying potential environmental or personal risks, including assessments for falls, use of bed rails, mobility, pressure area care, nutrition support, and necessary documentation completed. Where required, refer to the protection of vulnerable adult team suspected cases of elder abuse or neglect. Nursing staff must comply with all infection and prevention control measures.

Table 9.3 *(Continued)* Areas of responsibility

End-of-life care	There needs to be openness on the part of nurses and other healthcare professionals to discuss and support older people with decisions that they may have made with regards their own death. Consideration must be given to advance directives and 'living wills'. Nurses must be culturally sensitive to religious or spiritual needs, and have awareness of how these may impact upon attitudes to death and care of the person following death. Provision must be made to discuss personal wishes and preferences about end-of-life care.

The areas of nursing responsibility illustrated in Table 9.3 are recurrent themes in a number of the reports to which we have referred in this chapter (Magee et al. 2008; HCC, 2009; The Patients Association, 2009). They are therefore considered to be essential components of the nursing care provided to older people.

Student activity

Having reflected upon the key responsibilities in Table 9.3, consider the following questions.

- What does each of these responsibilities mean to you?
- How might you incorporate these in your practice when caring for older people in your care?

Arguably, all of these key responsibilities are fundamental when caring for older people in hospital—and indeed any—care settings. However, we would now like to focus upon the first three responsibilities, exploring the implications of these when providing care for older people. The other key responsibilities are addressed within earlier or subsequent chapters.

See Chapter 2 on privacy and dignity, Chapter 13 on nutrition and fluids, Chapter 16 on pain management, and Chapter 18 on end-of-life care.

Importance of communication

The importance of communication cannot be stressed enough. Often, key information can be gleaned through general conversation with the patient whilst delivering other elements of care, such as washing, dressing, feeding, or helping with moving and transferring. This highlights the need for the nurses to be interacting with the patients in their care whilst caring and not being distracted by colleagues. A patient's ability and often decreasing level of independence can be assessed by eliciting information about where the patient lives, whether they are alone or have a carer, whether they do their own shopping, drive, and attend day care, or whether they are completely independent and managed all of their affairs without any difficulties prior to admission.

Sometimes, the reason for admission to hospital is so catastrophic to an individual that it is immediately evident that the patient will require a change to their home circumstances on discharge. Although this is classed as a 'complex discharge', it is, in some respects, more straightforward to deal with, because it is usually obvious to the patient, family, and multidisciplinary team (MDT) that the change has to be made. The more difficult discharges to plan and coordinate are those cases in which the patient has deterioration in independence level that requires the input of carers and equipment to achieve a safe discharge.

Reflection point

At this point, it might be useful to reflect upon the case study relating to Charles' admission and identify what safeguards would need to be put in place to facilitate his safe discharge home.

Nutritional support

An important aspect of nursing care of older people is ensuring that their nutritional needs are assessed and supported (Magee et al., 2008; Heath and Sturdy, 2009). There is a wealth of research that indicates the health benefits of good nutrition. Therefore, nutritional support must be a priority when caring for older people. This is because some older people's nutritional status may be compromised through disease and disability. Sadly, evidence is still emerging that older people are developing malnutrition during their hospitalization (Age Concern, 2006). Developing malnutrition or going 'hungry in hospital' is not acceptable, because this is constitutes a form of institutional abuse. Therefore, nurses must introduce some system for assessing and alerting staff to the signs that an older person is at risk of developing malnutrition, or that they require assistance with eating and drinking.

Different strategies are being used, such as the 'red tray system', which notifies staff that a particular patient will need to be assisted and observed (Age Concern, 2006). Other strategies might include the use of non-obtrusive 'knife and fork' symbols placed in a visible point in the patient's bed area. Meal times need to be protected and any disturbances kept to a minimum, which will offer patients dedicated time in which to enjoy meals, and release staff to assist and observe.

See Chapter 13 on nutrition and fluids.

Preserving independence, individuality, and autonomy

Caring for older people is about offering support and encouragement, with the goal of preserving independence, individuality, and autonomy. One strategy that may help in this quest is never to lose sight of the fact that each older person has a life history—that is, a personal narrative or biography—with a wealth of experience and knowledge. It is easy to forget this in our fast-paced technological and medically focused caring environment.

On a cautionary note, there is also growing evidence that older people are less likely to complain about or criticize the care that they receive (HCC, 2007). Hospitals will need to be more proactive in seeking out older people's perceptions of the care received and delivered. It is imperative that all hospitals have older people represented on boards and forums, so that they have a voice and mechanism to present their concerns. Information detailing the role of the Patient Advisory Liaison Service (PALS) should be available in all hospitals. Staff at all levels should be supporting patients to access this service without fear of incrimination. These strategies will enable older people to feel empowered and more comfortable to raise any concerns that they may have about their hospital care.

In many hospitals, there is a dedicated team of healthcare professionals and a modern matron, or consultant nurse or therapist, whose sole responsibility is to champion and advocate for the rights of older people whilst receiving hospital care. In addition, hospitals are developing the role of the Protection of Vulnerable Adults (PoVA) lead, which is particularly important when issues of capacity are raised—for example, in older people with dementia or older people with learning disabilities.

See Chapter 2 on privacy, dignity, and adult protection.

Reflection point

- Evaluate your own attitudes to ageing and older people.
- Sign up to the Department of Health's Dignity Champion Programme online at http://www.dhcarenetworks.org.uk/dignityincare/index.cfm.
- Become an advocate for older people in your area.
- Challenge stereotypical attitudes to ageing and the older person.
- Always treat older people with respect and courtesy, and foster positive attitudes towards their care.

A skilled workforce

It would be a grave mistake to assume that nursing older people in hospital is no different from nursing any other client group. Yet older people should be afforded the same level of expertise and caring as any other group. We, therefore cannot discriminate and suggest that one group of patients is more deserving than another. However, the reasons why we have different specialities or wards is so that individual practitioners can develop their knowledge and expertise in a specific area. This principle applies to caring for older people. The NSFOP emphasizes that older people should be cared for by an experienced team of healthcare professionals with specialist knowledge and skills in gerontology, or gerontological nursing.

Kelly et al. (2005:16) define 'gerontological nursing' as:

A person centred approach to promoting healthy ageing and the achievement of wellbeing, enabling the person and their carers to adapt to health and life changes to face ongoing challenges.

This definition highlights that gerontological nursing requires specialist knowledge of the normal ageing process and the factors that may lead to a deviation from the norm. Consequently, in order that nurses can care for older people effectively within the hospital environment, there should be sufficient resources and a good skill mix among staff. This will necessitate excellent leadership and innovative practice.

Caring for older people is demanding and challenging, but ultimately rewarding. Anyone working within this speciality must reflect upon their own attitudes, values, and prejudices towards ageing and older people. Nursing older people requires empathy, compassion, and sensitivity, along with the ability to look beyond the medical diagnosis to the bigger picture.

Discharge planning

In 2001, the Department of Health committed itself to ensuring that, by 2004, every patient has a discharge plan developed from the start of their hospital admission. Planning for discharge at the point of admission is believed to be in the patient's, or older person's, best interest. Indeed, some would say that it should commence prior to admission and few would dispute the benefits. However, in practical terms, when an older person is admitted unwell, it is not usually identified as a priority to question them, their relatives, or their carers on discharge plans.

Patients, relatives, and carers have expectations in relation to a patient's discharge from hospital, including relating to factors such as being safe, and having the correct medications and discharge paperwork for any ongoing care. This care might involve the GP, community nurses, physiotherapists, occupational therapists, or anyone else in the MDT. The patient—or, more frequently, the relative or carer—has even more expectations with regard to choice of destination, and time of day and mode of transport with which they will leave hospital.

From the professional's perspective—that is, the perspective of the MDT—it is necessary to concur with the safe discharge elements and work to achieve this through regular MDT meetings or progress meetings. Such meetings would lead to the identification of any obstacles to early discharge or enable interventions to be implemented to prevent any delays. Although the MDT recognizes the importance of patient choice and aims to achieve this wherever possible, it has to be acknowledged that, sometimes, the requests and expectations of the patient and family maybe unrealistic, and may impact the service and operational ability of the organization, such as reduced bed availability.

Interface between health and social care sectors

A major consideration in the discharge of any older person from hospital is their destination—whether this is home, or intermediate or long-term care. The interface between acute and community/social sectors is pivotal in this process. Delays in discharge may arise because of a lack of capacity in these sectors, causing knock-on effects for the older person who, despite being medically well, remains in an acute hospital environment and faces the associated risks for an unnecessary period of time (NAO, 2003). These issues can be avoided by early planning, close communication with the discharge liaison team, and the appropriate involvement of the MDT, in consultation with the patient and primary carers.

Conclusion

This chapter suggests that most nurses working within a hospital environment will be caring for older people. Older people over the age of 65 are the primary recipients of hospital care. The chapter encourages anyone caring for older people to evaluate their own attitudes to ageing, so that the care that they provide is non-discriminatory. This chapter urges all caring for this vulnerable group to evaluate both traditional and contemporary practices, with a view to improving the organization and delivery of care.

The chapter is not revolutionary: it offers nothing new or innovative; rather, it simply encourages everyone to utilize the tools and skills already at their disposal. It advocates revisiting and reclaiming the fundamental aspects of care that seem to have been eroded and misplaced when caring for older people, such as courtesy, respect, and treating all older people as individuals in a dignified way.

Questions and self-assessment

Now that you have worked through the chapter, answer the following questions.

- From national surveys and reports, what have older people said about the care that they have received whilst in hospital?
- How is care organized and delivered to older people while in hospital?
- Identify the steps involved in discharging the older person from hospital.
- What key principles should underpin the care of older people in hospital?

Self-assessment

- Having read the chapter, how will you change your practice?
- Identify up to three areas relating to hospital care of the older adult in which you need to develop your knowledge and understanding further.
- Identify how you are going to develop this knowledge and understanding, and set deadlines for achieving this.

References

Acute Coordination Centre for the NHS Patient Survey Programme (2008) *The Key Findings Report From the 2008 Inpatient Survey*, available online at http://www.nhssurveys.org/Filestore//documents/Key_Findings_report_for_the_2008__Inpatient_Survey.pdf.

Age Concern (2006) *Hungry to be Heard: The Scandal of Malnourished Older People in Hospital*, London: Age Concern.

Castledine, G. (2002) 'Patient comfort rounds: A new initiative in nursing', *British Journal of Nursing*, 11(6): 407.

Castledine, G. (2005) 'Older people in acute hospitals need more care', *British Journal of Nursing*, 14(6): 351.

Cheek, J. and Gibson, T. (2003) 'Issues impacting on registered nurses providing care to older people in acute care setting', *Nursing Times Research*, 8(2): 134–49.

Chinn, M. and Spink, W. (2007) *Older People in the United Kingdom: Key Facts and Statistics 2007*, London: Age Concern Policy Unit.

Department of Health (2001) *National Service Framework for Older People*, London: DH.

Department of Health (2006a) *Dignity Challenge: High-quality Care Services that Respect People's Dignity*, London: DH.

Department of Health (2006b) *Dignity in Care: A Report on People's Views—What You Had to Say*, London: DH.

Department of Health (2006c) *Dignity in Care: Public Survey October 2006*, London: DH.

Department of Health (2008) *Health and Care Services for Older People: Overview Report on Research to Support the National Service Framework for Older People*, London: DH.

Department of Health (2009a) *Care and Compassion in the 21st Century*, Speech by the Rt Hon. Alan Johnson MP, Secretary of State for Health, NHS Chairs Conference, 28 January 2009, London: DH, available online at http://www.dh.gov.uk/en/News/Speeches/DH_093869.

Department of Health (2009b) *Dignity Map*, London: DH, available online at http://www.dhcarenetworks.org.uk/dignityincare/Topics/championresources/Dignity_Map/.

Health Care Commission (2006) *Living Well in Later Life: A Review of Progress against the National Service Framework for Older People*, London: Commission for Healthcare Audit and Inspection.

Health Care Commission (2007) *Caring for Dignity: A National Report on Dignity in Care for Older People While in Hospital*, London: Commission for Healthcare Audit and Inspection.

Health Care Commission (2009) *Investigation into Mid Staffordshire Foundation Trust*, London: Commission for Healthcare Audit and Inspection.

Heath, H. and Sturdy, D. (2009) *Nutrition and Older People*, London: RCN Publishing.

Hindle, A. (2008) Champions for Older People Programme', *Ageing & Health* [Journal of the Institute of Ageing and Health West Midlands], 16: 20–3.

Hweidi, I.M. and Al-Hassan, M.A.A. (2005) 'Jordanian nurses' attitudes towards older people in acute care setting', *International Nursing Review*, 22: 225–32.

Jones, J. (2005) 'Nursing older people in the acute care system: A clash of cultures or a time for nursing innovation?', *Australian Journal of Advanced Nursing*, 23(2): 4–5.

Kelly, T.B., Tolson, D., Schofield, L., and Booth, J. (2005) 'Describing gerontological nursing: An academic exercise or prerequisite for progress?', *International Journal of Older People Nursing*, in association with *Journal of Clinical Nursing*, 14(3a): 13–23.

Kratz, C.R. (1979) *The Nursing Process*, London: Baillière Tindall

Maben, J. and Griffiths, P. (2008) *Nurses in Society: Starting the Debate*, London: King's College London National Nursing Research Unit.

Magee, H., Parsons, S., and Askham, J. (2008) *Measuring Dignity in Care for Older People*, London: Picker Institute Europe for Help the Aged.

Narain, J. (2009) 'An Alzheimer's patient lies in a grubby hospital bathroom because of a shortage of beds: Will the elderly EVER be treated with dignity in Britain?', *Mail Online*, 14 January, available online at http://www.dailymail.co.uk/news/article-1114064/An-affront-human-dignity-Alzheimers-patient-left-grubby-hospital-bathroom-shortage-beds.html.

National Audit Office (2003) *Ensuring the Effective Discharge of Older Patients from NHS Acute Hospitals*, London: HMSO.

National Audit Office (2007) *Improving Services and Support for People with Dementia*, London: HMSO.

National Statistics (2010) *Ageing: Fastest Increase in the 'Oldest Old'*, available online at http://www.statistics.gov.uk/cci/nugget.asp?id=949.

Nursing and Midwifery Council (2007) *Essential Skills Clusters (Escs) for Pre-registration Nursing Programmes*, NMC Circular 07/2007, London: NMC.

Nursing and Midwifery Council (2009) *Guidance for the Care of Older People*, London: NMC.

Patients Association, The (2009), *Patients... Not Numbers, People... Not Statistics*, available online at http://www.patients-association.com/DBIMGS/file/Patients per cent20not per cent20numbers, per cent20people per cent20not per cent20statistics(1).pdf.

Rayner, C. (2009) 'Foreword', in The Patients Association, *Patients... Not Numbers, People... Not Statistics*, available online at http://www.patients-association.com/DBIMGS/file/Patients per cent20not per cent20numbers, per cent20people per cent20not per cent20statistics(1).pdf.

Royal College of Nursing (2008) *Defending Dignity Challenge and Opportunities for Nursing Royal College of Nursing*, London: RCN.

Sand, P.L., Wang, Y., McCabe, P.G., Jennings, K., Eng, C., and Covinsky, K.E. (2006) 'Rates of acute care admissions for frail older people living with met versus unmet activity of daily living needs', *Journal of American Geriatric Society*, 54: 339–44.

Online Resource Centre

You can learn more about hospital care for older people at the Online Resource Centre that accompanies this book: **http://www.oxfordtextbooks.co.uk/orc/hindle/**.

Part 4

Changes in the ageing process

Key medical disorders of older adults

Dr Jen Benbow and Professor Susan Mary Benbow

Learning outcomes

By the end of this chapter, you will be able to:

- understand the physiological changes associated with ageing and the psychosocial impact of long-term illness;
- understand some of the key health conditions commonly affecting the lives of older people, including the basic principles of diagnosis and management;
- understand the multiple roles that nurses can play in the assessment and management of patients with both acute and chronic medical problems;
- recognize the importance of listening to the individual's narrative in the formulation of their nursing care plan;
- identify ways of helping patients to manage their own health and to make their own treatment decisions, including some frameworks for holistic assessment of the older person;
- understand the complex interactions between the individual and their co-morbidities, medical therapy, and social environment; and
- recognize the importance of team working and how it benefits patient care.

Introduction

As we get older, we are more likely to develop health problems. Population estimates of the overall prevalence of chronic disease in older people differ due to the different methods used to collect data. A cross-sectional survey of community-dwelling adults aged over 65 found a 61.8 per cent incidence of self-reported long-standing illness (Ayis et al., 2003). A study in Ireland using pharmacy claims data found that 86 per cent of elderly people take three or more medications for chronic diseases (Naughton et al., 2006). Almost two-thirds of hospital beds in the UK are used by the over-65 age group (DH, 2001).

The increasing number of older people—particularly the very old—in society presents challenges for healthcare providers. In the future, there will be more people with multiple medical conditions and more taking a variety of different medications, with varying degrees of associated disability. We aim to show in this chapter how caring for these people can be complex, but that making a difference in older people's lives is also extremely rewarding.

People involved in caring for older people with medical problems have a responsibility to promote 'active ageing' (WHO, 2002). The word 'active' refers to continuing participation in all areas of life. People who suffer illness or disability can continue to be active in their contribution to their families, peers, communities, and nations. Medical problems need to be seen in context—that is, in terms of how they affect the individual, their family, and their life. Everyone is different, including in how they perceive 'health', and how they deal with and understand 'ill health'. The roles that people fulfil (for example, as parents, grandparents, friends, and neighbours) and their active participation are important in maintaining quality of life, whether or not they are living with illness or disability (ODPM, 2006). A common view of population ageing is that it will place an unprecedented demand on social and healthcare systems that will need to be paid for by a decreasing number of working-age people. This would place a significant brake on the economic development of all countries. There is nothing inevitable about this view of the future. If older people can remain healthy and if they live in an 'age-friendly' environment, there is no reason why they cannot continue to make a positive contribution until the very last years of life. There is already evidence from developed countries that older people today are healthier than previous generations, and that they want to remain socially engaged and productive (WHO, 2010).

This chapter is a summary of some of the major health conditions affecting older people—that is:

- diabetes;
- Parkinson's disease (PD);
- stroke;
- ischaemic heart disease (IHD);
- chronic heart failure (CHF);
- atrial fibrillation (AF);
- leg ulcers;
- chronic obstructive pulmonary disease (COPD);
- community-acquired pneumonia (CAP); and
- arthritis.

A brief summary of the diagnosis and nursing management of each condition is provided, and in areas in which a greater depth of knowledge may be required, the references offer a guide to finding more detailed sources of information.

Notable by their absence are some very important topics, including delirium and dementia, osteoporosis, falls and hip fractures, urinary tract infections, and constipation, all of which are covered in other chapters.

See Chapter 6 for more on falls, Chapter 11 for more on dementia, and Chapter 14 for more on elimination and incontinence.

Reflection point

As you read on, think about ways in which, as a nurse, you could promote 'active ageing' in a person with that particular condition.

What barriers does that condition pose and what would help the patient to overcome them?

Physiological changes of ageing

Figure 10.1 illustrates the physiological effects of ageing on the body.

Psychosocial aspects of chronic illness

In this chapter, we concentrate on physical illness and older adults. It is always essential to assess and treat illness in the context of an individual's life, and this means routinely considering the psychological and social aspects of every physical illness. Different people will have different priorities in managing their illness and will make different treatment decisions; the role of healthcare staff is to give them the information that they need, and to support them in finding the best way forward in their own unique and often complex circumstances—bearing in mind the options available to them and the evidence about how their illness might be managed.

The changes associated with ageing can impact on a person's concept of self: for example, changes in physical appearance due to increasing age can be particularly difficult for those who take a pride in their appearance, and therefore may affect their self-esteem and influence social aspects of their life. This, in turn, may affect mental health—for example, by precipitating anxiety or a depressive illness. Chronic illness has a major impact on all aspects of an individual's life and how people cope with this impact will depend on a range of factors, including their personality, what social/ family support they can draw on, their financial and living circumstances, and their ethnicity and religious faith. Since older adults may have age-related changes compounded by chronic illness and the social disadvantages associated with ageing, they are particularly at risk.

Chronic illness is known to be associated with reduced quality of life for many people, regardless of age. It is also a risk factor for depressive illness. The Social Exclusion Unit Report entitled *A Sure Start to Later Life* (ODPM, 2006) argues that increasing age is associated with exclusion from social relationships, service provision, and material consumption. Since 70 per cent of people aged over 65 report a long-standing illness (ODPM, 2006) and older people who perceive their health as poor are more likely to report a low quality of life, this suggests that older adults with physical health problems are at risk of multiple disadvantages.

There is a growing literature on the patient journey, which aims to study and learn from people's experiences with illness. Baker and Graham (2004) wrote poignantly about the 'long journey into the unknown' with Parkinson's disease. Simpson et al. (2005) wrote about rheumatoid arthritis and its impact. Dartington (2008) wrote about his wife's journey to death from dementia. Papers like these highlight the differing priorities of professionals and families, and the many ways in which chronic illnesses change people's lives. Simpson et al. (2005: 889) also illustrate the role of a nurse specialist in developing a relationship of trust and continuity, which includes '*a nurturing relationship with patients, offering empathy, encouragement, emotional support and hope*'.

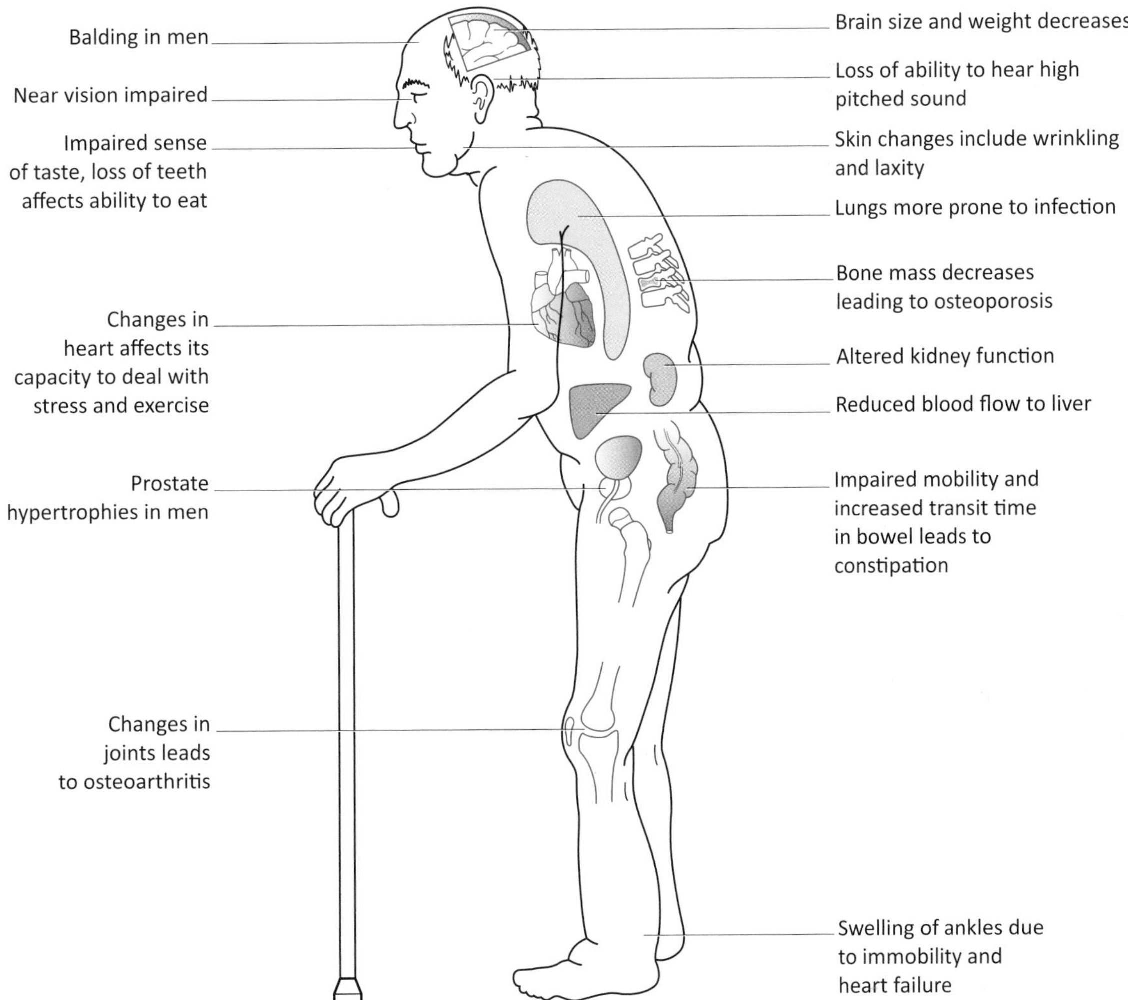

Figure 10.1 The physiological effects of ageing upon the body

This demonstrates how good relationships between patients and the professionals working with them (their travelling companions on the journey) go beyond the mechanics of care.

Maslow's hierarchy of needs

One useful framework for assessing the effects of illness is Maslow's 'hierarchy of needs' (Maslow, 1998), which is illustrated in Figure 10.2. This is presented as a pyramid, which has a broad base built of the physiological or bodily needs of life—that is, breathing, eating, drinking, excreting, sleeping, sexual expression, and maintaining homeostasis.

The next level up the pyramid (Level 2) can be described as 'safety', or 'security' needs; these address the security of the body, and include employment, resources, morality, the family, health, and property.

Above this, the third level is constructed of social, or 'love/belonging', needs—that is, friendship, family, and sexual intimacy—while the fourth level is 'esteem', or 'ego', needs, which include self-esteem/confidence/ achievement, plus respect of others and by others.

The pinnacle of Maslow's original pyramid (Level 5) is 'self-actualization'—that is, morality, creativity, spontaneity, problem-solving and acceptance.

Some people add 'spiritual needs' as an additional level at the tip of the pyramid.

The social role inventory

Another useful framework for considering the impact of an illness on a person's social life is the 'social role inventory' (O'Brien, 2006), which looks at:

- home and neighbourhood;
- family and friends (including sexual relationships);
- work;
- learning;

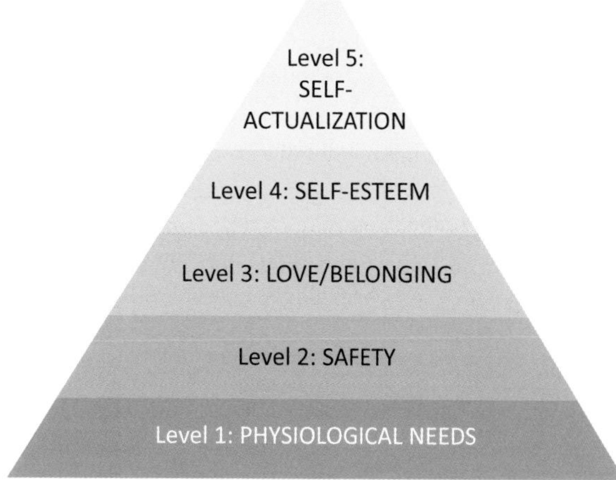

Figure 10.2 Maslow's hierarchy of needs
Source: Maslow (1943).

- spiritual and religious;
- citizenship;
- sports and fitness; and
- creative expression.

Assessing the impact of an illness on all of these areas of an individual's life may enable them to identify adverse impacts and to work out ways in which to function better—perhaps with support from family, friends, and/ or services.

The nurse also needs to consider the support, information, and contribution to quality of life that specific disease organizations can provide to individuals. They can also be a helpful reference point for the health professional. At the end of this chapter is a list of some of the key national websites. Nearly all of these will have local networks and support groups as well, so facilitating access can be very beneficial.

In this chapter, our focus is on the physical aspects of illness. In working with patients and families throughout a career in health care, we need to look more comprehensively at all aspects of their illnesses—that is, physical, mental, psychological, and social. Remember as you read this chapter that what is important to our patients and their families will not always be what we might expect.

> ***Student activity***
>
> Imagine that you are now aged 75. You have painful arthritis in a number of joints and are finding it difficult to get about even with a walking stick. Your eyesight is poor and your hearing is impaired.
>
> Reflect on the eight areas of the social role inventory.
>
> What do you think your priorities would be in each of these areas and how could you maintain your function?

Key endocrine conditions

The endocrine condition that you will come across most often in older people is diabetes. ('Endocrine' means that the condition is related to substances produced by glands within the body.)

Diabetes

What is diabetes?

Diabetes mellitus is one of the most common chronic medical conditions affecting older people. It is characterized by a raised level of glucose in the blood. Usually, when we eat food, the pancreas (a gland behind the stomach) releases insulin (the hormone that helps the body to use glucose efficiently) into the blood stream. This causes the glucose to move out of the blood (thereby decreasing the blood glucose level) and into cells, where it is broken down to produce energy.

There are two types of diabetes.

- **Type 1**—In this type of diabetes, the body is unable to produce any of its own insulin. People with this condition need to have regular injections of insulin to maintain control of the blood glucose level. It usually presents in young people.
- **Type 2**—In this type of diabetes, the body can still make some insulin, but not enough, or the insulin that it does produce does not work effectively (known as 'insulin resistance'). People with this condition do not always need insulin. Type 2 diabetes is more commonly seen in older people, so this will be the focus of this section (NCCCC, 2008c).

A normal fasting blood glucose level is between 4 and 6 mmol/l. A fasting blood glucose level of more than 7 mmol/l is diagnostic of diabetes.

Why is diabetes important?

It is important to treat diabetes in order to reduce complications that can dramatically reduce quality of life. There are microvascular complications (that is, involving *small* blood vessels), which include retinopathy (damage to the retina of the eye), neuropathy (damage to the nerves), or nephropathy (damage to the kidneys). These can have serious consequences including blindness, painful or numb hands and feet, foot ulcers, and kidney failure.

There are also macrovascular complications (that is, involving *large* blood vessels), such as peripheral vascular disease, strokes, and heart attacks.

Treatment of diabetes

A useful way of remembering the basic principles of diabetes management is to use the 'alphabet model' (Patel and

Morrissey, 2002). This can be a useful aide-memoire for patients and healthcare professionals alike.

A **Advice**—Advice should be provided about diet, exercise, weight loss, smoking cessation, and medication compliance.

B **Blood pressure**—The usual target blood pressure is 140/80 mmhg or lower. The target for those with kidney involvement is 125/75 mmhg.

C **Cholesterol**—The usual target is a total cholesterol of less than 5 mmol/l.

D **Diabetes control**—Large studies have shown that tight control of blood glucose levels is crucial in reducing complications (Diabetes Control and Complications Trial Research Group, 1993). HbA1c (glycosylated haemoglobin) should be checked every six months in stable patients.

NOTE: The HbA1c blood test is a measure of the amount of glycated haemoglobin in the blood. This gives a measure of the average blood sugar over the preceeding 8–12 weeks. In patients with high blood sugars, the quantity of glycated haemoglobin will be higher.

E **Eye screening**—Retinal screening should be performed annually.

F **Foot screening**—Feet should be formally checked annually, but patients should monitor themselves more regularly.

G **Guardian drugs**—Aspirin and some other medications are recommended for particular patients at greater risk of complications—for example, smokers.

Insulin and most oral hypoglycaemics should be given with meals. If not, they may cause the blood glucose to drop too low. This can be a problem when patients are admitted to hospital, because the amount of food and timing of meals may be different from their usual.

Diabetes care has changed considerably in recent years and has become much more nurse-led, with both diabetes specialist nurses, and community and practice nurses, playing central roles. The key to effective diabetes care is good communication and collaboration with the patient themselves, as well as effective coordination with other healthcare professionals involved. Diabetes care is truly multidisciplinary: potentially, dieticians, podiatrists, optometrist, ophthalmologists, physicians, general practitioners (GPs), and pharmacists are all involved. People make a big contribution towards their own care and may need encouragement to continue. Many older people with diabetes will have been managing themselves for years and will need little input. However, others may need significant involvement from nurses in particular. The goal is to empower the patient with the necessary knowledge, skills, and attitudes to lead a healthy life with diabetes. Where possible, encourage patients to check their own blood glucose levels (which is easily done with a simple finger-prick test) and to administer their own insulin. Studies have shown that nurse-led interventions, such as specialist nurse clinics, can improve outcomes in diabetes care (Davidson, 2003).

Issues particular to older people

Attempts to achieve tight blood glucose control can increase the risk of hypoglycaemia (the blood glucose going too low), which can contribute to confusion and falls, and affect quality of life. Older people are thought to be more at risk of hypoglycaemia and may be less likely to recognize the symptoms.

Signs and symptoms of hypoglycaemia include:

- confusion;
- sweating;
- hunger;
- tremor;
- weakness;
- fits;
- drowsiness; and
- falls.

In order to avoid hypoglycaemia, a more relaxed approach to blood glucose control is often preferred in older people (Mayes, 2000) with significant co-morbidities: the European Diabetes Working Party for Older People (2004) suggests a target fasting blood sugar of 5.0–7.0 mmol/l, or HbA1c of 6.5–7.5 per cent for older patients without significant co-morbidity. For frailer patients—particularly those with multisystem disease, care home residents, and those with dementia—targets should be a fasting blood sugar of 7.0–9.0 mmol/l, or HbA1c of 7.5–≤8.5 per cent. However, specific goals should be tailored to the individual and, in a fit, healthy older person with a reasonable life expectancy, aiming for tight control may still be appropriate to reduce the risk of complications (Benjamin, 2002).

NURSING PRACTICE INSIGHT: TREATING HYPOGLYCAEMIA

1. **If the patient is awake:**
   (a) **immediately give a sugary/glucose drink, such as Lucozade or milk (which will act quickly to bring up the glucose level, but will wear off quickly); and**
   (b) **follow this up with a long-acting carbohydrate such as toast, a sandwich, or plain biscuits.**
2. **If the patient cannot be woken, this is an emergency. Call for help immediately.**

Cognitive impairment and physical disability may affect a person's ability to check their own blood glucose, to take medication, or to administer insulin. They may be less likely to comply with lifestyle measures and may not recognize symptoms of hypoglycaemia. Some 10 per cent of patients living in care homes have diabetes (Bracewell et al., 2005). Many of these people will be dependent on carers for monitoring and medication, as well as for attending annual reviews, etc.

> **Student activity**
>
> During a placement in a nursing home, you meet a 92-year-old woman who has diabetes. She is also poorly mobile (because of arthritis) and forgetful. She is on a number of tablets for high blood pressure, heart problems, and arthritis, as well as oral hypoglycaemics. She has a large and loving family, who visit frequently and often bring her food as 'treats'. Her blood glucose is poorly controlled and the GP who saw her recently said that varying glucose levels were probably making her more confused.
>
> - What could you and the other staff in the nursing home do to help with this problem?
> - Which other services might be brought in to help this woman?

Key neurological conditions

Parkinson's disease and stroke are two key neurological conditions affecting older people.

Parkinson's disease

What is Parkinson's disease?

Parkinson's disease (PD) is one of the commonest neurological disorders affecting older people. It is a degenerative illness that gets more common with increasing age and affects:

- 1–2 per cent of people over the age of 65; and
- 5 per cent of people aged between 95 and 99 (De Rijk et al., 1995).

Parkinson's disease is caused by a progressive loss of nerve cells in the part of the brain known as the 'substantia nigra'. These cells are responsible for producing a chemical called 'dopamine', which influences areas of the brain that coordinate movement. With the loss of dopamine-producing cells, these parts of the brain are unable to function normally, causing the symptoms of PD.

There is no single reliable test with which to make the diagnosis of PD. The diagnosis is made based on the history with which the patient presents and typical examination findings. This can be particularly challenging in older people due to the common occurrence of co-morbidities, both physical and psychiatric—for example, sleep disturbance, fatigue, anxiety, and depression.

What are the symptoms of Parkinson's disease?

The main features of PD involve the motor (movement) system of the body and include:

- resting tremor—that is, shaking, or tremor, in a part of the body when it is not being used;
- rigidity—that is, stiff (or rigid) muscles, which can make everyday tasks uncomfortable or difficult; and/or
- bradykinesia—that is, a slowing of movement.

At first, the symptoms may be non-specific (Wilkinson and Lennox, 2005), but later on they can become more typical of PD, such as rest tremor, difficulty turning in bed, and a stooping, or shuffling, gait.

There are many other, non-motor, features of PD. Depression is very common, affecting about 30 per cent of people with PD (Slaughter et al., 2001; Veazey et al., 2005). Psychosis can occur—especially visual hallucinations. Dementia will develop in at least 50 per cent of people with PD: a Danish study found that 78 per cent of people with PD developed dementia over an eight-year period (Aarsland et al., 2003). Lewy body dementia is particularly associated with PD. Other features include urinary urgency, constipation, and erectile dysfunction. All of these symptoms can have a profound effect on a person's life and their ability to carry out activities of daily living.

See Chapter 11 for more on dementia, and Chapter 14 for more on elimination and continence.

> **Student activity**
>
> With the list of symptoms above in mind, can you imagine how this would affect your life? Write down the tasks that you might carry out on a typical day. Then reflect on which tasks you might find difficult if you were to have PD.
>
> - How might the disease affect your relationships with those close to you?
> - In what ways might these problems be overcome?

How is Parkinson's disease managed?

PD cannot be 'cured', but there are many treatments to help with symptoms and many services available to help to facilitate independent, active living (NCCCC, 2006b), including:

- patient education;
- PD nurse specialists (PDNSs);
- physiotherapy;

- occupational therapy;
- speech and language therapy;
- psychology/psychiatry;
- medications (for a good summary, see http://www.parkinsons.org.uk/), the two main groups of which are:
  - levodopa (in drugs such as Madopar or Sinemet)—a natural amino acid that the brain converts into dopamine, therefore replacing the missing chemical; and
  - other drugs that mimic the effects of dopamine on the brain (known as 'dopamine receptor agonists';
- surgical treatments, such as deep brain stimulation (only used if symptoms are not effectively treated with best medical treatment and other criteria are fulfilled); and
- palliative care, which should be provided at the end stage of PD.

PDNSs provide a range of specialist skills to people with the disease and their families, including education, support and advice, symptoms management, medicines management and assessment, and management of complications. Research has shown that provision of a specialist nursing service improves patients' sense of well-being with no increase in healthcare costs, and is valued by patients and families alike (Reynolds et al., 2000: Jarman et al., 2002).

Some patients will be on complex medication regimes that are reliant on medications administration at specific times. This is a particular area in which the role of the PDNS can be invaluable in educating individuals of the importance of medication timing and providing advice regarding strategies to facilitate this. Admission to hospital or a care home can often precipitate problems, because these facilities usually have set times for medication rounds. Anticipation of this can be a major source of stress for the individuals and their families or carers. Guidelines suggest that patients should have their medications at the appropriate time and that, in some cases, they should be permitted to self-administer (NCCCC, 2006b). Nursing staff should facilitate this. The perspective of the individual and their carer, where appropriate, should be sought and respected, because they may have been successfully managing their PD in the community for some time.

Sudden changes in PD medications can have serious consequences to the individual—particularly those with more advanced disease. PD medications should be adjusted only by, or after discussion with, a specialist in the management of PD (NCCCC, 2006b). Abrupt withdrawal of PD medications can be dangerous and should be avoided. In situations in which the patient cannot take their usual medications orally or is unlikely to be absorbing them—for example, in cases of gastroenteritis—this should be discussed with a specialist and alternative means of administration considered. The PDNS can play a central role in educating and supporting other healthcare staff in this respect.

See Chapter 7 on medication management.

Stroke

What is stroke?

A stroke is a brain injury caused by a sudden interruption of blood flow. Without blood flow, the brain cells become damaged or destroyed. Figure 10.3 shows how the fluid-filled spaces in the brain become larger to compensate for the loss of brain tissue following a stroke. The area of the brain in which the damage has occurred defines the pattern of symptoms experienced by the patient.

Stroke is the third commonest cause of death and the commonest cause of severe disability worldwide. The incidence of stroke increases with age, with 80 per cent of all events occurring in those over the age of 65 and 54 per cent in those over the age of 75 (Rothwell et al., 2005). Outcomes of stroke, including mortality rates, are worse in older people.

There are two types of stroke.

- **Ischaemic**—This is by far the commonest type, accounting for 85 per cent of strokes. It is caused by blockage of a blood vessel reducing blood flow to the area of brain supplied by that vessel.
- **Haemorrhagic**—This type of stroke is relatively uncommon, found only in 15 per cent of strokes. It is caused by a bleed into the tissue of the brain, usually because of a small ruptured aneurysm.

You may have heard the term 'mini-stroke'. This term is often used by laypeople to mean a transient ischaemic attack (TIA). A TIA presents as a stroke, but the interruption of blood supply is only transient, thus the symptoms resolve completely within 24 hours. In a stroke, symptoms persist longer than 24 hours and, in many cases, at least some element of *permanent* disability will result. It is, however, important to identify TIAs,

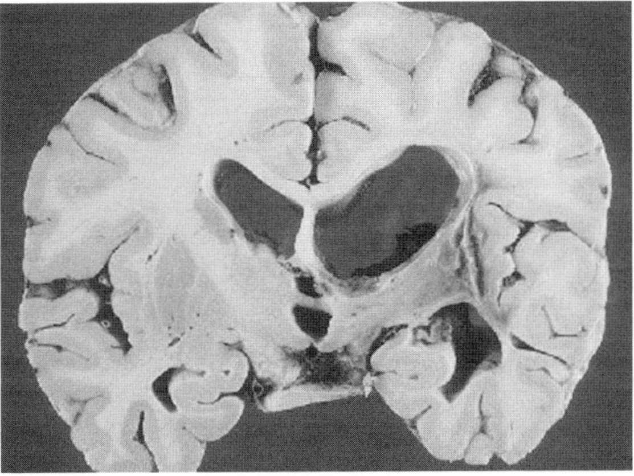

Figure 10.3 Photo showing how the fluid-filled spaces in the brain become larger following a stroke, which compensates for the loss of brain tissue
Source: By kind permission of the University of Manchester, Department of Pathology.

because they are a marker of risk for further cerebrovascular events (Coull et al., 2004).

The common symptoms caused by strokes include sudden onset of weakness (where this involves one side of the body, it is referred to as 'hemiparesis'), altered sensation, speech problems, swallowing difficulties, and visual problems.

NURSING PRACTICE INSIGHT: STROKES

The weakness experienced by the patient will be on the *opposite* side to that on which the stroke has occurred. This is because of the way in which the nerves connecting the limbs to the brain cross over in the spinal cord.

What is FAST?

The Stroke Association is campaigning to raise awareness of stroke and has been researching the use of 'FAST'—an acronym that paramedics use to facilitate the diagnosis of stroke in the community in order to speed up access to treatment and referral to a stroke unit, or accident and emergency (A&E).

FAST requires an assessment of three specific symptoms of stroke, as follows.

F **Facial weakness**—Can the person smile? Has their mouth or eye drooped?

A **Arm weakness**—Can the person raise both arms?

S **Speech problems**—Can the person speak clearly and understand what you say?

If the person has failed any one of these tests, it is:

T **Time to call 999**.

Stroke is a medical emergency, and by calling 999, you can help someone to reach hospital quickly and receive the early treatment that they need.

Further information can be found online at http://www.stroke.org.uk/campaigns/raising_awareness/act_fast.html

How can stroke be treated?

The treatment of people with stroke has advanced considerably in recent years. Key areas of treatment for ischaemic strokes are summarized below (NCCCC, 2008b); see also the *National Stroke Strategy* (DH, 2007).

1. Organization of stroke services
   - Patients with stroke should be cared for by a specially trained multidisciplinary team in a specialized stroke unit.
   - Caring for patients in a dedicated stroke unit can result in reduced rates of death, dependency, and need for institutional care (Langhorne et al., 1993).
   - Patients with TIA may not need hospital admission, but will need specialist assessment within 24 hours if they are at high risk of stroke, or one week if considered lower risk.
2. Assessment of acute stroke

   This involves:
   - imaging of the brain (usually a computed axial tomography, or CT, scan) within 24 hours of the event, or immediately if the patient fulfils certain criteria (see below);
   - an appropriately trained individual assessing the risk of aspiration and risk of malnutrition; and
   - assessing moving and handling needs, and the risk of developing pressure sores.
3. Acute interventions
   - Aspirin (300 mg) should be given as soon as possible after the acute stroke once a haemorrhage has been ruled out. Aspirin should also be given immediately to patients with suspected TIA who have a high risk of subsequent stroke.
   - 'Clot-busting' medication (thrombolysis) is sometimes given to appropriate patients within three hours of the onset of symptoms. Studies have shown that it is associated with reduced rates of death and dependency in the first three months (Wardlaw et al., 2003).
   - Normal blood glucose, arterial oxygen concentration, hydration, and temperature should be maintained.
   - To reduce the risk of disability or deformity, there needs to be careful limb positioning, and appropriate moving and handling. A full assessment is required prior to mobilization.
4. Rehabilitation

   This involves:
   - multidisciplinary team working, together with the patient, carer, and family using '*a shared philosophy and common goals*';
   - screening for depression and cognitive impairment;
   - physiotherapy, occupational therapy, and speech and language therapy assessments; and
   - monitoring nutrition, hydration, pressure areas, and bladder and bowel function.
5. Secondary prevention (to reduce the risk of further stroke)

   This involves:
   - lifestyle advice;
   - medications to treat high blood pressure and cholesterol; and
   - aspirin (or an alternative) for patients with ischaemic stroke or TIA.
6. Longer-term management

   This will involve encouraging independence.

Nursing roles are crucial in both the acute phase and more chronic phases of the treatment of stroke patients. In the acute situation, fast-tracking patients from A&E, rapid assessment for eligibility for thrombolysis, and appropriate monitoring should all either be instigated or coordinated by a specialist stroke nurse (Fitzpatrick and Birns, 2004).

Nursing stroke patients in the community involves educational activities (such as risk factor modification), participating in rehabilitation, assistance with various aids (for example, hoists), and coordination with social workers and healthcare professionals—in particular, occupational therapists, physiotherapists, and speech and language therapists.

Psychological support from nurses

In addition, nurses can play a key role in supporting the patient psychologically. Of all of the conditions in this chapter, stroke is the most acute cause of significant disability. Such a sudden change in physical ability, and loss of usual social roles and independence, can have a profound effect on the individual. They may no longer be able to live in their usual environment and their ability to communicate effectively may be impaired. This often has a significant impact on the lives of family members, who may suddenly be thrust into the role of carer. Rates of depression are high in both stroke patients and their carers (Pfeil et al., 2009). It is important that nurses are aware of this, and alert to the warning signs and symptoms. In addition, the nurse needs to provide support for families and carers, including carers' assessments.

See Chapter 5 for more on carers.

Key cardiovascular conditions

In the cardiovascular system, key conditions include ischaemic heart disease (IHD), chronic heart failure (CHF), and atrial fibrillation (AF).

Ischaemic heart disease

What is ischaemic heart disease?

Ischaemic heart disease (IHD) is caused by coronary artery atheroma—that is, plaques rich in cholesterol and other lipids (fats) on the inside walls of the blood vessels supplying the heart muscle (coronary arteries). These plaques obstruct blood flow to the heart muscle, thereby reducing the delivery of oxygen (see Figure 10.4). This can cause damage to—and even destruction of—the muscle cells (myocytes).

In practice, IHD manifests as two main clinical pictures, as follows.

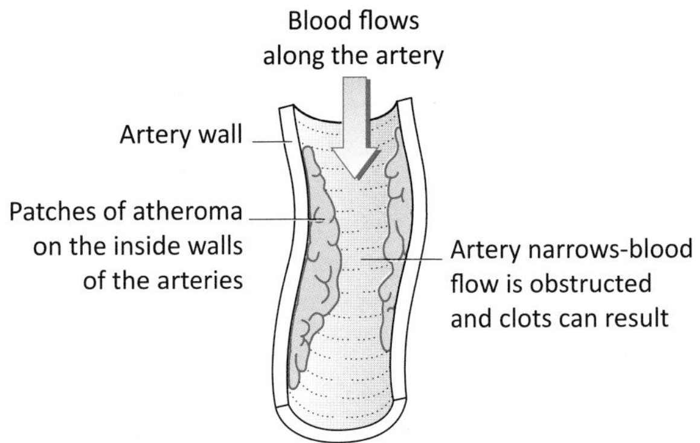

Figure 10.4 Coronary artery atheroma

1. **Angina pectoris**—usually known as 'angina'—is used to describe pain arising from the heart, usually when the blood supply to the heart muscle is temporarily compromised.
   - Usually, a heavy, crushing pain in the centre of the chest may 'radiate' down the left arm or up into the jaw.
   - Usually, angina comes on with exertion (may be as minimal as getting dressed) and goes away quite quickly with rest.
2. **Myocardial infarction (MI)**—often called a 'heart attack'—involves pain that is similar to that of angina, but more severe and lasts longer, and can happen at any time.
   - An initial sign, particularly for an older person, may be confusion.
   - Often, associated symptoms, such as sweatiness, nausea, vomiting, and shortness of breath, may present.
   - The person may look unwell, pale, clammy, and grey. They are often distressed and restless.

What are the risk factors for IHD?

There are many risk factors for IHD. Many of these are the same ones for stroke. They can be divided into two groups, as follows.

1. Intrinsic, **non-modifiable** risk factors
   - Increasing age
   - Gender—that is, it is overall more common in men, but in older people, the incidence is similar between genders
   - Family history
   - Ethnicity—that is, it is more common in people of Asian origin
2. **Modifiable** risk factors
   - Hyperlipidaemia
   - Smoking
   - Hypertension
   - Obesity
   - Diabetes
   - Physical inactivity

> ❖ ***Student activity***
>
> With these risk factors in mind, imagine that you are working on an acute admission ward. A 76-year-old man is admitted with an MI. He has recently remarried after being a widower for many years and is very worried about it happening again. He is overweight and has been a smoker since his 20s. Think about what he could do to try to cut down his risk for the future.
>
> - What advice would you give?
> - What services may be of benefit to him?

How is a myocardial infarction diagnosed and treated?

An MI can be diagnosed using electrocardiogram (ECG) tracings, which give an electrical printout of the heartbeat. Blood tests are used to help to confirm the diagnosis and to help to identify which patients are at the highest risk of having further problems.

The treatment given depends on the type of heart attack. All patients should be given 300 mg of aspirin immediately, as well as high-flow oxygen, where available. Other treatment may include analgesia (usually morphine) and medications, such as nitrates, to help to dilate the arteries to the heart.

In some cases, the patient may need to be taken immediately to a catheter laboratory for emergency unblocking of the particular artery/arteries involved. This treatment is now considered the best option to reduce the short-term and long-term complications of some forms of MI (Keely et al., 2003). In areas in which this is not available, or cannot be arranged quickly enough (usually within 90 minutes of symptom onset), 'clot-busting' medication (thrombolysis) may be given instead. The *National Service Framework for Coronary Heart Disease* (DH, 2000) set targets for administration of thrombolysis, which can be given up to 12 hours after the onset of symptoms, but is much more effective given within the first two hours. The key targets were that thrombolysis should be administered to all eligible patients within 60 minutes of calling for help (a 60-minute 'call-to-needle' goal) and that all patients should be treated within 30 minutes of arriving at hospital (the 'door-to-needle' time). Nurses play a pivotal role within the treating team in coordinating the rapid assessment and treatment of such patients.

How is ischaemic heart disease managed?

In managing IHD, there are two phases: acute management (as above); and long-term modification of risk factors to help to reduce the chance of future problems. This is achieved by taking various medications and through lifestyle advice, which should include:

- dietary advice;
- keeping alcohol consumption within recommended limits;
- increasing physical activity levels (ideally 20–30 minutes each day);
- smoking cessation; and
- weight reduction.

Most patients will have an angiogram to assess which arteries are blocked and how bad the blockage is. This will help to determine whether the measures mentioned above will be adequate on their own, or whether an angioplasty or coronary artery bypass graft (CABG) would be beneficial.

Issues particular to older people

Older people with IHD can have an MI without any chest pain. They may present without the usual symptoms—for example, with a fall or collapse, nausea, or confusion (Bayer et al., 1986). Therefore an MI must be considered in any acutely unwell older person. Painless MIs are also more frequently seen in people with diabetes.

NURSING PRACTICE INSIGHT: ISCHAEMIC HEART DISEASE

Because IHD can present without the usual symptoms, this diagnosis should at least be considered in any acutely unwell older person. Therefore, an ECG should be performed in all of these patients.

Lifestyle modifications may be more of a challenge for older people. In particular, other illnesses, such as arthritis or chronic obstructive pulmonary disease (COPD), may impact on ability to increase activity levels. Many medications for IHD cause complications and risks may be more pronounced in older people. For example, aspirin can cause gastrointestinal bleeding and antihypertensives may predispose patients to falls. These complications can occur in any patient, but will be more likely to occur in patients with other medical problems who are already taking multiple other medications, and so older people are at higher risk.

See Chapter 6 for more on falls and Chapter 7 for more on medication management.

Older age is a predictor of mortality in both acute and chronic IHD. Older people are more likely to benefit from so-called 'aggressive' interventions, such as CABG and angioplasty. One benefit of such interventions is the possible reduction in number, or dosage, of tablets that the individual needs to take. Nurses and other professionals caring for older people with IHD need to be strong advocates for their needs, and encourage evidence-based management.

Provision of information to the patient regarding treatment options is important, because they themselves may be reticent to accept more 'aggressive' forms of treatment due to lack of knowledge of the benefits and worries about adverse events.

Education and support for such patients, both in the acute and chronic stages of IHD, is a key role for nurses.

The British Heart Foundation provides helpful information on the different roles that nurses can play in caring for patients with IHD online at http://www.bhf.org.uk/.

Chronic heart failure

What is chronic heart failure?

Chronic heart failure (CHF) is a long-term condition that occurs when the heart does not pump enough blood around the body to meet its needs, usually because the heart muscle is damaged. The commonest reason for this is that the blood vessels supplying the heart are narrowed or blocked—that is, IHD.

Heart failure affects around 1 per cent of adults in their 50s. This figure rises to around 10 per cent of those in their 80s (Kannel and Belanger, 1991).

Typical symptoms of CHF are:

- getting short of breath either when exercising or at rest;
- ankle swelling;
- fatigue; and
- waking in the night gasping for breath or being unable to lie flat due to breathlessness.

People suspected of having CHF will have a chest X-ray and an ECG. An echocardiogram (echo) uses sound waves to show how the heart is pumping and to confirm the diagnosis of heart failure.

How is heart failure treated?

Treatment for CHF will include:

- Lifestyle changes to help the heart to pump more efficiently, including taking regular exercise, maybe attending a rehabilitation programme involving exercise, information and support, stopping smoking, attention to alcohol intake, and dietary advice (for example avoiding excessive salt intake).
- Helping people cope with their illness, for example, aids and equipment for the home.
- The usual drug treatments fall into three main groups
  - Diuretics (often called water tablets) reduce the amount of fluid in the body and help people breathe more easily.
  - ACEI (angiotensin converting enzyme inhibitors) help the heart to pump more blood and lower blood pressure.
  - Beta-blockers have been found to increase life expectancy for some people with CHF.
- Other drug treatments may include
  - Digoxin: a foxglove extract which improves the heart's pumping action
  - Nitrates which widen blood vessels to improve blood flow
- Surgical treatments are sometimes used, including:
  - Pacemakers which are implanted just under the skin and stimulate both sides of the heart to beat regularly and in synchrony with each other
  - Defibrillators which monitor the heart rhythm and can give it a small electrical shock if the rhythm becomes dangerously abnormal
  - Rarely specialist surgery might be considered
- Palliative care will be appropriate in the later stages.

(NCCCC, 2003).

Patient education (about the condition, its treatment, lifestyle advice, self-management, and monitoring), titration of medication dosage, and coordinating the involvement of other relevant professionals are key nursing skills. Studies have shown that such nursing interventions in the community can be effective in reducing admission to hospital in patients with heart failure (Blue et al., 2001).

Issues particular to older people

As with IHD, one of the commonest problems in older people is that they develop complications of their treatment. For example, the combination of diuretics and angiotensin converting enzyme inhibitors (ACEI) in susceptible people can lead to hypotension, dehydration, and kidney failure. This does not mean that such people should not receive these treatments, but it does mean that initial doses may need to be reduced and subsequent increases in dose be given only cautiously under close monitoring, often by a specialist heart failure nurse. The aim of treatment should be to achieve an acceptable quality of life for that individual with as few side effects as possible.

NURSING PRACTICE INSIGHTS: NURSING PRIORITIES

Nursing priorities for supporting older people with heart failure are:

- educating the patient, family, and carer on the condition, lifestyle, and self-management;
- reviewing medication dosages and raising awareness of adverse reactions;
- monitoring for dehydration and fluid overload, which will involve:
  - identifying whether there are mobility or incontinence issues that impact on the patient's ability to get drinks and go to the toilet;
  - undertaking regular fluid balance assessments—see Endacott et al. (2009);

- **coordinating care with other health professionals—particularly a specialist nursing heart failure team.**

See Chapter 7 for more on medication management, and Chapter 14 for more on elimination and continence.

Atrial fibrillation

What is atrial fibrillation?

Atrial fibrillation (AF) occurs when the electrical impulses controlling the heartbeat become disorganized, so that the heart beats irregularly and too fast. When this happens, the heart cannot pump blood efficiently round the body and the pulse becomes irregular. AF occurs more commonly with age, affecting fewer than 2 per cent of those under 65 years old, but around 6 per cent of those over the age of 65 (Feinberg et al., 1995). Initial screening for AF simply involves palpating the pulse. This should be a routine part of any relevant health check, particularly for nurses assessing older patients (Madoc-Sutton et al., 2009). If the pulse is irregular, an ECG should be performed to enable diagnosis.

Symptoms of AF may include:

- palpitations;
- chest pain or discomfort;
- shortness of breath;
- dizziness; and
- collapse or fainting.

Although severe symptoms can be life-threatening, most people with AF have only mild symptoms or even none at all. AF can come on suddenly, usually in response to an illness such as pneumonia (acute AF). It may be long-standing (chronic or permanent AF) or intermittent (paroxysmal AF). People with AF have at least a six-fold increased risk of stroke compared to those without (Peters et al., 2002). This is because the blood does not flow efficiently through the heart, predisposing to clot formation. If a clot dislodges from the heart, it can travel along the blood vessels to the brain and cause a stroke.

How is atrial fibrillation treated?

Treatment of AF aims either to control the heart rate (to prevent it beating too fast) or to restore the heart to a normal rhythm (either using medications or an electrical shock), as well as to reduce the risk of stroke and other complications (NCCCC, 2006a).

Anticoagulant drugs can be used to cut down the risk of clots forming if the benefits are thought to outweigh the risks of the treatment. Warfarin is considered the best treatment to reduce complications such as stroke. However, in some older people with medical problems or who are at risk of falls, this may not be considered the safest option. Sometimes, these patients may be prescribed aspirin instead.

Leg ulcers

Leg ulcers affect up to 3.5 per cent of people over the age of 65. It is important to identify the cause, because that will dictate the appropriate treatment. Most leg ulcers (90 per cent) are due to problems with the circulation, either venous (70 per cent), arterial (15 per cent), or a mixture of both (5 per cent). The remainder (10 per cent) have a non-vascular cause, which is not discussed here.

Returning blood to the heart (venous return) from the feet and legs is usually promoted by calf muscle contraction and one-way valves within the veins that prevent backflow of blood. When these mechanisms fail, or are inadequate, the deep veins cannot empty completely and high pressures (venous hypertension) develop. This can lead to distension and congestion of the superficial veins. Prolonged venous hypertension damages the skin and soft tissues making them susceptible to ulceration, which may be spontaneous or triggered by only minor trauma.

Grey-brown skin discolouration and hardening of the skin in the 'gaiter' area of the leg are typical changes found in chronic venous insufficiency. There is usually oedema and there may be varicose veins. Associated dermatitis (inflammation of the skin) may cause crusting, weeping, itching, and pain. Ulcers due to venous disease are usually quite shallow and tend to be located on the inner aspect of the ankle.

How are leg ulcers treated?

General measures for the treatment of venous ulcers include maintaining mobility, good nutrition, weight reduction if obese, and reducing risk of trauma to the feet by modifying falls risk factors. Good hygiene to the area must be maintained, as well as vigilance for signs of infection. Legs must be elevated when possible to reduce the oedema. Dry skin should be moisturized with a simple emollient.

See Chapter 6 on mobility and falls.

Student activity: Awareness of mobility and falls

Read Chapter 6 on mobility and falls so that you can understand how older patients can minimize their risk of falls whilst maintaining mobility in order to treat leg ulcers.

Multilayer compression bandaging should be used, provided that there is no evidence of arterial disease. There is reasonable evidence from trial data that venous ulcers heal more rapidly with compression than without. Multi-component bandaging systems containing an elastic component seem to be the most effective (O'Meara et al., 2009). These work by augmenting calf muscle pump action, reducing venous hypertension, and opposing leakage of fluid into the subcutaneous tissue, thus reducing oedema. In some cases, surgical intervention, such as skin grafting, may be required.

One of the main difficulties in the management of leg ulcers is the time that it takes for the ulcer to heal—often many months. A poor understanding of this by the patient and their carer may lead to poor compliance with therapy. Thus, education and clear communication is crucial, with careful explanation of the rationale behind treatment.

For other types of leg ulcer, many of the above principles still apply, but specific management targeted at the underlying cause may be needed. For example, if the ulcer is due to a blocked arterial supply, then a procedure to unblock the artery may be performed.

Key respiratory conditions

Chronic obstructive pulmonary disease

What is chronic obstructive pulmonary disease?

Chronic obstructive pulmonary disease (COPD) is a progressive lung condition primarily caused by damage due to smoking. The main symptoms are shortness of breath, wheezing, coughing, and sputum production. It can have a dramatic impact on quality of life and is the third biggest cause of death due to respiratory disease (after pneumonia and lung cancer). It is a common precipitant for admission to hospital, with about one in eight of all emergency admissions to hospital in the UK attributable to COPD.

It is diagnosed using spirometry (a type of breathing test). This can be difficult for some older people to perform either due to physical disabilities or, in those with dementia, due to cognitive problems.

How is COPD treated?

Medical management most frequently includes the use of inhalers and/or nebulizers to help dilate the airways (bronchodilators). Tablets are sometimes used regularly to help to thin secretions (mucolytics). Vaccinations (for influenza and pneumococcus) should be offered in primary care. Some people will require long-term oxygen therapy (there are strict criteria for who is eligible for this, one of which is that they must have stopped smoking). The Global Initiative for COPD (GOLD) has a useful 'pocket guide' to assessment and management of patients with COPD available online at http://www.goldcopd.com/

Further high-standard contemporary guidelines for COPD are available from the British Thoracic Society, online at http://www.brit-thoracic.org.uk/, and the National Institute for Health and Clinical Excellence (NICE) *Guidance for COPD*, available online at http://guidance.nice.org.uk/CG12

See the Online Resource Centre that accompanies this book for more on developments in relation to a UK National Clinical Strategy for COPD.

Behaviour change support delivered by nurses specifically employed to provide smoking cessation has been shown to increase rates of quitting (Rice and Stead, 2008). Nutritional advice, encouraging physical activity where possible, and breathing exercises are also important non-pharmacological measures. Pulmonary rehabilitation programmes have been shown to be effective in improving quality of life, reducing breathlessness, improving exercise capacity (Lacasse et al., 1996), and reducing use of health service resources. Opportunity to attend such programmes should be provided to all patients with moderate to severe COPD, if available.

Most exacerbations can be managed at home with nursing support, usually with increased use of nebulizers or inhalers, oral steroids, and sometimes oral antibiotics. Some areas have specialist COPD or respiratory nurses who provide care for older people with COPD and who will undertake assessments as required, depending on whether it is mild, moderate, or severe COPD. Rapid response teams or intermediate care teams may also intervene and provide support where there is an exacerbation. A study of older people with end-stage COPD living in the community (Thomas, 2009) found that changing activity, relaxation, and altering breathing pattern were strategies adopted by patients in addition to medications to manage their breathlessness. Nurses must work in partnership with the patient to identify strategies that have previously been effective for that particular individual and to incorporate them into their overall care plan.

Antibiotics are indicated for an exacerbation if it is associated with sputum that is more purulent than usual, suggesting the likelihood of a bacterial infection. If the sputum is not purulent, then antibiotics are not indicated unless there are signs of pneumonia, either clinically or on chest X-ray (NCCCC, 2010). In many of these cases, the infection triggering the exacerbation will be viral and therefore will not respond to antibiotic treatment. Nurses will need to be involved in patient education, because many will expect the prescription of an antibiotic even when it is not indicated. This is of particular importance in the light of growing evidence about the risks of antibiotic therapy (Linder, 2008). The decision whether or not to recommend antibiotics should be made on a case-by-case basis after a full medical assessment.

Treatment in hospital may be required for more severe exacerbations—in particular, if intravenous medication or breathing support, such as non-invasive ventilation (NIV), is required. In the terminal phase, the usual treatments may be less effective. Other medications, such as morphine and low-dose benzodiazepines, can ease the distress associated with breathlessness. Patients at this stage often require intensive psychological support and help with coping strategies. Respiratory nurses and palliative care services should be equipped to meet these needs, and the nurse–patient relationship may be more crucial than ever (Barnett, 2006).

Issues for older people

Breathlessness can be a very disabling symptom, not only because it limits physical activity, but also because it increases the risk of social isolation and depression. Care needs to be taken not to miss these problems—particularly in older people, who are already at greater risk.

NURSING PRACTICE INSIGHT: HOW NURSES CAN SUPPORT USE OF INHALERS

Many of the medications for COPD are given via inhalers. Some of these devices can be difficult to use, particularly for those with reduced manual dexterity (for example, arthritis, tremor, or poor coordination) or cognitive impairment. Nurses must assess patients' ability to use the device appropriately. There are different delivery devices available and it may be appropriate to seek specialist advice to find the most appropriate option for the individual.

Community-acquired pneumonia

Community-acquired pneumonia (CAP) is an important cause of morbidity, hospital admission, and mortality. The annual incidence in the community is 5–11 per 1,000 adult population. However, it is much more common in older people, with one study finding 34 cases per 1,000 population over the age of 75 (Jokinen et al., 1993). Patients living in long-term care facilities are particularly vulnerable: pneumonia accounts for 29 per cent of acute illness episodes in nursing-home residents (Zimmer et al., 1988).

How is it diagnosed and treated?

Pneumonia may be diagnosed on the basis of the history and physical examination alone.

Typical symptoms include:

- breathlessness;
- cough;
- fevers; and
- chest pain (which is worse on coughing and breathing in).

Tests may include blood tests, chest X-ray, oxygen saturations, and a culture of sputum samples.

The main treatment for CAP is with antibiotics. These may be given by mouth at home in those who are well with low risk of deterioration. These people should be advised to rest, to stop smoking, and to drink plenty of fluids. Simple painkillers may be needed if they have chest pain due to the pneumonia. Nursing assessment of these patients should include monitoring of vital signs, assessment and evaluation of mental, nutritional, and hydration status, and ensuring medication compliance (Ramsdell et al., 2005). Important goals include ensuring patient understanding of the condition and identifying signs of deterioration that may indicate necessity for hospital admission.

In those who are more unwell and have risk factors for poor outcome, intravenous antibiotics may be required from the outset, and whilst intravenous medications can be given in the community, admission to hospital may be necessary. High-risk patients may also require oxygen, chest physiotherapy, or even admission to the intensive care unit for assistance with breathing. If the illness is prolonged, nutritional support may be required.

Problems particular to older people

In the majority of older nursing-home patients, admission to hospital for treatment with pneumonia does not improve outcomes (Fried et al., 1995). They may be treated in the nursing home with oral, intramuscular, or even intravenous antibiotics. Given the hazards associated with hospitalizing frail older people and the financial implications, it seems reasonable to avoid doing so when there is no likely benefit. This may be the wish of the patient themselves or their carer. Careful monitoring—in particular of vital signs—is necessary to identify those at risk of deterioration and who may benefit from intensification of treatment in a hospital environment. Nurses should perform regular assessments, and provide support and information to the patient and their carer, as well as liaise with the GP as required.

Key musculoskeletal conditions

Arthritis

What is arthritis?

Arthritis simply means joint inflammation. There are many different types of arthritis, but the commonest two types are osteoarthritis (OA) and rheumatoid arthritis (RA). The burden of arthritis is significant: approximately 8 million people in the UK are affected by some form of the condition.

Osteoarthritis

Osteoarthritis is the commonest form of arthritis. Worldwide estimates suggest that 9.6 per cent of men and 18 per cent of women aged over 60 have symptomatic OA (Murray and Lopez, 1996). Older age is the strongest predictor for development of OA. It is more common in obese people and those who have participated in physically demanding activities or occupations.

It is caused by progressive destruction and loss of cartilage within the involved joint. This leads to attempts at repair, which can cause abnormal bony growth at the margins of the joint. The main consequence of this process is pain that is aggravated by movement and relieved by rest. The joints most often involved are some of the joints in the hands and the weight-bearing joints—that is, the vertebrae, hips, and knees.

Treatments for OA should be instigated after a holistic assessment has been carried out (NCCCC, 2008a). Occupational therapists and physiotherapists also need to be involved. Medical treatments are directed at pain control, initially with paracetamol and topical non steroidal anti-inflammatory drugs (NSAIDs). In younger patients, oral NSAIDs may be recommended for short periods of time. However, in older people, these are best avoided due to potential side effects.

Education, strengthening, low-impact exercises, and weight loss advice if the patient is obese are other recommended interventions that may be nurse-led. However, many of these goals may be limited in older people by other physical factors and co-morbidities. If pain or disability is severe, and cannot be controlled with these measures, joint replacement surgery may be required.

Rheumatoid arthritis

Rheumatoid arthritis is a less common condition than OA, affecting around 1–3 per cent of the population worldwide—but it can be very disabling. It is more common in women, and the incidence and prevalence increase with age, peaking at about 70 years old, and then declining.

RA is an autoimmune condition, which means that the body's immune system attacks the linings of the joints, causing them to become inflamed. RA, unlike OA, is a disorder that does not only affect the joints; it can also affect the eyes, the skin, the nerves, the lungs, and other organs. It can make the patient feel generally unwell, with fever, tiredness, and weight loss. The joints can be inflamed, painful, stiff, and swollen. This tends to be worse in the morning. Many joints can be involved, usually in a symmetrical pattern. Over time, with ongoing inflammation, the joints become permanently damaged and deformed.

Figure 10.5 shows that, despite their arthritis, some people can maintain or develop skills.

There are many medications that can be used to modify the underlying disease process to try to prevent long-term damage and deformity. These medications are often referred to as 'disease-modifying anti-rheumatic drugs' (DMARDs). However, because these drugs suppress the body's immune system, they make people more prone to infection.

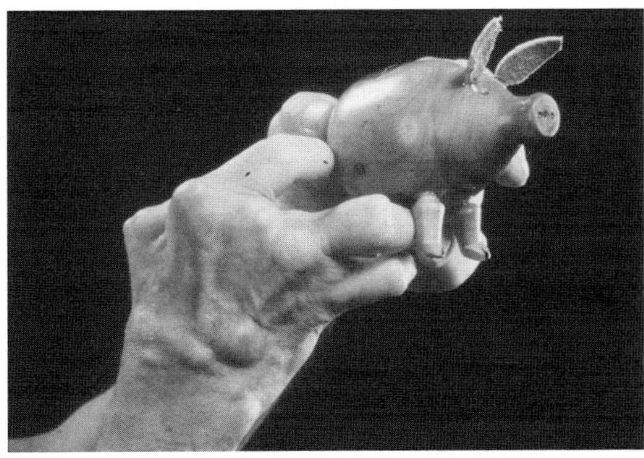

Figure 10.5 This photo shows the hands of a man with arthritis who, despite his condition, has carved the toy pig that he is holding
Source: By kind permission of Doncaster & Bassetlaw Hospitals and Garry Swann.

Impact of arthritis

The possible impacts of arthritis include:

- activities of daily living (ADLs) may be limited;
- physical disability and deformity;
- limitation of independence—particularly due to restriction of mobility;
- pain; and
- psychological/psychiatric consequences due to altered body image, loss of ability to work, reduced independence, and impact on relationships.

To assess the impact of arthritis, nurses need to foster active listening skills, be aware of the potential for psychological issues, and have knowledge of basic pain management (both non-pharmacological and pharmacological) (Read et al., 2001). Nurses need to be aware of the common limitations of ADLs encountered by people with arthritis, and facilitate access to necessary devices and adaptations in conjunction with occupational therapists (Swann, 2007). Facilitating access to national and local support networks or groups is another potential role. Wherever possible, self-management should be encouraged.

> ❖ ***Student activity***
>
> Do not forget to read about osteoporosis and hip fractures in Chapter 6 on mobility and falls.

Conclusion

Growing older brings with it an increased risk of ill health, disability, and dependency. However, this is not inevitable.

Healthcare providers can assist patients in modifying risk factors for disease, thereby promoting health and active ageing. The aim of this is not only to ensure a longer life, but also to improve or maintain functional level, to prevent disease, and to enhance well-being. Every individual is different and how these aims can be achieved will vary from person to person. Where an individual has multiple medical problems and is taking a number of different medications, promoting health and active ageing will be more complicated and varied.

To achieve these aims, nurses need to undertake a comprehensive assessment of each individual's needs, including medical problems, functional level, psychological issues, social circumstances, and living environment (Wieland and Hirth, 2003). Effective multidisciplinary team working is the foundation of this assessment, and depends on good awareness of the key issues and effective communication between all those involved in the person's care. The individual themselves must be involved in all aspects of care planning (where possible) and their views must be respected.

Questions and self-assessment

- Think about an older adult who has been in your care. How has ageing affected their physiological functioning?
- Consider how an older person living with long-term illness may want a nurse to help them to manage their own health and make their own treatment decisions. What are the fundamentals to achieving this?
- Identify a patient who has been in your care who has been diagnosed with more than one medical condition. How was the person's care individualized, taking into account the complex interactions between their health problems?
- What are the benefits of team working and how does it benefit patient care?

Self-assessment

- Having read the chapter, how will you change your practice?
- Identify up to three areas relating to key medical conditions in which you need to develop your knowledge and understanding further.
- Identify how you are going to develop this knowledge and understanding, and set deadlines for achieving this.

References

Aarsland, D., Anderson, K., Laresen, J.P., Lolk, A., and Kragh-Sørensen, P. (2003) 'Prevalence and characteristics of dementia in Parkinson disease: An 8-year prospective study', *Archives of Neurology*, 60: 387–92.

Ayis, S., Gooberman-Hill, R., and Ebrahim, S. (2003) 'Long-standing and limiting longstanding illness in older people: Associations with chronic diseases, psychosocial and environmental factors', *Age and Ageing*, 32: 265–72.

Baker, M. and Graham, L. (2004) 'The journey: Parkinson's disease', *British Medical Journal*, 329(7466): 611, available online at http://www.bmj.com/cgi/content/full/329/7466/611.

Barnett, M. (2006) 'Providing palliative care in end-stage COPD within primary care', *Journal of Community Nursing*, 20(3): 30–4.

Bayer, A.J., Chadha, J.S., Farag, R.R., and Pathy, M.S. (1986) 'Changing presentation of myocardial infarction with increasing old age', *Journal of the American Geriatrics Society*, 34(4): 263–6.

Benjamin, E.M. (2002) 'Case study: Glycaemic control in the elderly—Risks and benefits', *Clinical Diabetes*, 20(3): 118–22.

Blue, L., Lang, E., McMurray, J.J.V., Davie, A.P., McDonagh, T.A., Murdoch, D.R., Petrie, M.C., Connolly, E., Norrie, J., Round, C.E., Ford, I., and Morrison, C.E. (2001) 'Randomized controlled trial of specialist nurse intervention in heart failure', *British Medical Journal*, 323: 715–18.

Bracewell, C., Gray, R., and Rai, G. (2005) *Essential Facts in Geriatric Medicine*, Oxford: Radcliffe.

Coull, A.J., Lovett, J.K., and Rothwell, P.M. (2004) 'Population based study of stroke after transient ischaemic attack or minor stroke: Implications for public education and organization of services', *British Medical Journal*, 328: 326.

Dartington, T. (2008) 'Dying from dementia: A patient's journey', *British Medical Journal*, 337: a1712, available online at http://www.bmj.com/cgi/content/extract/337/sep25_1/a1712.

Davidson, M.B. (2003) Effect of nurse-directed diabetes care in a minority population', *Diabetes Care*, 26(8): 2281–7.

Department of Health (2000) *Coronary Heart Disease: National Service Framework for Coronary Heart Disease—Modern Standards and Service Models*, available online at http://www.dh.gov.uk/en/Publicationsandstatistics/Publications/PublicationsPolicyAndGuidance/DH_4094275.

Department of Health (2001) *National Service Framework for Older People*, available online at http://www.dh.gov.uk/en/Publicationsandstatistics/Publications/PublicationsPolicyAndGuidance/DH_4003066.

Department of Health (2007) *National Stroke Strategy*, available online at http://www.dh.gov.uk/prod_consum_dh/groups/dh_digitalassets/documents/digitalasset/dh_081059.pdf.

De Rijk, M.C., Breteler, M.M.B, Graveland, G.A., Ott, A., Grobbee, D.E., Van der Meche, F.G.A., and Hofman, A. (1995) 'Prevalence of Parkinson's disease in the elderly', *Neurology*, 45: 2143–6.

Diabetes Control and Complications Trial Research Group (1993) 'The effect of intensive treatment of diabetes on the development and progression of long-term complications in insulin-dependent diabetes mellitus', *New England Journal of Medicine*, 329: 977–86.

Endacott, R., Jevon, P., and Cooper S. (2009) *Clinical Nursing Skills: Core and Advanced*, Oxford: Oxford University Press.

European Diabetes Working Party for Older People (2004) *Clinical Guidelines for Type 2 Diabetes Mellitus*, available online at http://instituteofdiabetes.org/wp-content/themes/IDOP/other/diabetes_guidelines_for_older_people.pdf.

Feinberg, W.M., Blackshear J.L., Laupacis, A., Kronmal, R., and Hart, R.G. (1995) 'Prevalence, age distribution, and gender of patients with atrial fibrillation: Analysis and implication', *Archives of Internal Medicine*, 155: 469–73.

Fitzpatrick, M. and Birns, J. (2004) 'Thrombolysis for acute ischaemic stroke and the role of the nurse', *British Journal of Nursing*, 13(20): 1170–4.

Fried, T.R., Gillick, M.R., and Lipsitz, L.A. (1995) 'Whether to transfer? Factors associated with hospitalization and outcomes of elderly long-term care patients with pneumonia', *Journal of General Internal Medicine*, 10: 246–50.

Jarman, B., Hurwitz, B., Cook, A., Bajekal, M., and Lee, A. (2002) 'Effects of community-based nurses specializing in Parkinson's disease on health outcome and costs: randomized control trial', *British Medical Journal*, 324: 1072–5.

Jokinen, C., Heiskanen, L., Juvonen, H., Kallinen, S., Karkola, K., Korppi, M., Kurki, S., Rönnberg, P.R., Seppä, A., Soimakallio, S., Stén, M., Tanska, S. Tarkiainen, T., Tukiainen, H., Pyörälä, K., and Mäkelä, P.H. (1993) 'Incidence of community-acquired pneumonia in the population of four municipalities in eastern Finland', *American Journal of Epidemiology,* 137: 977–88.

Kannel, W.B. and Belanger, A.J. (1991) 'Epidemiology of heart failure', *American Heart Journal*, 121(3): 951–7.

Keely, E.C., Boura, J.A., and Grines, C.L. (2003) 'Primary angioplasty versus intravenous thrombolytic therapy for acute myocardial infarction: A quantitative review of 23 randomized trials', *The Lancet*, 361: 13–20.

Lacasse, Y., Wong, E., Guyatt, G.H., King, D., Cook, D.J., and Goldstein, R.S. (1996) 'Meta-analysis of respiratory rehabilitation in chronic obstructive pulmonary disease', *The Lancet*, 348:1115–19.

Langhorne, P., Williams, B.O., Gilchrist, W., and Howie, K. (1993) 'Do stroke units save lives?', *The Lancet*, 342:395–8.

Linder, J. (2008) 'Editorial commentary: Antibiotics for treatment of acute respiratory tract infections—Decreasing benefit, increasing risk, and the irrelevance of antimicrobial resistance', *Clinical Infectious Diseases*, 47: 744–6.

Madoc-Sutton, H., Pearson, E., and Upton, J. (2009) 'Pulse check as a screen for atrial fibrillation', *British Journal of Cardiac Nursing*, 4(9): 426–9.

Maslow, A.H. (1943) 'A theory of human motivation', *Psychological Review*, 50(4): 430–7.

Maslow, A.H. (1998) *Towards a Psychology of Being*, New York: John Wiley and Sons.

Mayes, M. (2000) 'Management of the older person with diabetes in the community', *British Journal of Community Nursing*, 5(9): 448–53.

Murray, C.J.L. and Lopez, A.D. (eds) (1996) *The Global Burden of Disease: A Comprehensive Assessment of Mortality and Disability from Diseases, Injuries, and Risk Factors in 1990 and Projected to 2020*, Cambridge, MA: Harvard School of Public Health, on behalf of the World Health Organization and The World Bank.

National Collaborating Centre for Chronic Conditions (2003) *Chronic Heart Failure: National Clinical Guideline for Diagnosis and Management in Primary and Secondary Care*, London: Royal College of Physicians, available online at http://www.nice.org.uk/guidance/index.jsp?action=download&o=29137.

National Collaborating Centre for Chronic Conditions (2006a) *Atrial Fibrillation: National Clinical Guideline for Diagnosis and Management in Primary and Secondary Care*, London: Royal College of Physicians, available online at http://www.nice.org.uk/nicemedia/pdf/cg036fullguideline.pdf.

National Collaborating Centre for Chronic Conditions (2006b) *Parkinson's Disease: National Clinical Guideline for Diagnosis and Management in Primary and Secondary Care*, London: Royal College of Physicians, available online at http://www.nice.org.uk/nicemedia/pdf/cg035fullguideline.pdf.

National Collaborating Centre for Chronic Conditions (2008a) *Osteoparthritis: National Clinical Guidelines for Care and Management in Adults*, London: Royal College of Physicians, available online at http://www.nice.org.uk/nicemedia/pdf/CG059FullGuideline.pdf.

National Collaborating Centre for Chronic Conditions (2008b) *Stroke: National Clinical Guideline for Diagnosis and Initial Management of Acute Stroke and Transient Ischaemic Attack (TIA)*, London: Royal College of Physicians, available online at http://www.nice.org.uk/nicemedia/pdf/CG68FullGuideline.pdf.

National Collaborating Centre for Chronic Conditions (2008c) *Type 2 Diabetes: National Clinical Guideline for Diagnosis and Management in Primary and Secondary Care (Update)*, London: Royal College of Physicians, available online at http://www.nice.org.uk/nicemedia/pdf/CG66diabetesfullguideline.pdf.

National Collaborating Centre for Chronic Conditions (2010) *Chronic Obstructive Pulmonary Disease: Management of Chronic Obstructive Pulmonary Disease in Adults in Primary and Secondary Care*, Update, London: Royal College of Physicians, available online at http://guidance.nice.org.uk/CG101.

Naughton, C., Bennett, K., and Feely, J. (2006) 'Prevalence of chronic disease in the elderly based on a national pharmacy claims database', *Age and Aging*, 35(6): 633–6.

O'Brien, J. (2006) *Reflecting on Social Roles: Identifying Opportunities to Support Personal Freedom and Social Integration*, available online at http://www.inclusion.com/socialroleinventory.pdf.

Office of the Deputy Prime Minister (2006) *A Sure Start to Later Life: Ending Inequalities for Older People—A Social Exclusion Unit Final Report*, available online at http://www.communities.gov.uk/publications/corporate/surestart.

O'Meara, S., Cullum, N.A., and Nelson, E.A. (2009) 'Compression for venous leg ulcers (review)', *The Cochrane Library*, 4, available online at http://mrw.interscience.wiley.com/cochrane/clsysrev/articles/CD000265/pdf_standard_fs.html.

Patel, V. and Morrissey, J. (2002) 'The alphabet strategy: The ABC of reducing diabetes complications', *British Journal of Diabetes and Vascular Disease*, 2: 58–9.

Peters, N.S., Schilling, R.J., Kanagaratnam, P., and Markides, V. (2002) 'Atrial fibrillation: Strategies to control, combat, and cure', *The Lancet*, 359: 593–603.

Pfeil, M., Gray, R., and Lindsay, B. (2009) 'Depression and stroke: A common but often unrecognized combination', *British Journal of Nursing*, 18(6): 365–9.

Ramsdell, J., Narsavage, G.L., and Fink, J.B. (2005) 'Management of community-acquired pneumonia in the home', *Chest*, 127: 1752–63.

Read, E., Mceachern, C., and Mitchell, T. (2001) 'Psychological well-being of patients with rheumatoid arthritis', *British Journal of Nursing*, 10(21): 1385–91.

Reynolds, H., Wilson-Barnett, J., and Richardson, G. (2000) 'Evaluation of the role of the Parkinson's disease nurse specialist', *International Journal of Nursing Studies*, 37: 337–49.

Rice, V.H. and Stead, L.F. (2008) 'Nursing interventions for smoking cessation', *Cochrane Database Systematic Reviews*, 2 January, Art. No. CD001188, available online at http://www2.cochrane.org/reviews/en/ab001188.html.

Rothwell, P.M., Coull, A.J., Silver, L.E., and Fairhead, J.F., Giles, M.F., Lovelock, C.E., Redgrave, J.N., Bull, L.M., Welch, S.J., Cuthbertson, F.C., Binney, L.E., Gutnikov, S.A., Anslow, P., Banning, A.P., Mant, D., and Mehta, Z. (2005) 'Population-based study of event-rate, incidence, case fatality, and mortality for all acute vascular events in all arterial territories (Oxford Vascular Study)', *The Lancet*, 366: 1773–83.

Simpson, C., Franks, C., Morrison, C., and Lempp, H. (2005) 'The patient's journey: Rheumatoid arthritis', *British Medical Journal*, 331: 887–9, available online at http://www.bmj.com/cgi/content/extract/331/7521/887.

Slaughter, J.R., Slaughter, K.A., Nichols, D., Holmes, S.E., and Martens, M.P. (2001) 'Prevalence, clinical manifestations, etiology and treatment of depression in Parkinson's disease', *The Journal of Neuropsychiatry and Clinical Neurosciences*, 13: 187–96.

Swann, J. (2007) 'Rheumatoid arthritis: Coping strategies', *Nursing and Residential Care*, 9(6): 269–72.

Thomas, L.A. (2009) 'Effective dyspnoea management strategies identified by elders with end-stage chronic obstructive pulmonary disease', *Applied Nursing Research*, 22: 79–85.

Veazey, C., Aki, S.O.E, Cook, K.F., Lai, E.C.. and Kunik, M.E. (2005) 'Prevalence and treatment of depression in Parkinson's disease', *Journal of Neuropsychiatry and Clinical Neurosciences*, 17: 310–23.

Wardlaw, J.M., del Zoppo, G., Yamaguchi, T., and Berge, E. (2003) 'Thrombolysis for acute ischaemic stroke', *Cochrane Database of Systematic Reviews*, 3, Art. No. CD000213, available online at http://www.cochrane.org/reviews/en/ab000213.html.

Wieland, W. and Hirth, V. (2003) 'Comprehensive geriatric assessment', *Cancer Control*, 10(6): 454–62.

Wilkinson, I. and Lennox, G. (2005) *Essential Neurology*, 4th edn, Oxford: Blackwell Publishing.

World Health Organization (2002) *Active Aging: A Policy Framework*, available online at http://whqlibdoc.who.int/hq/2002/WHO_NMH_NPH_02.8.pdf.

World Health Organization (2010) *Our Ageing World*, available online at http://www.who.int/ageing/en/.

Zimmer, J.G., Eggert, G.M., Treat, A., Brodows, B., and Hyg, M.S. (1988) 'Nursing homes as acute care providers: A pilot study of incentives to reduce hospitalizations', *Journal of the American Geriatric Society*, 36: 124–9.

For further reading and information

Endacott, R., Jevon, P., and Cooper, S. (eds) (2009) *Clinical Nursing Skills: Core and Advanced*, Oxford: Oxford University Press

http://guidance.nice.org.uk/CG12

http://www.arthritiscare.org.uk/

http://www.bhf.org.uk/

http://www.brit-thoracic.org.uk/

http://www.diabetes.org.uk/

http://www.goldcopd.com/

http://www.lunguk.org/

http://www.parkinsons.org.uk/

http://www.stroke.org.uk/

Online Resource Centre

You can learn more about the key medical disorders of older adults at the Online Resource Centre that accompanies this book:

http://www.oxfordtextbooks.co.uk/orc/hindle/

Dementia, mental health, and the older adult

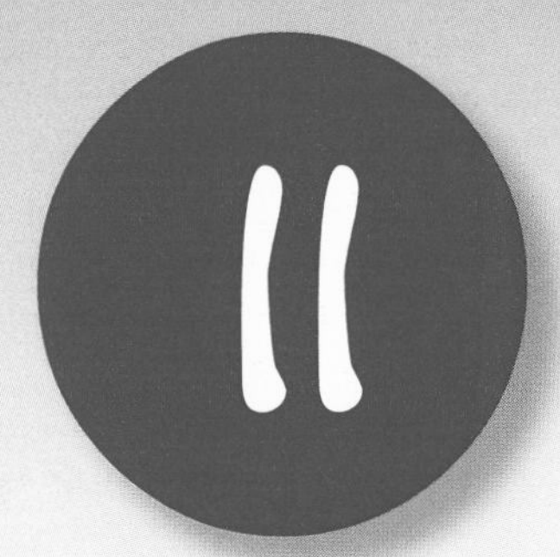

Alison Coates

Learning outcomes

By the end of this chapter, you will be able to:

- understand how mental health problems may affect older adults;
- appreciate the impact that dementia can have on an older person's life and the care that may be required;
- recognize key issues influencing the mental health of older adults;
- understand how mental health problems may be identified; and
- identify how the nurse could work effectively with older people with mental health problems in order to aid recovery and enhance quality of life.

Introduction

Nurses work with older people who have mental health problems in all clinical areas. It is estimated that 50 per cent of older people in general hospitals, 60 per cent of those in care homes, and 40 per cent of older people who consult their general practitioner (GP) have mental health problems (DH, 2007). Some of these older people will have had mental health problems all of their lives; others may have developed mental health problems following a particular event. They may have become depressed after bereavement, or may have developed mental health problems as a result of biological changes to their brain—for example, those people who have developed dementia. The UK government paper *Making Safeguarding Everybody's Business* (DH, 2005) states that older people with mental health care needs are entitled to the same standards of care as anyone else, that access to mental health services should not be based on age, and that their needs should be met whatever the health or social care setting. Support and advice should be sought by healthcare workers from specialist services such as psychiatric liaison teams or older people's mental health teams, so that they are able to meet the needs of older people with mental health problems in all settings.

A person's mental health is affected by complex interactions between the environment in which they live and their own response to that environment. There are different approaches—psychological, biological (medical), and social—concerning the cause and treatment of mental health problems. These approaches are useful in developing an understanding of how and why some older people develop mental health problems, and in identifying the most appropriate treatment approach (Norman and Ryrie, 2004). The nurse is an ideal healthcare professional to select from and work with these different approaches, and provide person-centred care. However, patients and relatives will describe their symptoms and problems from their own perspectives, and they may not use the same constructs or language as health professionals. You must also bear in mind that many people, including those who are from non-Western cultures, may have different health beliefs from those normally recognized and provided for within the National Health Service (NHS) (Holland and Hogg, 2001). Listening to the patient and carer is an important skill, and is key to developing an understanding of a patient's problems and working therapeutically. Because people's experience of mental health problems and their needs will be individual to them, care must be patient-centred and based on partnership working.

See Chapter 2 for more on working with people with different beliefs.

This chapter provides an overview of a large and complex subject. It will draw on different approaches to mental health, in order for the nurse to develop an understanding of the issues and to begin developing the core skills needed when working with older people who have mental health problems.

Dementia

Dementia is a generic term used to describe loss of intellectual functioning, including memory loss. Dementia is not a disorder confined to older people and younger people can be diagnosed, but the incidence of dementia increases with age.

Most older people do not have dementia, however, even in extreme old age. Approximately 1.3 per cent of the population aged 65–69 have dementia, and 32.5 per cent of the those over the age of 95 have dementia. However, this still means that 67.5 per cent of people over the age of 95 do not have dementia (Knapp et al., 2007). These figures currently suggest that approximately 684,000 people living in the UK have dementia; this constitutes 1.1 per cent of the entire population. However, a recent study has identified that the figures might actually be much higher than this, suggesting that approximately 820,000 people are currently suffering from dementia in the UK (The Alzheimer's Research Trust, 2010). With an increase of older adults in the UK, this figure is expected to rise to 1 million by 2025 (Knapp et al., 2007).

The UK government has issued a *National Dementia Strategy* (DH, 2009a). This outlines three key steps towards improving the quality of life for people with dementia and their carers:

- the need to ensure better knowledge about dementia;
- the need for people with dementia to be properly diagnosed and supported; and
- the need for services for people with dementia and their carers to meet their changing needs.

The National Audit Office (2010) estimates that providing care for people with dementia costs the NHS and social care services approximately £8.2 bn a year and this figure is increasing. Future funding to deliver the *National Dementia Strategy* is identified as needing to come from efficiency savings by keeping people out of acute hospital beds and by providing care for people in their own homes for as long as possible. Clearly, good nursing practice is important to the success of this strategy.

Causes and assessment of dementia and dementia-like syndromes

There are many different causes of dementia. The most common cause is the neurodegenerative condition Alzheimer's disease. Vascular dementia, which occurs as a result of damage to the brain following strokes or insufficient blood flow to the brain, is the second commonest cause. Other neurodegenerative diseases causing dementia include Lewy body dementia, which accounts for dementias including frontotemporal dementia, and neurological conditions, such as Parkinson's disease, Huntington's disease, and Creutzfelt–Jacob disease.

Table 11.1 illustrates the key causes of dementia and the percentage of dementia patients affected by them.

There are many other causes of dementia and dementia-like syndromes, including infections such as neurosyphilis, HIV, New Variant Cretzfeldt–Jacob disease, some metabolic disorders, and some vitamin deficiencies. Poisoning by carbon monoxide, metal poisoning, and alcohol trauma can all cause dementia. About 10 per cent of people have more than one form of dementia (Alzheimers Society, 2009).

Symptoms will vary depending upon the cause of the dementia, but the main symptom is always memory problems. Other symptoms may include behavioural and psychological changes, including depression, psychosis (hallucinations), sleep problems, aggression, communication problems, and wandering. Particularly at the later stages, the patient may also experience a loss of appetite, with associated loss of weight and vulnerability to infections, and incontinence. These problems lead to issues in managing activities of daily living, such as washing, dressing, and eating. People with Alzheimer's disease will often display problems in remembering words; they may also show diminished judgement (for example, wearing a thick coat in the summer); they may get confused when performing everyday tasks and be subject to mood changes. People with vascular dementia may display the same symptoms as those with Alzheimer's disease, but the progression of the disease happens in steps and people will notice that there are periods of stability followed by a sudden deterioration. The symptoms of Lewy body dementia include

Table 11.1 Causes of dementia and the percentage of dementia patients affected by them

Alzheimer's disease	62%
Strokes or insufficient blood flow to the brain (vascular dementia)	17%
Other neurodegenerative diseases (e.g. Lewy body dementia)	10–15%

hallucinations, tremors, and changes to the person's gait (walk) and they may be liable to falls.

People who are concerned about memory loss should be encouraged to seek help from their GP. For most people, this will be the first point of contact when memory problems are noticed. Because there may be other reasons for forgetfulness, it can be difficult to diagnose dementia—particularly in the early stages—and so specialist services are being developed. The UK *National Dementia Strategy* (DH, 2009b) identifies that all people with dementia should have access to a pathway of care that delivers a rapid and competent specialist assessment, and an accurate diagnosis that is sensitively communicated (DH, 2009b). A referral to a specialist memory service should be made, by which a thorough assessment will be undertaken, including a detailed personal history, a physical examination (to exclude treatable causes), and a mental health assessment, such as the 'mini mental state examination' (Folstein et al., 1975) and the six-item 'cognitive impairment test' (Katzman et al., 1983).

Further specialist investigations, such as a magnetic resonance imaging (MRI) or computerized tomography (CT) scan, may be required to rule out other cerebral pathologies and to help to diagnose the type of dementia that the person has. The function of specialist memory services will also include treatment and support, including information for carers and people with dementia, which should be of a high quality. It has also been recognized that carers and people with dementia need a named and known individual who they can approach for information and advice. The development of effective services for people with dementia is a UK government priority (DH, 2009a).

Working with carers

Family carers are identified as the most important resource for people with dementia (DH, 2009a). Carers should be treated with respect, their opinions should be sought, and care plans should be agreed with them.

Even if the person with dementia is in residential care, then their carers should still be consulted on areas of care, including diet, hygiene routines, normal sleep routine, and religious beliefs and observances. Carers should also be advised of advocacy and carer support groups, or support services such as the Admiral Nursing Service (a specialist nursing service offering support to the families of people with dementia).

Further information can be found online at http://www.fordementia.org.uk/.

See Chapter 5 for more on working with carers.

Providing nursing care

Care should be person-centred, and carers should be involved in assessing and care planning. Carers will be a source of information and support for the patient, and it is important that the nurse involves them, and respects their opinions and experience. Care should be based on the person's life history, personal and family circumstances, and preferences; in this way, person-centred care will be achieved. For most causes of dementia, there is no cure, although some medications may help to alleviate symptoms for patients in some cases. The National Institute for Health and Clinical Excellence (NICE, 2007) recommends that cognitive-enhancing medication be prescribed to those with moderate Alzheimer's disease. The overuse of anti-psychotic medication to control behaviour disturbance has been identified in a recent government report (DH, 2009c). Using medication to control behaviour in these incidences places the patient at risk and should not be used in place of good care.

Care should include ensuring that the patient has a meaningful activity programme and participates in activities, such as exercise groups and others tailored to what they enjoy (see Figure 11.1). NICE (2004) identifies that cognitive stimulation, in the form of activities that require some problem-solving, is beneficial.

NURSING PRACTICE INSIGHT: GETTING TO KNOW THE PEOPLE IN YOUR CARE

In order for the nurse to work effectively with a person with dementia and address their individual needs, there are some core skills that will help to improve the quality of care the patient receives.

Firstly, you need to know the person in your care, and this includes understanding something of their life history, skills, likes, and dislikes.

- What did they use to enjoy?
- What were their interests or hobbies?
- Were there things that the person did not like?

Any care should be person-centred, so knowing what sort of things the person enjoyed or disliked will help you to plan individualized care.

Working closely with carers will also help you to get to know a patient, and their particular likes and dislikes.

Communicate effectively

When caring for a person with dementia, it is critical that you communicate effectively. You should take every opportunity to talk with the patient even when carrying out routine tasks. You might also use these opportunities to find out more about the person for whom you are caring, because this will help reinforce their sense of identity and help you to provide person-centered care.

The following suggestions will help you to improve face-to-face communication.

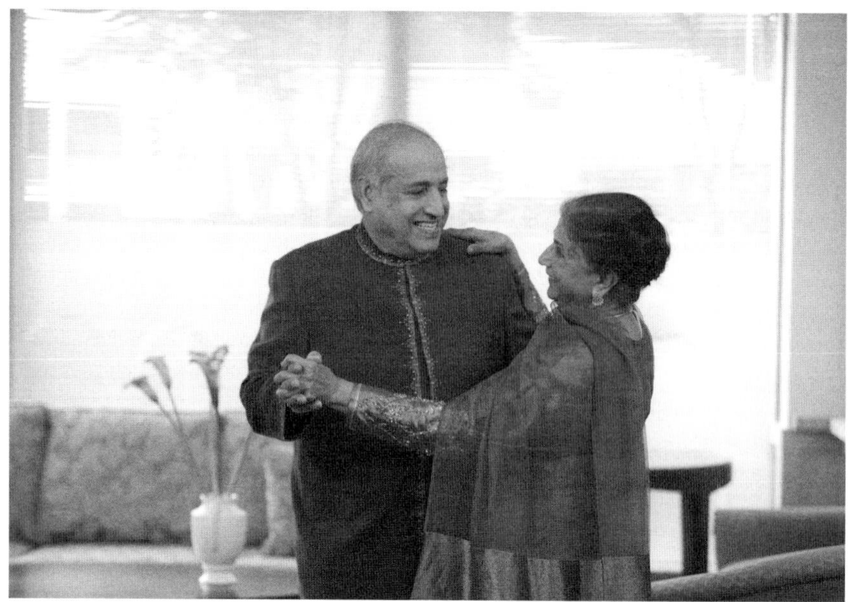

Figure 11.1 Life with dementia can still be active and enjoyable, provided that the right care is given
Source: © Photodisc.

- Approach the person from the front, so that they can see you.
- Use the patient's name as you address them, and introduce yourself by name and role.
- Use simple words and keep sentences short.
- Only ask one question at a time, and make sure that your voice is calm and reassuring.
- If the patient is having difficulties finding the right word, ask them to explain in a different way.
- If the patient has a hearing aid, make sure that they are wearing it and that is switched on.
- Make sure that the patient is wearing their glasses and dentures.
- Make conversation about things that the patient can remember—perhaps positive events from their past.

Non-verbal communication

When patients have limited verbal communication, their non-verbal communication becomes the main way in which you can understand their needs and feelings. In addition, your use of non-verbal communication can be key to successful interaction with a person with dementia.

The following are suggestions for how you might improve communication using and understanding non-verbal communication.

- Watch carefully and observe the patient's behaviour. Try to understand what the patient wants or needs. Someone who is wandering might be looking for the lavatory or be in need of reassurance. We all communicate through non-verbal signs, and the nurse needs to watch closely and try to interpret what the patient wants or is feeling. If a person becomes aggressive, then you should try to identify the cause of this behavior: for example, they may always have disliked pop music and the radio may have been left on with pop music playing.
- Show respect by giving time, attention, and kindness.
- Use non-verbal skills, such as smiling, so that the person knows that you are friendly.
- You may also find that it helps to show the person what you are about to do. For example, show them the blood pressure cuff before you ask them to put their arm out.

Environment

The impact of the environment should not be underestimated. When in an environment such as a hospital, even simple steps can make a difference, as follows.

- Make sure televisions are not left on all day reducing noise levels will reduce confusion and agitation.
- A calm environment with good lighting will help to reduce confusion and agitation.
- Keep the patient active by engaging with them in meaningful activity, such as asking them to help to lay the table at mealtimes or to water the plants.

Physical care

Finally, in addition to meeting any specific health needs that the patient may have, particular attention should be paid to ensuring that the patient's physical health needs are met. Often, the patient cannot meet these needs for themselves, so it is important that these needs are met by providing good care.

Of particular importance are the following matters.

- Ensure that the patient is safe from harm and cannot wander off unnoticed, or harm themselves by falling or coming into contact with harmful substances, such as boiling water.
- Ensure that adequate food and fluids are taken, and ensure constipation does not occur. Loss of appetite is a normal progression of the disease, so people with dementia may not experience hunger and thirst. It is the nurse's responsibility to ensure that patients receive an adequate diet and fluids; where there is dysphagia (that is, swallowing difficulties), a referral to a speech and language therapist is required.

See Chapter 13 on nutrition and fluids.

- Ensure that medical conditions are properly assessed and that care or treatment plans are followed.

Prevention

Nurses have a role to play in health promotion. Whilst dementia is a progressive condition, there is growing evidence that a healthy lifestyle, including not smoking, taking exercise, eating well, and keeping mentally active, may help to protect against dementia (Alzheimer's Society, 2009).

Delirium (acute confusional state)

Delirium is a symptom arising due to the direct physiological consequence of a medical condition, substance intoxication, or substance withdrawal. About a third of cases of delirium are preventable.

Older people are more susceptible to delirium than younger people and it is estimated that 30 per cent of older people admitted to acute medical wards are acutely confused (British Geriatric Society, 2006). Delirium is not confined to people in hospital and older people may develop delirium in their own homes. Some people are more susceptible to developing delirium and these include people who have coexisting conditions (British Geriatric Society, 2006), such as:

- depression;
- dementia;
- severe illness;
- physical frailty;
- visual impairment;
- people on multiple medications (polypharmacy);
- people with infections;
- renal impairment;
- alcohol excess; and
- people in hospital awaiting surgery—in particular, for fracture of the neck or femur.

Those at risk should be identified and prevention strategies implemented to reduce the risk of developing delirium. If delirium does occur, then the patient with delirium may have visual hallucinations, and they may be irritable, aggressive, or frightened; others may be quiet and display a 'flat effect' in their mood. Patients who develop delirium have longer lengths of stay in hospital than non-delirious patients and have high mortality rates.

For a diagnosis of delirium, the patient must display the following four symptoms:

- a disturbance of consciousness;
- a change in cognition;
- a disturbance that develops over a short period of time; and
- evidence from the history, physical examination, or laboratory findings that the disturbance is caused by direct physiological consequence of a medical condition, substance intoxication, or substance withdrawal.

Providing nursing care

A full history and physical assessment, including referral for further tests, should be carried out to determine the underlying cause of the problem in order for medical treatment to be prescribed. Medication may be prescribed to sedate the patient in some clinical areas such as intensive care, but should be kept to a minimum dose, and reviewed and discontinued as soon as possible.

Reducing the likelihood that an older person will develop delirium

Nurses need to ensure that older people in hospital do not receive poor care resulting in delirium. When nursing someone who is at risk of developing delirium, the nurse should ensure that the patient:

- takes adequate diet and fluids;
- avoids constipation;
- receives sufficient central nervous system (CNS) oxygen;
- experiences undisturbed sleep;

- is given good lighting;
- keeps orientated, by reminding them of the day and time (usually informally, such as things like 'It's quiet for a Monday', or similar);
- is encouraged to remain mobile and active;
- wears any hearing aids and spectacles;
- is given adequate pain analgesia; and
- receives visits from family and friends.

These measures will help to reduce the risks of developing delirium.

Helping older people to cope if they do develop delirium

If a person does develop delirium, then, in order to support the patient, the nurse should ensure that the measures above are maintained. In addition, the following measures can help.

- Communicate clearly, keeping messages simple. Introduce yourself by name and role, and explain what you are going to do or what you want the patient to do.
- Minimize the number of staff involved and try to ensure that only familiar people work with the patient.
- Maintain a calm environment, and ensure that televisions and radios do not disturb patients.
- Spend time with the patient and ensure that they do not feel isolated. Engage in simple conversation that will orient them within their environment.

Case study

Mrs Savage is a 98-year-old lady who has lived alone since her husband died 20 years ago. With a little help from family, friends, and neighbours, she maintains her independence, and she retains an interest in reading and current affairs.

One night, at 3 a.m., Mrs Savage was found out in the street in her nightdress shouting; the police were called and she was taken to hospital. On arrival, she was very tired, confused, and agitated; her neighbour, who accompanied her to the hospital, said that this behaviour seemed to have come 'out of the blue'.

The admitting nurse carried out a routine urine test using a urine multistick and found that Mrs Savage had a urine infection. With antibiotic treatment, the urine infection cleared and Mrs Savage's behaviour returned to normal.

Depression

Depression in older adults has been identified by the *National Service Framework for Older People* (NSFOP) (DH, 2001) as being an area needing special attention; it is estimated that between 10 per cent and 15 per cent of adults over the age of 65 suffer from depression (DH, 2001). Depression is the most common mental health problem in older adults.

All people experience a low mood at times, but this does not mean that they will be diagnosed with depression.

Be aware of the general moods of your patients. If a patient who is usually very chatty and content becomes quiet and withdrawn for a sustained period of time (see Figure 11.2), raise your concerns with your mentor and discuss whether the patient should be assessed for depression.

For a diagnosis of depression to be made, an assessment will seek to establish the symptoms, the duration, and the intensity. The Geriatric Depression Scale (GDS) (Sheikh and Yesavage, 1986) may be used as a screening device. A short example of the format and type of questions are given in Table 11.2; the full assessment is available online at http://www.stanford.edu/~yesavage/GDS.html

The reasons why older people are vulnerable to depression may be linked to several factors. The *Health Survey for England* (DH, 2007) found that those reporting depression were most

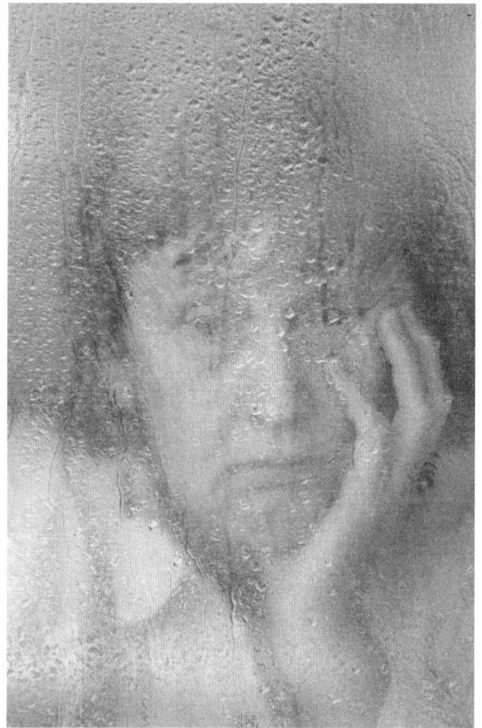

Figure 11.2 Be on the lookout for patients becoming quiet and withdrawn
Source: © Photodisc.

Table 11.2 Extract from Geriatric Depression Scale (GDS)

Choose the best answer for how you have felt over the past week:	Response
1. Are you basically satisfied with your life?	YES / NO
2. Have you dropped many of your activities and interests?	YES / NO
3. Do you feel that your life is empty?	YES / NO
4. Do you often get bored?	YES / NO
5. Are you in good spirits most of the time?	YES / NO
6. Are you afraid that something bad is going to happen to you?	YES / NO
7. Do you feel happy most of the time?	YES / NO
8. Do you often feel helpless?	YES / NO

Answers in bold indicate depression. Although differing sensitivities and specificities have been obtained across studies, for clinical purposes, a score of more than 5 points is suggestive of depression and should warrant a follow-up interview. Scores of more than 10 points are almost always indicative of depression.

- Source: Sheikh and Yesavage (1986).

likely to report long-standing illness and be from low-income household—particularly those in receipt of benefits dependent upon disability or means testing. Other factors include loneliness and bereavement. Depression may also be associated with medication being taken for physical health problems, such as cardiovascular disease, gastrointestinal disorders, hormone treatments, and many other medical conditions.

Providing nursing care

Psychological therapies—such as cognitive behavioural therapy (CBT), which aims to help people to change how they think (cognitive) and what they do (behaviour)—are effective for people with depression and may be of benefit to older depressed people (Wilson et al., 2008). The depressed person may need social support, such as help in claiming benefits. Support from family and friends may need to be established, and the patient may benefit from being put in contact with a social or support group. A person who is depressed following bereavement may benefit from attending a support group for bereaved people; alternatively, they may be encouraged to re-establish an interest or hobby.

Antidepressant medication is effective in the treatment of depression with older people, but care must be taken because of the possible side effects, such as sedation (making falls more likely) or impaired sexual functioning (Healy, 2009). Mottram et al. (2006) recommend selective serotonin reuptake inhibitors (SSRIs) as an effective treatment for depression in the older adult. However, it is important to consider whether the person is also being treated for other medical conditions. NICE (2009) guidelines make recommendations concerning different types of antidepressant for people who are being treated with long-term medical conditions.

Electroconvulsive therapy (ECT) is sometimes used in cases of severe depression—for example, when the patient is not eating or drinking, when there is a high suicide risk, or when antidepressant medication has not worked.

NURSING PRACTICE INSIGHT: DEPRESSION

- Spend short periods with the patient throughout the day. Your presence will be valued, so sitting in silence is not wasting time. Do not force cheerfulness and avoid platitudes such as 'Cheer up—things aren't that bad'. Use simple, concrete words, because the person's concentration and understanding will be slow. Listen to what the person is saying and watch for covert messages about suicide (see below). Severely depressed people will not want, or be able, to join in group activities, so spend time on a one-to-one basis with the person. As the patient's mood improves, they may be able to join in small group activities.
- Ensure that the patient gets adequate food and fluid; this may include high-protein fluids and frequent prompting may be needed. Small, frequent snacks will be better received than large meals. Monitor for constipation and assist with personal hygiene if necessary.
- Relatives may be asked to provide objects of personal comfort, such as slippers or photos.

Suicide

Although suicide rates have fallen in recent years, they remain high, with older men being most at risk (NMHDU, 2009). Identifying those at risk is an important factor in reducing suicide rates. The Royal College of Psychiatrists (2003) identified that social isolation, including living alone, was a risk factors. Other risk indicators include the following.

- Verbal
  - Expressing the wish to die
  - Talking about future events as if the patient will not be around to participate
- Behavioural
  - Hoarding medication
  - Making or changing a will
  - Putting one's affairs in order
  - Attending religious establishment or re-establishing religious faith
  - Self-neglect

- **Situational and symptomatic**
  - Sudden change in circumstances, such as the death of a close relative, retirement, or diagnosis of serious illness
  - Presence of depression (highly significant)
  - Sudden recovery from depression
  - Change in sleep and eating habits
  - Tension agitation or guilt
  - Isolating oneself

The *National Suicide Prevention Strategy for England* (DH, 2002a) identified that there was a need for better assessment and management of depression amongst older people.

Dementia and depression

Dementia and depression are commonly associated, but can be difficult to diagnose, because some of the symptoms of depression and dementia are the same—for example, forgetfulness. The coexistence of both conditions occurs frequently, and the existence of depression may make the dementia worse and increase the confusion, because the person is struggling with two sets of problems.

Depression with dementia is associated with a more rapid decline in function—particularly in relation to the activities of daily living—increased possibility of physical aggression, and higher likelihood of transfer to residential care. Assessment tools, such as the Cornell Scale for Depression and Dementia, may be used (Alexopoulos, 2002). Because people with dementia may give unreliable answers, the assessment is carried out using two semi-structured interviews: one with an informant (for example, a carer); and one with the patient. If there are any discrepancies, then the carer and patient are re-interviewed. Observation is also important, because the assessor's clinical impression forms part of the assessment.

Anxiety disorders

Generalized anxiety state

Anxiety often accompanies depression, although the two conditions may exist separately. Generalized anxiety disorder (GAD) is the most common anxiety disorder in older people and refers to anxiety that is not attached to a specific event or object. Anxiety can often accompany depression and dementia, although it may also exist on its own.

The symptoms of anxiety are varied and can be grouped as follows.

- **Mental state**
  - Worry
  - Poor concentration
  - Dissociative symptoms—that is, feeling disconnected from their environment
  - Fear (of going 'mad' or losing control)
- **Autonomic arousal**
  - Increased heart rate
  - Palpitations
  - Tremor
  - Muscle tension
  - Sweating
  - Nausea
  - Chest discomfort
  - Hyperventilation
- **Other**
  - Irritability
  - Poor sleep
  - Obsessions

Phobias

A phobia occurs when people have feelings of anxiety attached to a particular situation or object, even though they know that the situation or object cannot harm them. Anxiety is experienced when facing or anticipating a particular situation or object. Anxiety can be so great that the person experiences a panic attack.

The *International Classification of Diseases 10* (WHO, 2003) identifies three groups of phobia:

- agoraphobia;
- social phobia; and
- specific (isolated) phobias.

Agoraphobia includes the fear of going in public places and travelling alone. Social phobias include the fear of other people's scrutiny, leading to the avoidance of social situations, and specific phobias include specifics such as fear of closed spaces, heights, flying, blood, and certain animals. These phobias can result in avoidance behaviour and some people rarely get anxious if they can avoid the situation or object that they fear. However, avoidance can also lead to social isolation and loneliness. Phobic anxiety and depression often coexist.

Obsessive compulsive disorders

Obsessive compulsive disorders include obsessive thoughts and compulsive acts. Obsessive thoughts may take the form of endless rumination over usually unpleasant thoughts or images. Sometimes, people can see so many alternatives in a situation when a decision is to be made that they are unable to make it. Depression and obsessive ruminations are frequently linked. Compulsive acts usually involve repeated checking or ritual acts, such as washing hands. People rarely develop obsessive compulsive disorders in older age, but symptoms can come and go throughout life, and stress and life changes may exacerbate the condition.

Somatoform disorders

Somatoform disorders is a term that refers to patients who have frequently changing physical symptoms, but despite extensive investigations being carried out, nothing is found to be wrong with them. Anxiety and depression are often present. Sheehan et al. (2002) found that older people's somatoform symptoms decrease when anxiety and depression are treated. However, because older people do have more physical health problems, it can be difficult to separate often intertwined symptoms.

Providing nursing care

Medication in the form of anxiolytics may be prescribed to treat the symptoms of anxiety. Benzodiazepines may be prescribed, but they often cause confusion and sedation, which increase the possibility of falls. The risks to the older patient have to be considered against the possible benefits. Antidepressants may be prescribed and are often considered the treatment of choice for older people. NICE (2004) identifies that CBT is effective for people with anxiety.

NURSING PRACTICE INSIGHT: ANXIETY DISORDERS

When caring for an older person with an anxiety disorder, listen to the patient and acknowledge their anxiety. Be careful not to undermine the patient's feelings by telling them that they have nothing to worry about.

Relaxation techniques may benefit some people. There are many different techniques, but, in essence, the patient is taught to relax each major muscle group in turn and focus on their breathing, while listening to calming music. These simple-to-learn techniques can be of benefit to some patients.

A daily routine and activities that prevent a constant focus on problems can also help to reduce anxiety problems. Some anxious patients may have difficulty sleeping, so ensuring a peaceful environment is important.

Self-help advice and support in taking regular exercise may be of value, as might dietary advice concerning the elimination or reduction of caffeine and alcohol.

Bipolar affective disorder

Most older people who have a diagnosis of bipolar affective disorder (formerly known as 'manic depression') have had the diagnosis for many years. However, some 8–10 per cent of admissions to psychiatric hospitals are of older people for this condition (Depp and Jeste, 2004).

With bipolar disorder, people's moods move between depression and elation (mania). The symptoms of depression have been described above; with mania, the person's behaviour and mood is elated, and their behaviour is often extremely reckless. For example, they may become sexually disinhibited or overspend on a huge scale. Their speech is often very fast, they are full of energy, and they sleep very little. They may feel very important and have ideas of grandeur, and they may also be irritable or aggressive. When in a manic state, people with bipolar disorder may have delusions (fixed false beliefs) and hallucinations (often, they hear voices).

The diagnosis of bipolar disorder depends upon there being an episode of both depression and mania.

Providing nursing care

A number of different drugs may be prescribed for patients with bipolar disorder and some people may be prescribed more than one. Antipsychotic medication may be prescribed—particularly when the person is in a manic state. Lithium may be prescribed both to control the mania and as a mood stabilizer, and other medication may also be prescribed. Antidepressants may be given to treat the depression, and benzodiazepines prescribed short-term to deal with periods of mania and accompanying agitation.

Doses of medication for older people are lower than those given for younger people and particular care needs to be paid to people who are prescribed lithium, because toxicity can develop, so careful monitoring is required (Healy, 2009).

NURSING PRACTICE INSIGHT: BIPOLAR AFFECTIVE DISORDER

During periods of mania, the nurse may need to protect the person from engaging in hazardous behaviours.

Ensure that the older person gets adequate food and fluids.

As the mania subsides, people can often be embarrassed by their behaviour and support will be needed.

Schizophrenia

Most older people diagnosed with schizophrenia will have had the diagnosis for much of their adult life.

However, Arunpongpaisal et al. (2003) estimate that at least 0.1 per cent of the world's older population have a diagnosis of schizophrenia that started late in life. Late-onset schizophrenia is considered to start after the age of 40 and 'very late-onset schizophrenia-like psychosis' after the age of 60 (Howard et al., 2000). People who are diagnosed with 'very late-onset schizophrenia' tend to be female, have some sensory impairment (such as poor sight or poor hearing), often be socially isolated, and be poor.

For those people who have had a diagnosis of schizophrenia for much of their adult lives, the nurse should be aware that they are likely to have concurrent physical health problems. Social exclusion and poverty will have contributed to health problems—in particular, many people with serious mental health problems smoke, and are therefore likely to have high rates of respiratory and cardiovascular diseases. For these reasons, older people with schizophrenia are a particularly vulnerable group.

The symptoms of schizophrenia can be divided in to **positive** and **negative** symptoms.

- **Positive symptoms (that is, an excess or distortion of normal functions)**
  - Delusions (a fixed false belief)
  - Hallucinations (auditory, visual, smell, tactile (touch), and taste)
  - Thought disorder
- **Negative symptoms (that is, a loss of normal functions)**
  - Flat mood
  - Poverty of speech
  - Inability to experience pleasure
  - Lack of motivation

With late-onset schizophrenia and very late-onset schizophrenia, the main differences from schizophrenia seen in younger people tend to be that the delusions are often persecutory and that sufferers may, for example, be convinced that people are entering their home or stealing from them. Hallucinations may also be more sensory. The negative symptoms of schizophrenia are rarely present.

Providing nursing care

Treatment for schizophrenia-type disorders will include medication with antipsychotic medication, although with much lower doses than those given for younger adults. Antipsychotic medication can cause serious side effects and clients should be closely monitored (Healy, 2009). Specific psychological treatments, such as CBT with particular focus on delusional beliefs, may be appropriate. Social support, such as help with claiming benefits, may be required, alongside establishing support from friends and relatives, if possible. The person may benefit from attending a day centre for social activities to reduce social isolation.

NURSING PRACTICE INSIGHT: WORKING WITH OLDER ADULTS SUFFERING FROM DELUSIONS

When working with people suffering from delusions, the nurse should not reinforce those delusions by agreeing—but neither is it useful to argue. Focus on concrete realities. So, for example, if the patient says 'I don't want to talk to that nurse today, because she's planning on hurting me', the nurse might respond: 'The nurse has come to see you to discuss how you're feeling today. Perhaps you'll feel like speaking to her tomorrow'.

Provide structure for the patient by spending regular time with them. Practical support may be needed by protecting the person from harming themselves or others. Ensure that they have adequate food, fluids, and rest.

Case study

Mrs Carter is a widow aged 74 and has lived on her own for 12 years. She spent her working life in various jobs in factories and lives in a council house. She has a limited income and very little social life. She has three adult children, a son and two daughters, who left home for university and did not return to live in the area when they completed their studies. Her children do speak with her on the phone, but visit irregularly.

Mrs Carter's son had recently become concerned by some of the things that his mother had been saying on the phone. One evening, he received a phone call from the police to say that they had arrested his mother following a disturbance. She had thrown paint over her neighbour's car and broken the windscreen wipers, because she was angry about what they had been broadcasting about her on national television.

Following a mental health assessment, Mrs Carter was admitted to a mental health hospital and treated with a low dose of antipsychotic medication. She returned home four weeks later with support from the mental health team.

Alcohol

The problem of alcohol abuse among older people is an issue of growing concern. Older people are more likely to drink regularly and, in 2003, UK government figures showed that 28 per cent of men and 15 per cent of women aged 65 and over drank on five or more days in the week compared to 11 per cent of men and 7 per cent of women aged 16–24 (Evans et al., 2003).

About a third of older people with an alcohol problem have developed the problem in later life; others have grown old with an existing drink problem. Older people may develop problem drinking after bereavement, or due to social isolation and loneliness. In moderation, alcohol can improve the quality of people's lives, because it is often a social activity. However, due to the physiological changes occurring with age, older people are more susceptible to the effects of alcohol. Medication prescribed for other health problems may be affected by alcohol and the impact of balance being affected by alcohol may cause more damage than it would for younger people if a fall occurs. Alcohol may also make other problems worse, such as incontinence, insomnia, forgetfulness, and depression.

Identifying that an older person has a drinking problem can be difficult. If an older person lives alone and is not in work, then there may be fewer opportunities for identifying the problem. Screening tools for hazardous drinking including 'AUDIT', developed by the World Health Organization (WHO), and 'CAGE', which may be in use in the clinical area (McKenzie et al., 1986).

Providing nursing care

Care will be dependent on individual assessment, and may include detoxification and withdrawal; this would be carried out in hospital, although withdrawal from alcohol may also be an unexpected result of admission to hospital for other health problems. Medication during this period might include benzodiazepine and vitamin replacements. Not all problem drinkers are physically addicted to alcohol and many may benefit from interventions that aim to reduce alcohol intake. Referral to specialist alcohol misuse services should be made when hazardous drinking is identified. Support such as that provided by groups such as Alcoholics Anonymous may also be beneficial.

NURSING PRACTICE INSIGHT: DRINK PROBLEMS

It is important that nurses treat people with drink problems with the same respect as they do any other patient. Because most people with a drinking problem already feel bad about their behaviour, it is important that the nurse demonstrates a non-critical manner towards the patient with drink problems. This can help the patient to feel positive about effecting a change in their life.

Conclusion

Older people's mental health is often a complex interaction between their physical, psychological, and social environment. As the number of older people statistically increases, so too will the number of older people who have mental health problems. Nurses need to be prepared to respond positively to older adults with mental health problems, and they have an important role to play in the provision of care and the development of services.

Questions and self-assessment

Now that you have worked through the chapter, answer the following questions.

- Think about a situation in which you were involved in a mental health assessment of an older adult.
  - How might age have had an impact on the person's presentation of mental health problems?
  - How should age taken into consideration when care is planned?
- When working with a client who has been diagnosed with dementia:
  - what skills should you use to communicate effectively?
  - how would you demonstrate respect and maintain dignity of the person in your care?
  - how might you involve the patient's carers or relatives in assessment and care planning?
- Identify an older person with whom you have worked who developed delirium.
  - What changes in the person's behaviour made you suspect delirium?
  - What actions might the nurse take to reduce the likelihood of delirium occurring?

Self-assessment

- Having read the chapter, how will you change your practice?
- Identify up to four areas relating to older adult mental health in which you need to develop your knowledge and understanding further.
- Identify how you are going to develop this knowledge and understanding, and set deadlines for achieving this.

References

Alexopoulos, G. (2002) *The Cornell Scale for Depression in Dementia*, available online at http://www.afmc.us/Documents/quality_improve/depression/CornellScaleGuidelines.pdf.

Alzheimer's Research Trust, The (2010) *Dementia 2010*, available online at http://www.dementia2010.org/.

Alzheimer's Society (2009) *What is Dementia?*, available online at http://www.alzheimers.org.uk/site/.

Arunpongpaisal, S., Ahmed, I., Aqeel, N., and Paholpak, S. (2003) *Antipsychotic Drug Treatment for Elderly People with Late-onset Schizophrenia*, available online at http://www.cochrane.org/reviews/en/ab004162.html.

British Geriatric Society (2006) *Guidelines for the Prevention, Diagnosis and Management of Delirium in Older People in Hospital*, available online at http://www.bgs.org.uk/.

Department of Health (2001) *National Service Framework for Older People*, London: DH, available online at http://www.dh.gov.uk/prod_consum_dh/groups/dh_digitalassets/@dh/@en/documents/digitalasset/dh_4071283.pdf.

Department of Health (2002a) *National Suicide Prevention Strategy for England*, London: DH, available online at http://www.dh.gov.uk/en/Publicationsandstatistics/Publications/PublicationsPolicyAndGuidance/DH_4009474.

Department of Health (2002b) *The Single Assessment Process: Guidance for Local Implementation*, London: DH, available online at http://www.dh.gov.uk/en/SocialCare/Chargingandassessment/SingleAssessmentProcess/index.htm.

Department of Health (2005) *Making Safeguarding Everybody's Business*, London: DH, available online at http://www.dh.gov.uk/en/Consultations/Closedconsultations/DH_4114901.

Department of Health (2007) *The Health Survey for England 2005: Health of Older People*, London: DH, available online at http://www.dh.gov.uk/en/Publicationsandstatistics/PublishedSurvey/HealthSurveyForEngland/Healthsurveyresults/DH_635.

Department of Health (2009a) *Living Well with Dementia: A National Dementia Strategy*, London: DH, available online at http://www.dh.gov.uk/en/Publicationsandstatistics/Publications/PublicationsPolicyAndGuidance/DH_094058.

Department of Health (2009b) *Report on the Prescribing of Anti-psychotic Drugs to People with Dementia*, London: DH, available online at http://www.dh.gov.uk/en/Publicationsandstatistics/Publications/PublicationsPolicyAndGuidance/DH_108303.

Depp, C. and Jeste, D. (2004) 'Bipolar disorder in older adults', *Bipolar Disorders*, 6(5): 343–67.

Evans, O., Singleton, N., Meltzer, H., Stewart, R., and Prince, M. (2003) *The Mental Health of Older People*, London: HMSO.

Folstein, M.F., Folstein, S.E., and McHugh, P.R. (1975) 'Mini-mental state: A practical method for grading the cognitive state of patients for the clinician', *Journal of Psychiatric Research*, 12: 189–98.

Healy, D. (2009) *Psychiatric Drugs*, London: Churchill Livingstone

Holland, K. and Hogg, C. (2001) *Cultural Awareness in Nursing and Health Care*, London, Arnold.

Howard, R., Rabins, P.V., Seeman, M.V., and Jeste, D.V. (2000) 'Late-onset schizophrenia and very-late onset schizophrenia-like psychosis: An international consensus', *American Journal of Psychiatry*, 157: 172–8.

Katzman, R., Brown, T., Fuld, P., Peck, A., Schechter, R., and Schimmel, H. (1983) 'Validation of a short orientation-memory-concentration test of cognitive impairment', *American Journal of Psychiatry*, 140: 6.

Knapp, M., Comas-Herrer, A., Somani, A., and Banerjee, S. (2007) *Dementia International Comparisons Summary Report for the National Audit Office*, London: Personal Social Services Research Unit.

Mackenzie, D.M., Langa, A., and Brown, T.M. (1996) 'Identifying hazardous or harmful alcohol use in medical admissions: A comparisons of AUDIT, CAGE and BRIEF MAST', *Alcohol and Alcoholism*, 31(6): 591–9.

Mottram, P., Wilson, K., and Strobl, J.J. (2006) 'Antidepressants for depressed elderly',. *Cochrane Database of Systematic Reviews*, 1: Art. No. CD003491, DOI: 10.1002/14651858.CD003491.pub2, available online at http://www2.cochrane.org/reviews/en/ab003491.

National Audit Office (2010) *Improving Dementia Services in England: An Interim Report*, available online at http://www.nao.org.uk/publications/0910/improving_dementia_services.aspx.

National Institute for Health and Clinical Excellence (2004) *Clinical Guidelines for the Management of Anxiety*, available online at http://www.nice.org.uk/.

National Institute for Health and Clinical Excellence (2007) *Dementia: The NICE–SCI Guidelines on Supporting People with Dementia and Their Carers in Health and Social Care*, available online at http://www.nice.org.uk/nicemedia/pdf/CG42Dementiafinal.pdf.

National Institute for Health and Clinical Excellence (2009) *Depression in Adults with a Chronic Physical Problem: Treatment and Management*, available online at http://www.nice.org.uk/.

National Mental Health Development Unit (2009) *National Suicide Prevention Strategy: Annual Report on Progress 2008*, available online at http://www.nmhdu.org.uk/silo/files/national-suicide-prevention-strategy-for-england--annual-report-on-progress-2008.pdf.

Norman, I. and Ryrie, I. (2004) *The Art and Science of Mental Health Nursing*, Maidenhead: Open University Press

Royal College of Psychiatrists (2003) *Suicide in the Elderly*, available online at http://www.rcpsych.ac.uk/default.aspx?page=0.

Seehham, B., Philpot, M., and Banerjee S. (2002) 'Attributions of physical symptoms in patients of old age psychiatry services', *International Journal of Geriatric Psychiatry*, 17: 61–4.

Sheik, J.I. and Yesavage, J.A. (1986) 'Geriatric Depression Scale (GDS): Recent evidence and development of a shorter version', *Clinical Gerontologist*, 5: 265.

Wilson, K.C.M,, Mottram, P.G., and Vassilas, C.A. (2008) 'Psychotherapeutic treatments for older depressed people', *Cochrane Database of Systematic Reviews*, 1: Art. No. CD004853, DOI: 10.1002/14651858.CD004853.pub2, available online at http://www2.cochrane.org/reviews/en/ab004853.html.

World Health Organization (2003) *International Classification of Diseases and Related Health Problems 10*, available online at http://www.who.int/classifications/icd/en/.

Online Resource Centre

You can learn more about mental health and older people at the Online Resource Centre that accompanies this book:
http://www.oxfordtextbooks.co.uk/orc/hindle/

Learning disabilities and the older adult

Kim Scarborough

Learning outcomes

By the end of the chapter, you will be able to:

- understand what is meant by 'learning disabilities', and how patients and families view themselves;
- consider the right, values, and principles that underpin services for older people with learning disabilities;
- discuss the impact on older people's health of having a learning disability and the associated health risks;
- develop an awareness of the barriers experienced by older people with learning disabilities and how you might remove or reduce them;
- develop awareness of accessible information and be able to identify where such resources are found; and
- reflect on how nursing practice may need adapting to meet the needs of patients with learning disabilities.

Introduction

In many parts of the world, improvements in medicine and living conditions have meant that people are living longer and this includes people with learning disabilities (LD). Older people with LD have greater health needs than the general population. They have a higher incidence of epilepsy, physical disability, mental illness, and sensory loss (DH, 2001c), and physical illnesses can go undiagnosed, resulting in unmet health needs (DH, 2001c). Baxter et al. (2006) identified unmet health needs as including diabetes, hypertension, asthma, and cardiac and mental problems, while Lennox et al. (2007) added untreated sensory loss.

Poor diagnosis is linked to communication difficulties, poor health education, unequal access to health care, inadequate education of health professionals, and prejudice (DRC, 2004). The increased prevalence of certain illnesses in people with LD, coupled with these diagnosis issues, has lead to people with LD being four times more likely to die of a preventable cause than people without (Hollins et al., 1998). The *Death by Indifference* report (Mencap, 2007) recorded how Ted, a 61-year-old man with LD, had health needs that were unmet. Ted died because of what Mencap considered to be institutional discrimination within the National Health Service (NHS) against people with LD. The ensuing inquiry called for people with LD to receive equal access to health care without discrimination (Michael, 2008). Nurses have a role in making this happen.

Older people with LD can and do live full and active lives. They develop similar health issues as the general population, but morbidity and mortality rates differ (Hollins et al., 1998). Janicki et al. (1999) identified that, in the late 1970s, the average age at death for people with LD was 59 years old (54 years old for people with Down's syndrome). Today, people with LD who do not have the complex health needs associated, for example, with Down's syndrome will have life expectancy approaching that of their non-disabled peers (Janicki et al., 1999). Indeed, Hogg and Lambe (1998) reported that 50 per cent of people with LD will have a normal lifespan. However, people with Down's syndrome do experience earlier death, with average age of death being 57 years old for women and 54 years old for men—although people can survive into their 60s and 70s (Janicki et al., 1999).

Prevalence of LD is similar in North American, Australian, and European populations, as is increased longevity

(Emerson et al., 2001). Emerson et al. (2001) estimate that there are 1.2 million people with LD in the UK. There are generally more males than females, with the majority having mild to moderate LD.

Terminology

Learning disabilities are referred to by different terms. In the UK, the term 'learning disabilities' is used; internationally, the term 'intellectual disabilities' is accepted. This chapter will use the term 'learning disabilities' (LD), which is defined as having:

A significant intellectual impairment [...] with deficits in social functioning or adaptive behaviour [...] which is present from childhood.

(Emerson et al., 2001: 5)

Although the World Health Organization (2007) refers to 'mental retardation', many people with learning disabilities and their families consider this an offensive term. Self-advocates (that is, people with LD taking control of their own lives) often refer to themselves as having 'learning difficulties' and older family carers sometimes use the older term 'mental handicap'. Inappropriate language can cause barriers between the nurse, service user, and carer.

Definitions are challenged by people with LD. This is what are self-advocate says about learning disabilities:

Definitions of learning difficulties are based on the medical model of disability. They are about deficits and lack of abilities. We do not agree with these definitions. We think that definitions should be based on the social model. This means that it is how society treats a person that disables them. If people are given information in a way they understand they can make decisions, if the environment is accessible everyone can use it. If people do not judge people but get to know the person they can be part of their community. Learning difficulties means a person needs support to learn, time to understand, people who have empathy, money to get good support and to be accepted for who they are.

(Hyde, 2008)

Selman (2004) discusses the traditional, medical, social, and integrative models of disability.

Learning disabilities can be further subcategorized into 'mild', 'moderate', 'severe', and 'profound' (see Table 12.1). But accurately assessing the level of an individual's LD is complex, because people with LD have communication difficulties.

The British Institute of Learning Disabilities (BILD) offers further discussion of these categories online at http://www.bild.org.uk/05faqs_7.htm

Table 12.1 Subcategories of learning disabilities and possible impact on life

Mild and moderate learning disabilities	Severe and profound learning disabilities
• Specific communication needs • Health needs • Sensory impairments • Own home—independent living • Job • Married with a family • Some literacy skills • Minimum or specific support needs	• Complex communication needs • Complex associated health needs • Multiple sensory impairments • Physical impairments • Social and leisure needs • Support to build and maintain relationships • High support needs

Rights and principles

The *Montreal Declaration on Learning Disabilities* (Montreal PAHO/WHO Collaborating Centre, 2004) affirms that people with LD have the same rights and freedoms as all human beings, and states universal values that underpin society. The United Nations (UN) General Assembly published its Convention on the Rights of Persons with Disabilities in 2007. These reflect the values and principles present in many governmental and UK LD papers, such as *Valuing People* (DH, 2001c) and *Valuing People Now* (DH, 2009).

More information on the rights and principles outlined in these papers is presented in Box 12.1.

Upholding these values and principles is crucial in providing good health care. Their subjugation has contributed to poor health and the early death of individuals with LD (Mencap, 2007; Michael, 2008). Equality of treatment does not necessarily mean the 'same' treatment, and both Michael (2008) and the Disabilities Right Commission (2006) mention 'reasonable adjustment'. Reasonable adjustment means adapting how you communicate, giving information differently, supporting decision-making and consent, and giving the individual more time.

NURSING PRACTICE INSIGHT: UPHOLDING VALUES AND PRINCIPLES

As a nurse, you need to ensure that your ways of working are adjusted to ensure that older people with LD experience equal health outcomes. As a nurse, you have a professional responsibility to treat people with dignity and respect (NMC, 2008).

Box 12.1 Rights and principles

The Montreal Declaration on Intellectual Disabilities (Montreal PAHO/WHO Collaborating Centre, 2004) acknowledged cultural differences and stated the universal values of:

- dignity;
- self-determination;
- equality; and
- justice for all.

The UN Convention on the Rights of Disabled People (UN, 2007) stated principles of:

- respect and dignity;
- autonomy;
- choices;
- non-discrimination;
- equality;
- inclusion;
- participation; and
- accessibility.

The UK government's *Valuing People* (DH, 2001c) stated key principles of:

- rights;
- independence;
- choice; and
- inclusion.

Communication strategies and people with learning disabilities

Effective communication is essential in ensuring high-quality health care (Balandin and Hemsley, 2008) and is an essential skill for nurses (NMC, 2007). Because communication difficulties are a characteristic of people with LD, the nurse needs strategies that can be used to promote communication and understanding by removing barriers, and developing their skills and knowledge.

Common communication difficulties in health settings include the person with LD having:

- poor literacy skills;
- a limited vocabulary;
- poor comprehension and memory;
- ill health, impeding communication because of:
  - pain;
  - anxiety;
  - depression;
- a sensory loss impacting on communication;
- no understanding of the communication system (see box 12.2);
- atypical non-verbal language, such as (in relation to autism) limited eye contact;
- speech impediments; and
- the need for extended time in which to process language—meaning that they will perceive people as 'butting in'.

Nursing staff, meanwhile, may:

- not actively listen to individuals;
- not value information from carers;
- only pretend that they understand the individual;
- have poor skills in making information accessible;
- not be able to use a range of communication systems;
- lack experience and confidence;
- be under time constraints, resulting in rushed contacts;
- use jargon;
- be unaware of their own non-verbal language;
- have their own prejudices and discriminatory practices; and
- have only a limited understanding of capacity, consent, and best interest principles.

Within the healthcare environment, communication takes place in a variety of ways, with an expectation that it will be understood and no adjustment will be necessary. However, many of the ways in which we communicate may present barriers to people with LD, as Table 12.2 demonstrates.

Communication aids

People may use augmentative and alternative communication (AAC) methods, which are a range of low-tech and high-tech systems, strategies, and devices that either replace or enhance verbal communication. Although there is no expectation that nurses are skilled in all AACs, an awareness that they exist and a desire to develop skills should the need arise is required. The learning disabilities nurse is expected to have a deeper understanding of AACs.

Common AACs include:

- total communication (individual communication plan)—that is:
  - eye contact (eye pointing);
  - body language; and
  - gesture;
- communication passports (individual communication plan);
- real objects (for example, give your cup = get a drink);

Table 12.2 Barriers to effective communication experienced by people with learning disabilities

Communication system	Examples	Barrier	Strategies to overcome barrier
Written communication (Letters and pamphlets)	• Letters • Appointment details and instructions • Appointment cards • Information pamphlets • Health education materials • Specific health advice, including medication regimes and side effects	Complex information and complex language	Small amounts of information per short sentence Use pictures, photographs, photo stories Telephone call or text message on day of appointment
		Style and size of font	Large font (14 pt at least)
		Jargon	Telephone call to confirm letter received and understood
		Complex information	Bullet-pointed instructions
		Poor handwriting	Word process information to make it easy to read Develop accessible recording systems for people to track self-care
		Too much information on the page	Use accessible materials describing common illnesses and medication, and how to self-care (For examples, see websites)
		Not supported with pictures	Large card with graphics with picture of appointment location, date written '12 September 2008' (not '12.9.08'), photograph of clock set to time of appointment
Spoken communication (Initial)	• Booking in at reception	Limited time and noisy environment	Make space and time to talk in a quieter area
		System of queuing and waiting not flexible	Flexibility as to where the person should wait, how they will be called for their appointment, and length of wait
Written communication (Signage)	• Called for appointment • Use signage to find way	Signs use only words	Staff to escort people who are unable to read or follow directions
		Small signs	Photos on staffs doors
		Verbal directions complex	Colour-coded directions and rooms
		Staff rushed, with limited awareness of learning disabilities	Participate in awareness training
Spoken communication (Main)	• Verbal conversations about health and well-being	Negative past experiences not considered and uncertainty not catered for	An opportunity to visit health premises when well and ask questions about the environment Accessible documentation about environment Access plan for people who find new environments very challenging Break instruction into small steps Use gestures and give demonstrations to support understanding
		Use of health vocabulary including jargon, which may not be understood	Objects, your drawings, and photographs of body parts, including body map to which individual can refer Use Easy Read, with no jargon, and use different words if the person does not understand you
		Assuming that when a person says 'OK', it means that they understand	Use alternative and augmentative communication if used by individual (see website)
		Talks to carer due to limited verbal communication and appears to ignore the individual	Always talk to individual, but you may also need to use good observation skills and involve carers in health appointments
		Limited time to discuss health and treatment options	Allow double appointments or longer discussion time to discuss health and explore options

- objects of reference (for example, give a piece of towel = go swimming);
- photographs (for example, use photo to replace words and as prompts), including:
  - picture exchange communication systems; and
  - personal photos;
- picture charts (for example, pictures to represent a day's activities);
- alphabet charts (that is, point and spell);
- symbols, including:
  - Makaton; and
  - BLISS;
- sign language, including:
  - British sign language;
  - Makaton; and
  - finger spelling;
- TEACCH (that is, systems to provide structure in autism);
- computers, including:
  - for use with alphabet or picture charts; and
  - voice synthesizers;
- the written word—specifically, large fonts, and usually used with pictures or symbols.

See the Online Resource Centre that accompanies this book for more on finger spelling and examples of other AACs

Student activity

Have you used any AAC or seen a method used?

People with mild–moderate LD who have limited or no support rely on the nurse's communication skills to meet their information needs. Health information is often inaccessible (ECNI, 2007), but there are steps that can be taken to make information more accessible, including:

- lots of white space on the page;
- sans serif (that is, plain) fonts, such as Arial or Comic Sans;
- minimum 14-pt type size;
- pictures that are relevant, clear, and enhance understanding;
- easy words;
- bullet points; and
- colour, if possible.

Consent

Because informed consent is central to providing nursing care (NMC, 2008), the nurse is required to assume that everyone can give consent, and to develop skills to communicate and provide information in a way that enables understanding. Nurses must understand the consent laws of their country. Generally, consent is about decisions made following the presentation of information in a way that a person can understand, allowing time for questions and exploration of treatment options, and supporting the individual to reach their own decision. Capacity to consent should be assumed in people with LD, but for some individuals, capacity may need to be assessed.

When an adult is considered unable to give consent, it is good practice to involve advocates and significant others in making health decisions. However, it is the clinician who makes the final decisions based on the best interest of the individual. The UK Department of Health (2001b) has produced a document entitled *Seeking Consent: Working with People with Learning Disabilities*, which clarifies the points introduced above.

See Chapter 4 for more on the law and older people.

Life experiences

People with LD are now living ordinary lives, and many adults have jobs, get married, and have families. However, older people with LD may have had different life experiences from their non-disabled peers that have resulted in barriers to health, including the following.

- Segregated education with limited chances to learn to read, and an inability to use computers or the telephone, can result in poor access to health information. Individuals may have reduced health vocabulary. Limited health education or negative experiences of healthcare provision means that older people with LD may fail to recognize, or ignore, signs and symptoms of illness, resulting in late detection of treatable illnesses. These individuals need nurses with excellent observation skills, who listen and with whom they can develop a trusting relationship.
- Communal living carries its own risks: for example, an increased risk of having experienced abuse (Respond, 2007). Never having married or had children limits the number of family members who 'keep an eye' on people as they age. This increases vulnerability to abuse in care settings (Respond, 2007).

See Chapter 5 for more on care settings and adult protection.

- Many older people with LD live with ageing parents as their main carers. As parents develop age-related health problems, roles may be reversed, with people with LD becoming their parents' carers. Concern over the future can affect all of the family, and if a parent dies, the individual may experience loneliness when they live on their own.

With changes in education, employment, access to information, and support to be independent, such as travel training and supported living, these barriers are being reduced. During any period of transition, the nurse needs to understand the older person's life and give support as appropriate to the individual.

Causes of learning disability, and effect on health and ageing

Because older people with LD are not a homogeneous group, understanding the differences in health and ageing is complex. With this in mind, it is essential to work in person-centred ways during assessment, planning, implementing, and evaluating health interventions. Having a learning disability increases health risks (DH, 2001c), but does not mean that ill health is inevitable. Most people with LD will not have a diagnosis of the cause of the LD, but if a specific diagnosis is made, it can highlight susceptibility to specific health issues—for example, a person with Down's syndrome is at higher risk of thyroid problems. Some common diagnoses linked to having LD are listed in Box 12.2. Diagnoses such as cerebral palsy or foetal alcohol syndrome may not result in the individual having a learning disability, but higher risks of co-morbidity exist. A diagnosis such as Down's syndrome can result in mild to profound disabilities. Therefore, a diagnosis does not indicate the level of LD.

Box 12.2 Diagnoses linked to possible learning disabilities

- Autism
- Cerebral palsy
- Down's syndrome
- Fragile X
- Patau's syndrome
- Rett's syndrome
- Williams syndrome
- Prader-Willi syndrome
- Tuberous sclerosis
- Foetal alcohol syndrome
- Cockayne's syndrome

NURSING PRACTICE INSIGHT: DO YOUR RESEARCH

If you know the specific diagnoses of an individual's learning disability, access websites maintained by support groups such as SCOPE (cerebral palsy) or Down's syndrome associations, which provide excellent information on associated health risks.

Common higher health risks for people with learning disabilities

People with LD have a higher risk of developing a range of health problems (see Box 12.3 below). Many will age earlier than their non-disabled peers (Hatzidimitriadou and Milne, 2005). The primary causes of death among the UK's general population are heart disease and cancer. The primary cause of death in people with LD is respiratory disease; the secondary cause is heart disease, and deaths from cancer are rising with increased life expectancy (Hollins et al., 1998). People with LD have a higher risk of developing dementia, with the mean age at onset being 67 in people with LD and 53 in people with Down's syndrome.

Box 12.3 Health risks for older people with learning disabilities

Hatzidimitriadou and Milne (2005)

- Dementia
- Heart disease
- Alzheimer's
- Mental ill health—particularly depression and anxiety
- Sight and hearing impairment
- Pulmonary disease
- Rheumatic illness
- Arthritis

Janicki et al. (2002)

- Falls
- Obesity

Barr et al. (1999)

- Dental decay (untreated)

Van Shrojenstein Lantiman-de Valk et al. (1997)

- Epilepsy
- Gastric and oesophageal problems

Aspray et al. (1998)

- Osteophrosis

To manage higher health risks, health screening is essential in monitoring health because people with LD may not be able to self-report health changes (DHA, 2007; NHS, 2008). In the UK, health screening occurs at GP surgeries and includes:

- **A review of physical and mental health with referral through the usual practice routes if health problems are identified:**
  - **health promotion**

- chronic illness and systems enquiry
- physical examination
- epilepsy
- behaviour and mental health
- specific syndrome check

- **a check on the accuracy of prescribed medications**
- **a review of coordination arrangements with secondary care**
- **a review of transition arrangements where appropriate.**

(NHS, 2008: 5–6).

Some people with LD have a health action plan (HAP) (that is, an individual plan explaining a person's health needs) or a care plan. These may contain health information, records of health appointments or medication, and health goals, as well as instructions for providing person-centred care. These can be a useful resource not only for providing consistency across health settings, but also for discussing health with an individual. An HAP may also contain information about health risks associated with specific diagnoses.

Dementia and people with learning disabilities

People with LD have a higher incidence of dementia and it occurs at an earlier age—for example, at age 50–64, 13 per cent in the LD population compared with only 1 per cent in the non-LD population have dementia (Kerr, 2007). Diagnosis can be complex due to deterioration being attributed to LD unless a baseline assessment has been completed for comparison. The mini-mental state examination (MMSE) used to assess indicators for dementia is not reliable with this group, so the 'dementia in mental retardation' (DMR) and 'dementia scale for Down's syndrome' (DSDS) are effective tools for all people with LD (Strydom and Hassiotis, 2003).

With early detection, appropriate support and education can be given to the individual, their carers, and co-residents, making it more likely that they can remain at home rather than move to an older person's facility (Wilkinson et al., 2004).

Down's syndrome

Down's syndrome is a well-researched genetic condition caused by differences in chromosome pair 21. Individuals are predisposed to a range of associated health risks (Box 12.4), with increased age related to higher risks of dementia and thyroid disease. The Alzheimers Society (2010) reports that 54.5 per cent of people with Down's syndrome have dementia at age 60–69 years. At autopsy, all people with Down's have brain changes typical of Alzheimer's, but not all individuals develop the characteristics associated with Alzheimer's whilst alive.

Diagnosing dementia in people with Down's is hampered further because thyroid disease can be misdiagnosed as normal old-age decline or dementia and left untreated (Kerr, 2007).

Box 12.4 Health risks associated with Down's syndrome (Prasher and Janicki, 2002)

- Heart problems
- Respiratory illness
- Thyroid disease
- Sight impairment and cataracts
- Ear infections and hearing impairment
- Atlanto-instability
- Obesity
- Alzheimer's
- Depression
- Eczema

Regular health screening for the health issues identified in Box 12.4 should be completed. Baseline assessments for dementia should be completed around the person's 35th birthday, because people can develop Alzheimer's as young as the age of 40. The 2gether NHS Foundation Trust (2006) uses the DMR as one screening tool in its care pathway (see Figure 12.1) and, once referred, people are screened every five years to detect, for example, Alzheimer's disease.

Cerebral palsy

Cerebral palsy (CP) has no single cause and is not a cause of learning disabilities, but people with learning disabilities can have CP. Possible causes include maternal infection during pregnancy, premature birth, abnormal foetal brain development, and trauma at or shortly after birth. The outcome is that messages from the brain to the body are impaired.

People with CP experience early onset of ageing (Hogg et al., 2000). As individuals with LD and CP age, they experience musculature and skeletal deterioration due to the long-term effects of living with physical disabilities. Common problems associated with ageing with CP need to be carefully managed, and include pain, incontinence, arthritis, spasms, gastrointestinal problems, and epilepsy (Scope, 2007).

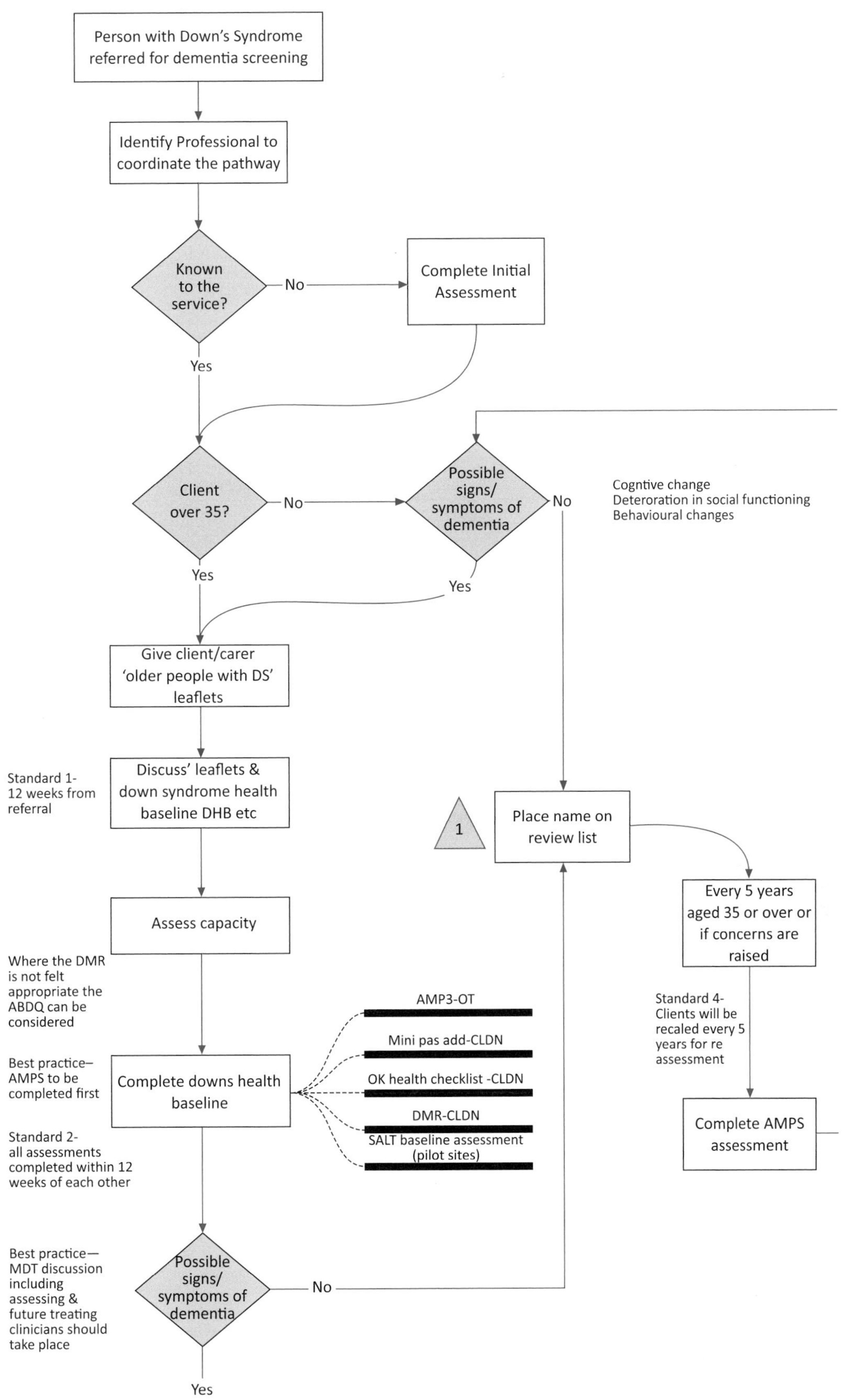

Figure 12.1 Care pathway for dementia and people with Down's syndrome
Source: 2gether NHS Foundation Trust (2006).

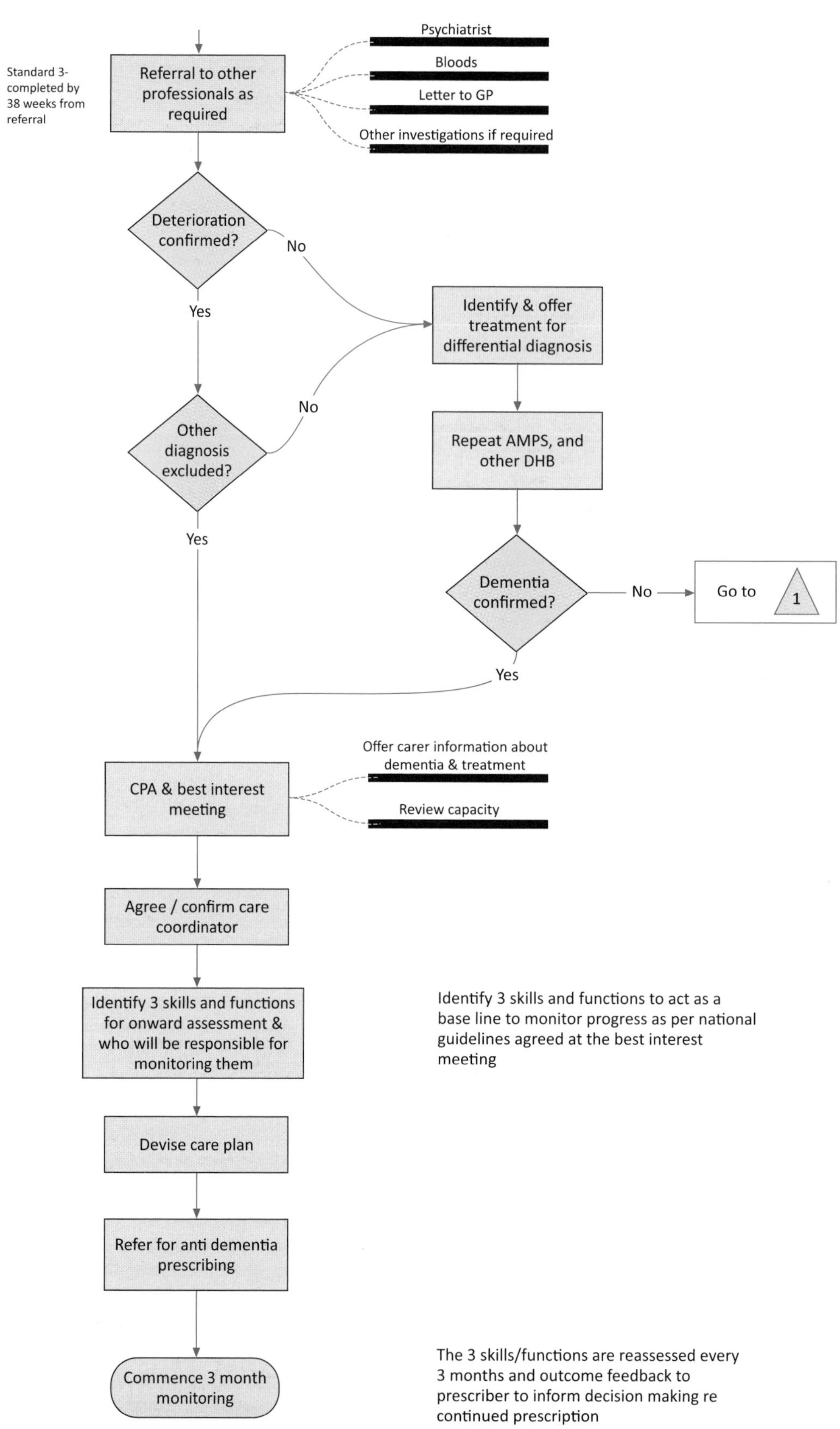

Figure 12.1 *(Continued)* Care pathway for dementia and people with Down's syndrome
Source: 2gether NHS Foundation Trust (2006).

Significant issues for people with CP discussed by SCOPE (2007) include polypharmacy, poor posture, and dysphagia.

- Polypharmacy occurs when people receive medication for muscle tightness, pain, constipation, epilepsy, and gastrointestinal problems. Health assessments should include a full medication review to ensure that the side effects of taking multiple drugs are not negatively impacting on the individual's life.
- Poor postural management leads to deterioration in body symmetry. This can be managed with safe sleeping, swallowing, moving, and seating positions agreed in a person-centred physiotherapy plan. This often requires specialist equipment and the nurse needs to understand its correct use. Increasingly, families and carers are experts in relation to posture management and the 'I Got Life' self-care package is an excellent resource (PCSP UK Ltd, 2006). When people with CP experience skeleton and muscle changes, their health becomes compromised. As the spine develops a scoliosis, the spinal cord can be compressed and the risk of pressure sores increases (Rapp and Torres, 2002). Such complex changes increase the risk of pain, urinary infections, and skin problems.
- Dysphagia can occur, resulting in repeated chest infections as food and drink is aspirated. Any swallowing difficulties need rapid assessment by the speech and language therapist, who is able to develop safe eating and drinking protocols for the individual. There has been an increase in the use of enteral nutrition, and this is contributing to improvements in nutrition and hydration for people with dysphagia.
  See Chapter 14 for further information on enteral feeding.

NURSING PRACTICE INSIGHT: MAINTAINING POSTURAL CARE

If your patient has physical impairments, ask if they have a postural care plan, or a safe eating and drinking plan. If they have one, ask the carers to explain it to you, so that you give consistency in maintaining postural care.

Pain management

Health screening should include pain monitoring and management. It is a myth that people with LD have high pain thresholds compared to the general population. Accepting behaviour change (which may occur because the person is in pain, but cannot express this in any other way) as something that happens because the person has LD is known as 'diagnostic overshadowing' (that is, when presenting symptoms are considered part of their learning disability). Negative assumptions about disability and ageing prevent changes being fully investigated, resulting in appropriate assessment and treatment not being undertaken. Diagnostic overshadowing and myth can result in inadequate pain control.

Good communication and observation skills, and the involvement of people who know the individual with LD, improve pain management (Kerr et al., 2006). A useful tool for monitoring distress and identifying possible causes, such as pain, is the Disability Distress Assessment Tool (DISDAT) (St Oswalds Hospice NTW NHS, 2005).

Health initiatives and meeting the needs of people with learning disabilities

National Service Frameworks (NSFs) and health guidance may make reference specifically to meeting the needs of older people with LD, but this is not always explicit. While *Our Health, Our Care, Our Say* (DH, 2006) refers to health inequalities and people with LD, the *National Service Framework for Older Persons* (NSFOP) (DH, 2001a)—especially Standard 6 on 'Falls'—does not discuss issues of falls and people with LD. Diagnostic overshadowing can result in people thinking that it is normal for older people with LD to fall, so having their needs stated is important in overcoming these issues. Specific needs, such as earlier ageing, including sight impairments, effects of epilepsy, and higher risk of osteoporosis, and difficulties in self-reporting for older people with LD are also not considered explicitly in the NSFOP (Aspray et al., 1998).

The nurse's role in supporting people with LD to have equal access to health services may mean speaking up for individuals and ensuring that their needs are not forgotten.

Challenges in services for older people with learning disabilities

Learning disability services are changing with the reduction of institutional care, and increase in community and person-centred care. Papers have been produced worldwide driving change for older people with LD, but few come with the necessary resources to implement change (Bigby, 2008). Meanwhile, people with LD are ageing and health staff are unprepared for how their needs can be meet (DRC, 2006; Michael, 2008).

Nursing

The challenge is to ensure that health staff are skilled in delivering equitable care, and the *Healthcare for All* report (Michael, 2008) recommended that LD training be made compulsory in all pre- and post-qualified nurse education programmes. In addition, the role of the LD nurse in co-working with other health professionals to support equality of health outcomes for people with LD means that the LD nurse needs to develop skills in interprofessional working and teaching.

Person-centred planning

Older people with LD often live with family members. Services for people with LD are a mix of specialist LD services, older person's services, primary care, and community health services. Ensuring that people receive the service most appropriate for them can be problematic, resulting in reduced quality of life (Wilkinson et al., 2004). The use of best practice in person-centred planning (that is, planning based on principles of inclusion from the social model of disability) in placement planning helps to overcome these problems (SCIE, 2005). This involves the individual, family members, friends, and services in developing a plan of what the person wants and needs as they age. Such person-centred planning empowers individuals to get the life that they want.

Specialist services for people with learning disabilities

A range of specialist services exist for people with LD in the UK, although the milder the LD, the less likely the person is to be in contact with services.

- Community learning disability teams (CLDTs)

  These include specialist nurses, consultants, speech therapists, occupation therapists, physiotherapists, psychologists, social workers, and others who provide support to individuals and families, and increasingly to healthcare professionals and support staff.

- Specialist support teams

  These teams usually specialize in specific areas, such as challenging behaviour, mental health support, and profound disabilities. In Ireland, there are older people's teams being developed.

- Liaison nurses

  These LD nurses are employed to improve access to primary and secondary care, and can be involved in admissions and discharge planning.

Although ageing earlier, people with LD report the importance of continuing to have meaningful day occupation (FPLD, 2002). This is easier if they remain in a locality with which they are familiar. Wilkinson et al. (2004) discuss models of service provision, from 'ageing in place', to 'in-place progression', and finally 'referral out'.

- Ageing in place means supporting the individual with LD to stay in their own home, whether that is independent living accommodation, the family home, or residential care. This is the preferred model.
- Progression in-place means staying with the same service provider, but moving to an area able to provide more intensive support.
- Referral out means being referred to older people services and is the least preferred option.

It is important that, whichever option is taken, the older person maintains relationships with friends and family, and, wherever possible, stability in occupation.

Case study

Clare is a 62-year-old lady with Down's syndrome. Clare has come to accident and emergency (A&E) after a fall. The care staff where she lives have reported that she has started wandering around, appears more confused, and that her behaviour has changed. Clare seems upset and uncooperative.

- What might be causing Clare to be upset and uncooperative?
- Outline possible communication strategies that might be useful.
- What might Clare have in place to help in her initial assessment?
- List who might be involved in an initial assessment.

Clare's parents visit her in hospital, where she is booked for a hip X-ray. They report that she has not had a physical examination for at least four years, but did have a dementia screen four years ago and everything was fine. They say that Clare is not her 'usual self' and seems unhappy.

- Describe the possible causes of Clare's change in behaviour.
- How will you identify higher risks of health issues for Clare?
- What advice might you give care staff about health screening as Clare ages?

A staff nurse with whom you are working thinks that Clare is being awkward. She says that all older people with Down's syndrome are uncooperative and that there is nothing wrong with Clare.

- How might diagnostic overshadowing impact on Clare's health care?
- List people to whom you would go for support if you were to feel that diagnostic overshadowing or negative attitudes existed.

- List five practical things that you could do when caring for an individual with learning disabilities to improve communication.
- Look at your list and identify one thing that you need to learn to implement your list and make an action plan to meet your learning needs.

Conclusion

People with learning disabilities have higher health needs than their non-disabled peers and experience health inequalities. Upholding people's rights by ensuring that nurses work within the values of dignity, self-determination, equality, and justice will do much in removing such inequalities. Effective communication is the key to good health, and the promotion of self-care and consent. Nurses are well placed to support individuals to better understand their health, and to develop skills and confidence to use the healthcare provision that is available for all.

Questions and self-assessment

Now that you have worked through the chapter, answer the following questions.

- Think about the language of disability. Why is it important to use the same language as the family or individual uses to describe themselves?
- Identify possible barriers experienced by people with learning disabilities when accessing health care.
- What is 'diagnostic overshadowing'?
- Explain how diagnostic overshadowing can impact on an older person with learning disabilities.
- State four differences in life experiences that can result in health inequalities for people with learning disabilities.
- List five higher health risks that people with learning disabilities experience.
- Describe useful communication strategies when working with people with learning disabilities.

Self-assessment

- Having read the chapter, how will you change your practice?

References

2gether NHS Foundation Trust Gloucestershire (2006) *Downs Syndrome and Dementia Screening Pathway*, Gloucester: 2gether NHS Foundation Trust.

Alzheimer's Society (2010) *Learning Disabilities and Dementia*, available online at http://alzheimers.org.uk/site/scripts/documents_info.php?categoryID=200137&documentID=103&pageNumber=1.

Aspray, T.J., Francis, R.M., Thompson, A., Quilliam, S.J., Rawlings, D.J., and Tyrer, S.P. (1998) 'Comparison of ultrasound measurements at the heel between adults with mental retardation and control subjects', *Bone*, 22(6): 665–8.

Balandin, S. and Hemsley, B. (2008) 'Intellectual disabilities, ageing and communication', Systematic review paper presented at the International Association for the Scientific Study of Intellectual Disability (IASSID) Congress, Cape Town, *Journal of Intellectual Disability Research*, 52(8/9): 642.

Barr, O., Gilgunn, J., Kane, T., and Moore, G. (1999) 'Health screening for people with learning disabilities by a community learning disability service in Northern Ireland', *Journal of Advanced Nursing*, 29: 1482–91.

Baxter, H., Lowe, K., Houston, H., Jones, G., Felce, D., and Kerr, M. (2006) 'Previously unidentified morbidity in patients with intellectual disability', *British Journal of General Practice*, 56: 93–8.

Bigby, C. (2008) 'Comparative issues in the development of policy and programmes for people with intellectual disabilities who are ageing: The state of the science', Paper presented the International Association for the Scientific Study of Intellectual Disability (IASSID) Congress, Cape Town, *Journal of Intellectual Disability Research*, 52(8/9): 624.

Department of Health (2001a) *National Service Framework for Older People*, London: DH, available online at http://www.dh.gov.uk/prod_consum_dh/groups/dh_digitalassets/@dh/@en/documents/digitalasset/dh_4071283.pdf.

Department of Health (2001b) *Seeking Consent: Working with People with Learning Disabilities*, available online at http://www.dh.gov.uk/en/Publicationsandstatistics/Publications/PublicationsPolicyAndGuidance/DH_4007861.

Department of Health (2001c) *Valuing People: A New Strategy for Learning Disability for the 21st Century*, London: HMSO.

Department of Health (2006) *Our Health, Our Care, Our Say*, available online at http://www.dh.gov.uk/prod_consum_dh/groups/dh_digitalassets/@dh/@en/documents/digitalasset/dh_4127459.pdf.

Department of Health (2009) *Valuing People Now: A New Three-year Strategy for People with Learning Disabilities*, available online at http://www.dh.gov.uk/prod_consum_dh/groups/dh_digitalassets/documents/digitalasset/dh_093375.pdf.

Department of Health and Ageing (Australia) (2007) *Medicare Health Assessment for People with Intellectual Disabilities*, available online at http://www.health.gov.au/internet/main/publishing.nsf/Content/3D3DA75E129B47A6CA25771F000B63EA/$File/6461%281004%29%20Medicare%20Health%20Assessments%20Factsheet%206-%20Intellectual%20Disability%20SCREEN.pdf.

Disability Rights Commission (2004) *You Can Make a Difference: Improving Hospital Services for Disabled People*, available online at http://www.dh.gov.uk/en/Publicationsandstatistics/Lettersandcirculars/Dearcolleagueletters/DH_4084243.

Disability Rights Commission [now Equality and Human Rights Commission] with the Sainsbury Centre for Mental Health (2006a) *Formal Investigation into the Physical Health Experienced by People with Mental Health Problems and People with Learning Disabilities*, available online at http://www.scmh.org.uk/results.aspx?cx=016848078521504535379%3Avigfmqlo5rg&cof=FORID%3A11%3BNB%3A1&q=Formal+Investigation+into+the+Physical+Health+Experienced+by+People+with+Mental+Health+Problems+and+People+with+Learning+Disabilities%2C&sa.x=33&sa.y=11&sa=Search.

Duff, M., Hoghton, M., Scheepers, M., Cooper, M., and Baddeley, P. (2001) 'Helicobacter pylori: Has the killer escaped from the institution? A possible cause of increased stomach cancer in a population with learning disabilities', *Journal of Intellectual Disability Research*, 45: 219–25.

Emerson, E., Hatton, C., Felce, D., and Murphy, G. (2001) *Learning Disability: The Fundamental Facts*, London: Mental Health Foundation.

Equality Commission Northern Ireland (2007) *Formal Investigation: The Accessibility of Health Information in Northern Ireland for People with a Learning Disability*, Belfast: ECNL.

Foundation for People with Learning Disabilities (2002) *Today and Tomorrow: Report of the Growing Older with Learning Disabilities Programme*, London: FPLD.

Hatzidimitriadou, E. and Milne, A. (2005) 'Planning ahead: Meeting the needs of older people with intellectual disabilities in the UK', *Dementia*, 4: 341–55.

Hogg, J. and Lambe, J. (1998) *Older People with Learning Disabilities: A Review of the Literature on Residential Services and Family Care Giving*, London: Mental Health Foundation.

Hogg, J., Lucchino, R., Wang, K., Janicki, M.P., and Working Group (2000) *Healthy Ageing: Adults with Intellectual Disabilities—Ageing and Social Policy*, Geneva: WHO.

Hollins, S., Attard, M.T., von Fraunhofer, N., McGuigan, S., and Sedgwick, P. (1998) 'Mortality in people with learning disability: Risks, causes and death certification findings in London', *Developmental Medicine and Child Neurology*, 40(1): 50–6.

Hyde, T. (2008) *People with Learning Difficulties as Health Trainers*, Paper presented at Galaxy of Health Trainers Conference, Taunton, March.

Janicki, M.P., Dalton, A.J., Henderson, C.M., and Davidson, P.W. (1999) 'Mortality and morbidity among older adults with intellectual disability: Health services considerations', *Disability and Rehabilitation*, 21(5/6): 284–94.

Janicki, M.P., Davidson, P.W., Henderson, C.M., McCallion, P., Taets, J.D., Force, L.T., Sulkes, S.B., Frangenberg, E., and Ladrigan, P.M. (2002) 'Health characteristics and health service utilization in older adults with intellectual disabilities living in community residences', *Journal of Intellectual Disabilities Research*, 46(4): 287–98.

Kerr, D. (2007) *Understanding Learning Disability and Dementia*, London: Jessica Kingsley.

Kerr, D., Cunningham, C., and Wilkinson, H. (2006) *Responding to the Pain Experiences of People with Learning Difficulties and Dementia*, York: Joseph Rowntree Foundation.

Lennox, N., Bain, C., Rey-Conde, T., Purdie, D., Bush, R., and Pandeya, N. (2007) 'Effects of a comprehensive health assessment programme for Australian adults with intellectual disability: A cluster randomized trial', *International Journal of Epidemiology*, 36(1): 139–46.

Mencap (2007) *Death by Indifference*, available online at http://www.mencap.org.uk/case.asp?id=14970.

Michael, J. (2008) *Healthcare for All: Independent Inquiry into Access to Healthcare for People with Learning Disabilities*, Commissioned by Department of Health, available online at http://www.dh.gov.uk/prod_consum_dh/groups/dh_digitalassets/@dh/@en/documents/digitalasset/dh_106126.pdf.

Montreal Pan American Health Organization/World Health Organization Collaborating Centre (2004) *Montreal Declaration on Intellectual Disabilities*, available online at http://conferencemontreal2004paho-who.com/english/declaration.htm.

National Health Service (2008) *Clinical Directed Enhanced Services (DES) Guidance for GMS Contract: Delivering Investment in General Practice—Appendix 3*, London: NHS.

Nursing and Midwifery Council (2007) *Essential Skill Clusters Pre-registrations*, London: NMC.

Nursing and Midwifery Council (2008) *The Code: Standards of Conduct, Performance and Ethics for Nurses and Midwives*, London: NMC.

PCSP (UK) Ltd (2006) *I Got Life! Families in Control: Complex and Continuing Healthcare Needs*, available online at http://www.posturalcareskills.com/.

Prasher, V.P. and Janicki, M. (2002) *Physical Health of Adults with Intellectual Disabilities*, Oxford: Blackwell.

Rapp, C. and Torres, M (2002) Cerebral Palsy in Prasher, VP. Janicki, M. (2002) *Physical Health of Adults with Intellectual Disabilities*, Oxford: Blackwell.

Respond (2007) *People with Learning Disability: An Ageing Population*, available online at http://www.respond.org.uk/support/resources/articles/people_with_learning_disabilities-_an_ageing_population.html.

Scope (2007) *An Introduction to Ageing and Cerebral Palsy*, Milton Keynes: Scope.

Selman, K. (2004) 'Trends in rehabilitation and disability: Transition from a medical model to an integrative model', *Disability World*, 22, available online at http://www.disabilityworld.org/01-03_04/access/rehabtrends1.shtml.

Social Care Institute for Excellence (2005) *Practice Guide 04: Adult Placements and Person-centred Approaches for People with Learning Disabilities*, London: SCIE.

St Oswald's Hospice, Northumberland Tyne and Wear NHS (2005) *The Disability Distress Assessment Tool (DISDAT Tool)*, available online at http://www.mencap.org.uk/document.asp?id=1476&audGroup=&subjectLevel2=&subjectId=&sorter=1&origin=pageType&pageType=112&pageno=&searchPhrase=.

Strydom, A. and Hassiotis, A. (2003) 'Diagnostic instruments for dementia in older people with intellectual disability in clinical practice', *Ageing & Mental Health*, 7(6): 431–7.

United Nations (2007) *Convention on the Rights of People with Disabilities*, available online at http://www.un.org/disabilities/default.asp?navid=13&pid=150.

Van Shrojenstein Lantiman-de Valk, H., Van den Akker, M., Maaskant, M., Havenman, M., Urlings, H., Kessels, A., and Crebolder, H. (1997) 'Prevalence and incidence of health problems in people with intellectual disability', *Journal of Intellectual Disability Research*, 41(1): 42–51.

Wilkinson, H., Kerr, D., Cunningham, C., and Rae, C. (2004) *Support for People with Learning Difficulties in Residential Settings Who Develop Dementia*, York: Joseph Rowntree Foundation.

World Health Organization (2007) *International Statistical Classification of Diseases and Related Health Problems (ICD 10)*, 10th Revn, available online at http://www.who.int/classifications/apps/icd/icd10online/.

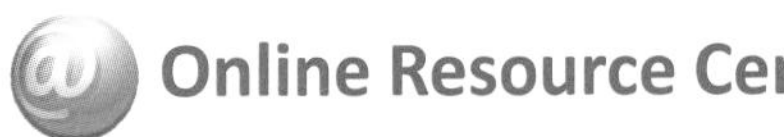

Online Resource Centre

You can learn more about learning disabilities and older people at the Online Resource Centre that accompanies this book:

http://www.oxfordtextbooks.co.uk/orc/hindle/

Nutrition and fluids

June Copeman

Learning outcomes

By the end of this chapter, you should be able to:

- use the Eat Well Plate to encourage healthy eating among older people;
- appreciate the importance of nutritional screening and dietary assessment, and their role in the detection of malnutrition;
- understand why older people may be at risk of developing malnutrition, the negative consequences, and the interventions to prevent malnutrition;
- adopt a systematic approach to nutrition interventions for individual clients, including those with multiple eating difficulties; and
- identify physical signs of dehydration, their possible consequences, and implement practical steps to ensure that an older person is hydrated.

Introduction

Nutrition is the study of food—its composition, selection, consumption, and utilization within the body. It considers the impact of the types and quantities of food eaten on the individual and their general health.

Being 'nutritionally healthy' means that someone is eating a sufficient variety and quantity of food and drink to meet their nutritional needs. If someone consumes too much or too little over a period of time, this nutritional balance is disturbed, and the person either becomes overweight or underweight and malnourished.

Food and nutrition is important in all stages of life, and is key to health, healing, and general well-being, but many older people are not able to consume an adequate variety of food to ensure optimal nutritional health. This situation is influenced by economic, social, and physical factors, such as low income, poor housing, chronic disease, and restricted support networks.

In spite of repeated government initiatives, reports, research, nutrition interventions, and media stories, there are a significant number of older people in the UK who continue to be malnourished (DH, 1992; Lennard-Jones, 1992; Bond, 1997; HAS, 1998; DH, 2000; DH, 2001b; Age Concern, 2006; NICE, 2006a).

The role of the nurse in prioritizing nutrition in the care of patients has been highlighted in the Royal College of Nurses (RCN) campaign *Nutrition Now*, launched in 2008 (RCN, 2008) with the following core messages.

- Nutrition and hydration are essential to care, as vital as medication and other types of treatment.
- It is our responsibility as members of a multi-disciplinary team to ensure patients in our care have the right nutrition and hydration at the right time.
- Working practices that prioritize nutrition and hydration can overcome the challenges that stand in the way of excellence.

Nutrition consequences of normal ageing

Ageing is associated with a degeneration of functional capacity in all parts of the body and at all levels of organization within

Table 13.1 Age-related changes impacting on nutrition

Change related to ageing	Consequence/risk	Impact on nutrition or hydration
Reduction in ratio of lean body mass to fat	Lower basal metabolic rate Deterioration in muscle function affecting physical fitness and strength and respiratory and circulatory systems	Reduced energy requirements Reduced ability to shop and prepare food
Increased rate of bone resorption	Reduction in bone strength and mass with increased risk of osteoporosis (see National Osteoporosis Society online at http://www.nos.org.uk/)	Requirement to consume adequate calcium
Atrophy of the mucosal and muscle layers throughout the gut, shorter intestinal villi	Less surface area for absorption of nutrients Increased susceptibility to intestinal infections Reduced gut motility Reduction in gastric acid secretion	Risk of nutritional deficiencies Constipation Reduced iron absorption
Reduced efficiency of immune system	Increased susceptibility to infection and delayed recovery	
Decrease in senses of smell, taste, and sight	Reduced enjoyment of food Increased risk of consumption of stale food	Increased salt intake

Source: Webb and Copeman (1996).

the body, from cells to complete organ systems. The rate of this degeneration varies between parts of the body and between people, being influenced by genetic and environmental factors. Table 13.1 outlines age-related changes of particular importance to the general nutrition of older people.

Hydration and fluid consequences of normal ageing

Mild dehydration is common among older people and is often not recognized or considered significant (Hodgkinson et al., 2003), yet it impairs cognitive function, causes headaches, tiredness, alertness, and dizziness (Rogers et al., 2001; Wilson and Morley, 2003), and increases the risk of falls (DH, 2001c).

Potential causes of dehydration can be attributed to normal ageing, illness, or institutional factors (see Table 13.2).

People with dementia or those who have experienced a stroke also have a reduced thirst sensitivity, so they may be particularly at risk of dehydration unless formal monitoring of fluid intake is initiated.

Possible physical signs of dehydration include a dry-coated tongue, dry mucous membranes in the mouth and nose, and a lack of saliva, making masticating food more difficult. Frequent episodes of constipation and elimination of a small volume of urine can also be signs of dehydration. Other consequences of an inadequate fluid intake and the consequent dehydration include altered cardiac function and electrolyte imbalance, loss of skin elasticity, and increased risk of pressure ulcers. Globally, dehydration increases the length of hospital stay and impacts negatively on mortality rates.

Table 13.2 Some potential causes of dehydration

Causes of dehydration	Mechanism
Loss of elasticity and thinning of the skin Central heating	Increased water loss via skin
Reduction in thirst receptors Confusion, dementia, depression Drowsiness Immobility Lack of staff to offer drinks Drinks inaccessible or served at wrong temperature Inadequate monitoring of fluid intake	Inadequate fluid intake
Impaired continence or reduced ability to get to a toilet easily	Reluctance to drink
Deterioration in renal function (plasma renal flow and glomerular filtration rate)	Reduced ability to concentrate urine or eliminate waste products
Medication, such as diuretics or laxatives	Increased fluid loss

Nutritional status of older people

A comprehensive study of the nutritional status of people over the age of 65 in the UK was carried out in 1998 as a specific programme of the National Diet and Nutrition Survey (Finch et al., 1998). This indicated that, generally, older people in the UK are adequately nourished, although analysis of the dietary data found that the intake of non-starch polysaccharides (NSP) (dietary fibre) was low, and that the intakes of saturated fatty acids, salt, and table sugar were high. Dietary intakes of iron and vitamin C (ascorbic acid) were adequate, but blood analysis indicated that a significant percentage of people were anaemic with low-serum ascorbic acid levels. Reduced absorption, achlorhydria (that is, reduced acid in stomach), and slow bleeds in the gastrointestinal tract may all contribute to anaemia. The body has increased requirements for vitamin C during stress, infection, injury, and for wound healing, so these factors may influence the haematological data.

The average energy intake of individuals on a low income and/or receiving means tested benefits was lower, as were the intakes of protein, NSP, and vitamin C. People living in institutions were most likely to be malnourished, with one in six people living in care homes being underweight, while two-thirds of the free-living group were overweight or obese. People with no natural teeth, as a subgroup, experience difficulties due to their poor dental health and oral function, which reduces the range and variety of food eaten (Steele et al., 1998)

Nutritional requirements and nutritional guidelines

Nutrient and energy requirements for healthy people are defined in the *Dietary Reference Values* (DRVs) adjusted for subgroups (age and sex) within the population (DH, 1991). These figures, expressed in terms of nutrients, assume that the range of requirements for any particular nutrient within a healthy population follows a normal distribution pattern—that is, they are statistical estimates. The DRVs defined four terms, as follows.

- **Safe intake**—This term is used to give an indicative intake when there is insufficient information to estimate more accurately. The amount is sufficient for everyone, but not so large as to cause undesirable side effects.
- **Reference nutrient intake (RNI)**—A figure relating to protein, a vitamin, or a mineral, this is the amount sufficient for about 97 per cent of the population.
- **Lower reference nutrient intake (LRNI)**—For protein, a vitamin, or a mineral, this is the amount sufficient for only 3 per cent of the population who have low needs.
- **Estimated average requirement (EAR)**—Generally used for energy, this figure refers to the point at which approximately half the population subgroup will need more and half less.

Table 13.3 shows the EAR for energy for males and females according to their age.

The DRVs can be used for:

- labelling purposes, as a basis for providing information about the nutrient content of food;
- the provision of food supplies and institutional catering, where the meal service should provide sufficient nutrients to meet the requirements for most of the target population; and
- assessing diets of individuals and groups.

NOTE: The DRVs are intended for use for groups of people and therefore caution should be exercised if used to assess the adequacy of a reported diet. The aggregation of individual food intakes from a group of people will diminish the day-to-day variability, therefore the group mean will more typically measure habitual food intake. If the habitual intake for a particular nutrient is below the LRNI, it is unlikely that the individual is consuming sufficient to maintain function; if the intake is above the RNI, it is unlikely that they are deficient in that nutrient.

The Nutrition of Elderly People (DH, 1992) accepted the recommendations of the previous year (DH, 1991), highlighting

Table 13.1 EAR for energy according to age and sex

Age in years	Weight		Estimated average requirements (EAR)	
	Male kg	Female kg	Male MJ/d (kcal/d)	Female MJ/d (kcal/d)
51–59			10.60 (2550)	8.00 (1900)
60–64	74.0	63.5	9.93 (2380)	7.99 (1900)
65–74	71.0	63.0	9.71 (2330)	7.96 (1900)
75+	69.0	60.0	8.77 (2100)	7.61 (1810)

Source: DH (1991; 1992).

the need for more research to explore the specific nutrients requirements for older people. There is no evidence for most nutrients of additional needs in old age, therefore the DRVs are the same throughout adulthood, with the exception of vitamin D. The panel recommended an increased allowance for vitamin D, because the declining renal function leads to diminished metabolism of vitamin D and reduced calcium absorption. For housebound individuals with restricted access to sunlight, supplementation is recommended.

The reduction in lean body mass with age results in a decline in basal metabolic rate (that is, the amount of energy required by the body at rest); combined with an illness or disability by which physical activity is limited, this leads to a reduction in energy expenditure.

The panel recognized the need to encourage older people to consume sufficient food energy, so that nutrient needs can simultaneously be met. It therefore encouraged some physical activity to stimulate energy expenditure when possible.

Nutritional guidelines: healthy eating—the 'Eat Well Plate'

The DRV information has been translated into nutritional guidelines as the basis for healthy eating for the UK population. Pictorially, this is presented as the 'Eat Well Plate' (FSA, 2008), as illustrated in Figure 13.1.

The plate visualizes the proportion of food from each food group needed to construct a healthy diet. This means that about a third of daily foods should be derived from starchy carbohydrate foods, such as bread, potatoes, rice, and pasta, and a further third from fruit and vegetables. If energy requirements are reduced because less physical activity is undertaken, it is important to reduce the quantity of fats and sugars eaten, so that unnecessary weight is not gained.

Table 13.4 provides practical key messages and recommendations for each food group.

Fluid

A fluid intake of between 1.5 l and 2 l is an initial target, with between six and eight drinks offered during the day (see Table 13.5). Organizational issues regarding access to sufficient fluids must be identified and addressed, such as how frequently clients are offered a drink, and whether clients require assistance or reminders to reach and consume fluid.

Fresh drinking water should be available throughout the day in an accessible format, and individuals should be encouraged to consume a glass with a meal and to sip fluid at intervals throughout the day.

Water UK (2005) has produced guidance on hydration and older people in care homes, and a *Hydration Best Practice Toolkit for Care Homes* that can be found online at http://www.water.org.uk/home/water-for-health/older-people. The toolkit includes best practice and practical tips that are supported by medical evidence on the requirements of good hydration in older people.

NURSING PRACTICE INSIGHT: ENCOURAGING DRINKING

- Water is more appealing when served fresh and cool. It thus should not be left in open jugs.
- Citrus fruits, such as a slice of lemon, can make a drink of fresh water more attractive.
- Many people prefer to drink little and often, so water should be accessible at all times.
- Frail and vulnerable older people can lose their thirst response and taste sensation, so the nurse should be encouraging the older person to drink and not take it for granted that an older person knows when they need to drink.
- Good hydration should be promoted to the carers and families, as well as the patient—particularly where a lack of adequate fluids can contribute to illness.
- Offer drinks with and after food—for example, water with meals, tea/coffee afterwards.
- Ensure drinks are in reach and in an appropriate cup/beaker.
- If the patient is experiencing altered taste, offer drinks with a sharper taste or savoury drinks.
- Involve family and friends at all times in ascertaining patient preferences/giving drinks.
- Ensure that the older person is in a correct position to drink.
- Persevere and demonstrate patience and a calm approach.

Mediterranean diet

There is significant evidence that adherence to a 'Mediterranean diet' has health benefits; the Eat Well Plate is a modification of this for the UK.

A meta-analysis exploring adherence to the Mediterranean diet, and the incidence of disease and mortality in prospective studies (12 studies with 15,742,999 subjects) concluded:

Greater adherence to a Mediterranean diet confers a significant protection for overall mortality (9 per cent), as well as cardiovascular disease mortality (9 per cent) and incidence of cancer (6 per cent) and degenerative diseases' (13 per cent reduction in risk of Parkinson's disease and Alzheimer's disease).

(Sofi et al., 2008).

The eatwell plate

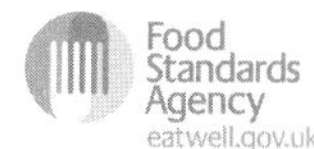

Use the eatwell plate to help you get the balance right. It shows how much of what you eat should come from each food group.

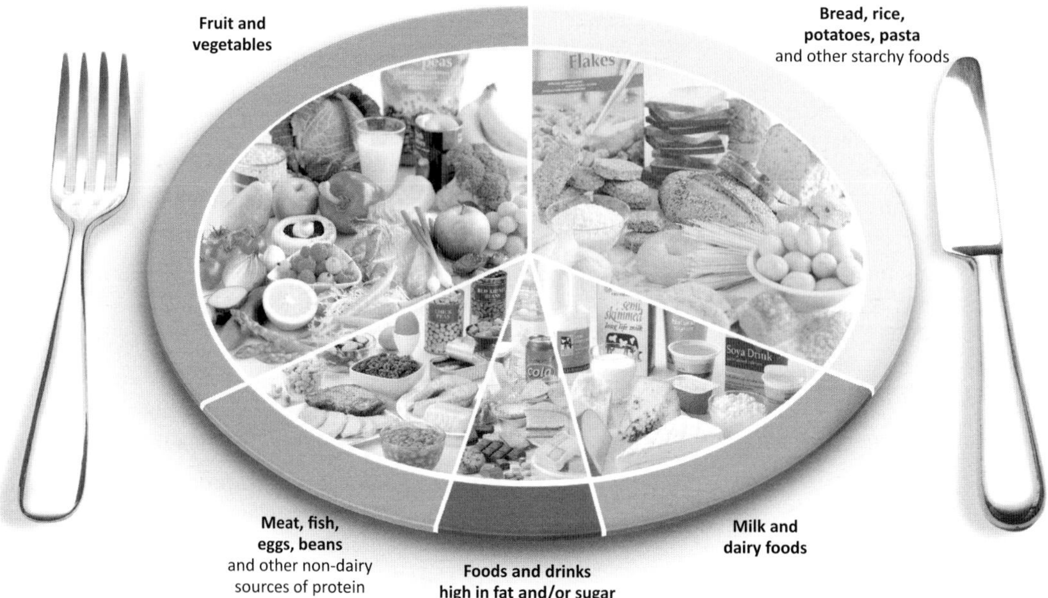

The **eatwell plate** shows how much of what you eat should come from each food group. This includes everything you eat during the day, including snacks.

So, try to eat:

- plenty of fruit and vegetables
- plenty of bread, rice, potatoes, pasta and other starchy foods – choose wholegrain varieties when you can
- some milk and dairy foods
- some meat, fish, eggs, beans and other non-dairy sources of protein
- just a small amount of foods and drinks high in fat and/or sugar

Look at the eatwell plate to see how much of a whole day's food should come from each food group and try to match this in your own diet.

Try to choose options that are lower in fat, salt and sugar when you can.

For more information on eating a healthy diet, visit: **eatwell.gov.uk**

Figure 13.1 The Eat Well Plate
Source: FSA (2008) © Crown Copyright.

King et al. (2007), using a sample from the *Atherosclerosis Risk in Communities* survey (15,708 participants), prospectively showed that middle-aged people who newly adopted a healthy lifestyle—involving five or more fruit and vegetables per day, regular exercise, a body mass index (BMI) of 18.5–29.9 kg/m^2, and no smoking—experienced a prompt benefit of lower cardiovascular disease and reduced mortality. Therefore, it is important to assure mature individuals that 'it is never too late to change'.

Promote healthy active life

During retirement, people experience many of the chronic lifestyle conditions common to middle-aged adults, such as obesity, diabetes, hypertension, cardiovascular disease, and cancers.

Table 13.2 Key messages for each section of the Eat Well Plate

Food group	Message	Recommendations
Bread, rice, potatoes, pasta, and other starchy foods	Eat plenty Starchy foods should make up a third of food intake	Increase proportion of wholemeal, wholegrain, brown or high-fibre versions Minimize added fats
Fruit and vegetables	Eat plenty At least five portions a day	Eat a wide variety
Milk, cheese, yoghurt and fromage frais Also included are calcium-enriched soya products	Eat some equivalent to 1 pt milk per day Choose lower fat alternatives whenever possible	Choose semi-skimmed or skimmed milk, low-fat yoghurts/fromage frais, lower-fat cheese
Meat, fish, eggs, beans, and other non-dairy sources of protein, i.e. nuts, beans and pulses soya, tofu, quorn	Eat some Choose lower-fat alternatives whenever possible	Aim for at least two portions of fish a week, including a portion of oily fish (i.e. fresh tuna, salmon, herring, mackerel, sardines trout, pilchards)
Food and drinks high in fat and/or sugar Margarine, butter, other spreads and oils Chocolate, cakes, biscuits, pastries, ice cream, crisps Rich sauces and gravy Soft and fizzy drinks, sweets, jam, and sugar	Eat only a small amount	Keep spreads and oils to low amounts

Obesity

The risk of obesity in older adults is greater due to the decline in metabolic rate, a loss of mean body mass, and reduced activity levels. As activity levels decrease, weight gain may exacerbate. Being overweight and obese is a serious health risk, reducing life expectancy, increasing the likelihood of developing other chronic diseases, and impacting on quality of life. The prevalence of obesity is 28 per cent in people aged 65–74 and 24 per cent in those aged over 75 (Health and Social Care Information Centre, 2009).

Tackling obesity is a complex issue that generally involves altering eating habits, increasing physical activity, and general adjustments in lifestyle. Effective weight loss requires motivation and permanent changes in eating habits and lifestyle. Considerable health benefits can be achieved by only a moderate (5–10 per cent) loss in weight; it is therefore important to encourage a slow, steady weight loss as appropriate (NICE, 2006b). A reduction in energy needs to be achieved without compromising the nutritional quality of the diet and thus older people who need to lose weight need to be supported with careful guidance.

There is a need to get the balance right with eating and exercise, and maintaining a balanced lifestyle includes healthy eating with a physical exercise programme, where possible (Denny, 2008; Shepherd, 2009). The recommendation is that older adults in good health should achieve 30 minutes of moderate-intensity exercise five days a week (DH, 2004).

See Chapter 6. on mobility and falls.

Table 13.3 A suggested day's fluid intake (with additional water offered)

Time of day	Beverage	Volume in ml
Early morning	Tea	150
Breakfast	Tea	150
	Fruit juice or water	100
Mid-morning	Tea/coffee/milky drink	200
Lunch-time	Soup/water	200
	Tea/coffee after meal	150
Mid-afternoon	Tea/water	150
Evening meal	Tea/coffee with meal	150
Supper/evening drink	Tea	150
Bedtime	Milky drink	200
TOTAL		1,600

Malnutrition

Age Concern (2006), in its major report *Hungry to be Heard*, raised the profile of older people and the risk of malnutrition, and stated that patients aged over 80 admitted to hospital are five times higher prevalence of malnutrition than those under the age of 50, and that as many as four out of ten older people admitted to hospital have malnutrition on arrival.

Malnutrition occurs when the body does not receive sufficient energy and nutrients over a period of time to meet physiological requirements, with resulting weight loss. This inadequate nutritional intake leading to undernutrition (malnutrition) is often not recognized—any weight loss being mistaken for a consequence of the ageing process or the impact of disease (McWhirter and Pennington, 1994; Edington et al., 1996; Elia, 2003; Stratton et al., 2004). Gradual weight loss may not be noticed, or may be masked by loose-fitting clothing, and therefore opportunities for early intervention may be missed. Obesity can also mask malnutrition if the quality of the diet is poor.

The causes of malnutrition are complex, and can be due to a range of social, economic, physiological, and physical factors, including disease. At a simplistic level, people lose weight for four reasons:

- a reduced food intake, either planned or incidental;
- increased energy requirements due to infection, disease, or trauma;
- increased physical activity; and
- impaired absorption, so that the food eaten is not available to the body.

It is therefore important to identify the contributing factors—often a combination of illness and a reduction in food consumed, with the disease precipitating a reduced food intake or vice versa, leading to a vicious downward spiral in nutritional health.

Frail older people are more at risk of malnutrition because they are reliant on others to provide their supply of food and drink, or because they have a reduced appetite due to chronic and/or acute illness, with symptoms of anorexia and nausea, or they may be depressed due to changing circumstances, such as bereavement.

Consequences of malnutrition can be significant, affecting the individual physically and psychologically, leading to greater risk of mortality, increased morbidity, a longer hospital stay, and increased probability of readmission (see Table 13.6).

Age Concern (2006) set out seven steps (see Box 13.1) to be taken in all health and social care institutional settings.

Table 13.6 Physical and psychological consequences of malnutrition

Physical consequences	Psychological consequences
Weight loss	Apathy
Muscle wasting	Depression
Loss of subcutaneous fat	Weakness
Delayed wound healing	Fatigue
Increased risk of infection	Anorexia
Nutritional deficiencies	
Reduced mobility	
Increased likelihood of cardiac failure	
Slower recovery from illness	

Box 13.1 The seven steps for *Hungry to Be Heard*

Step 1: Listening to older people, their relatives, and carers

Older people must be consulted about hospital menus, and their meal requirements and preferences, and hospitals must respond to what they are told.

Step 2: All ward staff must become 'food aware'

Ward staff need to take responsibility for the food needs of older people in hospital.

Step 3: Hospital staff must follow professional codes

Hospital staff must follow their own professional codes and guidance from other bodies.

Step 4: Assessing signs of malnourishment

Because 40 per cent of older people are malnourished on admission to hospital, all patients should be weighed and their height measured on admission.

Step 5: Introduce 'protected mealtimes'

Protected mealtimes should be introduced to ensure that older patients are given appropriate assistance to eat meals when needed and sufficient time in which to eat their meals.

Step 6: Implement a 'red tray' system

Older people who need help with eating should be identified on admission and their meal placed on a red tray to signal the need for help.

Step 7: Use volunteers where appropriate

Where appropriate, hospitals should use trained volunteers to provide additional help and support at mealtimes.

Nutrition screening and nutrition assessment

Screening has been defined as '*the organized attempt to detect, among apparently healthy people in the community, disorders or risk factors of which they are unaware*' (Hubley and Copeman, 2008). The American Society for Parental and Enteral Nutrition (ASPEN) defines nutritional screening as a process to identify an individual who is malnourished or who is at risk of malnutrition, to determine whether a detailed nutrition assessment is indicated (Teitelbaum et al., 2005).

Nutrition screening involves obtaining information in a systematic way about:

- current and previous food intake;
- recent weight change;
- appetite;
- swallowing and chewing ability;
- medical and physical condition, including medication; and
- mental
- socio-economic state.

The National Institute for Health and Clinical Excellence (2006b) estimated that only 30 per cent of patients were screened on admission to hospital prior to issuing its guidance *Nutritional Support for Adults* (NICE, 2006a).

Screening tools should be quick and easy to use, valid for the client group, and should identify those at risk of undernutrition. They should be used with all new admissions to any health and social care setting within 24 hours, and the information obtained acted upon. Screening should be repeated at regular intervals in line with the organization's policy, so that the changing pattern in eating and drinking, and therefore nutritional risk of the individual, is noted (DH, 2001a; DH, 2001b; DH, 2001c; DH, 2007). Screening tools should be carefully evaluated, with reference to the population to be screened, the setting in which the screening will be done, availability of valid and reliable nutrition screening tests, and cost, including time requirement to administer (Charney, 2008).

A review of nutritional screening tools identified tools as designated for use with an older population, but noted that many have not been subjected to evaluation (Green and Watson, 2006). The Malnutrition Universal Screening Tool (MUST) was developed by the Malnutrition Advisory Group—a standing committee of the British Association of Parenteral and Enteral Nutrition (BAPEN)—for use in all healthcare settings. It is a five-step screening tool that has been adopted across the UK to identify adults, who are malnourished, at risk of malnutrition (undernutrition), or obese (Malnutrition Advisory Group, 2003). This tool uses BMI, weight loss, and clinical condition to assign a score that indicates risk.

See the Online Resource Centre that accompanies this book for more on MUST.

Individuals being screened are likely to fall into three categories of nutritional risk: 'no risk'; 'some risk'; or 'high risk'. Those with some risk should be encouraged to eat and drink with the support of modified menus and/or supplements. Those with high risk should additionally be referred for further specialist nutritional assessment.

Assessment

Webster et al. (2009) note how 'screening' and 'assessment' are often used interchangeably—but it is important to distinguish that 'screening' identifies the potential or actual risk, while 'assessment' allows the clinician to gather more detailed information to determine whether there is actually a nutritional problem and its severity.

Nutritional assessment involves collecting:

- anthropometric (that is, physical) measurements, such as weight, weight change, height, mid-arm circumference, skin-fold thickness, waist circumference, and hand grip, which are then interpreted into percentage weight loss, BMI, and percentage body fat;
- biochemical and haematological data, such as blood cell count, electrolytes, and haemoglobin levels;
- observations of any physical and/or clinical changes, based on the standard global assessment (see Box 13.3); and
- notes on any dietary changes, including appetite, current and typical food intake, meal patterns, type of food, and personal food likes and dislikes.

Box 13.2 Five steps in using MUST

- **Step 1**: Measure height and weight, and determine BMI
- **Step 2**: Note percentage unplanned weight loss and score using tables provided.
- **Step 3**: Establish acute disease effect and score.
- **Step 4**: Add scores from steps 1, 2, and 3 together to obtain overall risk of malnutrition.
- **Step 5**: Use management guidelines and/or local policy to develop care plan.

(Malnutrition Advisory Group, 2003).

Box 13.3 Observation of physical and/or clinical changes

General appearance	Listless, apathetic, irritable
Sensory function changes	Taste, smell, vision, hearing
Mouth	Lips = dry and scaly Tongue = swollen, atrophy, dry, changes to colour particularly if purple Dentition = untreated dental needs, absent teeth, ill-fitting dentures Oral infections Gums that bleed
Skin	Discoloured, dry, scaly, pale
Gastrointestinal	Anorexia, indigestion, constipation/diarrhoea

How to assess what someone is eating and drinking

It is important to determine what an individual is eating and drinking, in terms either of their 'current food intake', 'typical food intake', and/or 'past food intake'. There are a variety of techniques used to assess dietary intake, depending on the purpose and level of detail required, but this should always commence with a discussion with the older person.

The most detailed form involves weighing and measuring all food and fluid consumed, but this is time-consuming, intrusive and may modify food intake.

A food diary involves noting everything eaten and drunk, with detailed descriptions, over a set time period, such as three or four days, to obtain a contemporary record. In institutional settings, a food and fluid chart may be employed to note food offered, and food wasted, with descriptions of quantity and type.

More commonly utilized are fluid balance charts.

See Chapter 14 for an example of one chapter fluid balance chart, together with a food diary.

A 24-hour recall is useful to assess meal patterns and food choices. An individual is questioned to remember what they have consumed during the previous 24 hours, using prompts such as time of day, and probing about the type and quantity of different items. This method depends on memory and the reliability can therefore vary, but it does not directly influence food choice, as contemporary collections may do. It is useful to obtain information about meal patterns and types of food, rather than quantity consumed.

Assessing the nutritional intake of frail older people and/or those with cognitive impairment can pose particular challenges. They may not prepare their own food and may therefore be unclear of the composition of mixed dishes. Loss of short-term memory impairs the ability to recall food eaten and food declined, and physical disability prevents the individual keeping a written record. The involvement of carers (formal and non-formal) is critical in discovering what food has been offered and, more importantly, what has been eaten.

The European Society for Parenteral and Enteral Nutrition (ESPEN) suggests that nutritional assessments should be conducted by an '*expert clinician, nutrition nurse or dietician*' (Lochs et al., 2006). Therefore, the local policies may determine criteria or scores from the nutritional screen that warrant referral to a specialist.

Food selection, choice, and consumption

Factors influencing food selection, choice, and consumption are complex and change over time. During old age, social, psychological, and economic influences combine with a person's physical state of health and environment to determine what an individual eats and drinks at any point in time. Some factors that may limit food choice and dietary intake are listed in Box 13.4. The nurse, in conversation with an older person, will be able to assess which of these factors are relevant and decide whether referral to other services, such as occupational therapy, are required.

For further information, see the Disabled Living Foundation (DLF) online at http://www.dlf.org.uk/

Box 13.4 Factors that may limit food choice and dietary intake

Psychosocial factors

- Loneliness
- Bereavement
- Restricted income
- Anxiety, depression
- Not inclined to cook
- Former/current food habits
- Religious beliefs
- Previous food experience
- Education
- Restricted social network
- Cooking for friends or eating alone
- Cultural traditions

Economic and environmental factors

- Limited cooking facilities
- Inadequate food storage
- Lack of cooking skills
- Time available
- Access to food supply
- Budgeting skills
- Individual food likes and dislikes

Health factors

- Arthritis in hands affecting ability to hold cooking utensils
- Limited mobility affecting ability to stand or move around kitchen to prepare food
- Visual impairment
- Ill-fitting dentures
- Cognitive impairment
- Dementia

Webb (2002) developed a framework for food selection to explain in a hierarchical way how availability influences food choice and consumption.

1. Food to be physically available
2. Economic availability
3. Cultural acceptability—that is, religious beliefs and cultural experiences
4. The gatekeeper—that is, the person who controls access to food within the household
5. Personal choice

Decisions made at each stage sequentially limit the range of food available for the next stage. This framework can be utilized with older people living in their own homes to determine whether food is really accessible.

Table 13.7 poses some possible questions that can be used to explore how much influence an individual has over their food choice and so help carers to begin to understand problems that exist. This framework can be adapted to explore issues in hospital or other health and social care settings.

Table 13.7 Assessing influence over food choice

For an older person living in their own home	In hospital, or other health and social care setting, including organizational influences
Physical: How mobile are you? Do you use a stick or walking aid? Can you visit the supermarket independently? Can you carry your own shopping? Do you need assistance? Do you prepare your own meals? Have you any visual impairment that disrupts food preparation? Do your cooking facilities restrict you?	**Physical environment:** Dining arrangements; seating arrangements; height of chair related to table; position of client in chair; meal out of reach; meal not visible to client; inappropriate cutlery; distraction of noise and smells; unnecessary activities during meal times; insufficient time to eat meals (rushed); poorly cooked food served at the wrong temperature with no choice of food or portion size; no assistance with eating and drinking. **Physical personal:** Inability to remove packaging used for some items, e.g. bread roll in cellophane, cheese in plastic wrapper; inability to chew; poorly fitting dentures; swallowing difficulties, so fearful to eat and drink; impact of ill health on appetite and mood; in pain; side effects of medication.
Economic: Is food affordable on your income? Does the price influence type and/or variety of what you can buy? Do you purchase special offers?	**Economic:** Food budget of organization; cost of different food items; poor-quality food ingredients; boring menu cycle with limited choice; lack of staff time; insufficient staff to assist clients to eat and drink.
Cultural: How do your religious beliefs influence what you eat? Are there any food items that you avoid due to religious beliefs?	**Cultural:** Is food item recognizable from the menu description? Does the menu cater for cultural and religious expectations? Are eating companions acceptable? Are washing arrangements appropriate to fulfil religious obligations prior to eating?
Gatekeeper: Who decides what food is in your home? If you do not shop, who does the shopping and what do they purchase? Who decides which food to buy? Do you prepare a shopping list? Can you influence the food purchased or cooked food delivered?	**Gatekeeper:** Variation in intergenerational food habits influencing menu selection; timing of meals offered; arrangements for hot drinks before, with, or after meals; access to drinks at other times; impact of other activities on meal times; stereotypical food likes assumed within organization; badly cooked and presented food; food safety versus patient choice; range of food items that can be brought in by family and friends.
Personal: How do your personal likes and dislikes affect your food choice? Are you still able to eat your favorite foods? When did you last try a new food?	**Personal:** Food likes and dislikes; taste preference; food combinations offered; time of meal service different from previous experience.

Strategies to improve the nutrition intake in individuals

In 2006, NICE (2006a) recommended the use of oral nutrition support for malnourished older patients in hospital and in the community. The systematic review undertaken by Vanderkroft et al. (2007) exploring the effectiveness of interventions in hospital in-patients concluded that the use of oral supplements could promote weight gain and increase lean body mass, but that there was a need to ensure that prescribed supplements were actually consumed.

It appears that encouraging older people to increase their dietary intake when their appetite is diminished due to illness-related malnutrition is important, but that the practical realities mean that generating robust randomized control trial data is difficult. Current good practice is therefore to continue to encourage older people with a diminished appetite to increase their nutritional intake.

After nutritional screening to identify a problem, and dietary assessment to identify which factors are limiting food selection and food intake, the next step involves making any physical adjustments to ensure that the client is positioned in the best way so that they can eat and drink in a comfortable, safe manner. When someone requires assistance with eating and drinking, this should be offered discreetly in a targeted manner. Individuals with cognitive impairment may need reminders to prepare a meal or repeated prompting to eat each mouthful. Further steps to increase intake may include the following.

Supplementing a poor food intake

Before considering the use of prescribed oral nutritional supplements, efforts should be made to increase the intake of someone with a poor appetite using foods.

Small servings and snacks

It is important not to overwhelm someone with main meals that are too large, because it is widely recognized that small portions served attractively are more likely to be eaten. Easy-to-eat snacks may be preferred to a main meal, such as a corned beef sandwich, or cheese and crackers. Small quantities of food and drink throughout the day—that is, 'little and often', such as a full-fat milky drink mid-morning, or a piece of cake, scone with jam, or whole-milk yoghurt mid-afternoon—can increase the nutritional intake of an individual.

Enriching food

If someone is only consuming a small quantity of food, every mouthful must count, therefore additional energy and nutrients should be incorporated without increasing the bulk of the original food.

Possibilities include:

- margarine or butter added to vegetables and potatoes;
- butter or margarine spread more thickly on bread, toast, and crackers;
- evaporated milk or jam/honey added to milk puddings;
- full-fat milk fortified with milk powder;
- sugar added to food as a sweetener; and/or
- cream or butter added to soups.

Prescribed oral nutrition supplements

Supplementary products are designed to give extra protein, energy, and other nutrients in powder, liquid, or dessert forms, and are available in a range of savoury and sweet flavours, including:

- 'milk-based' drinks (sip feeds), with or without fibre;
- 'juice-based' drinks (sip feeds);
- fortified desserts;
- energy and/or protein supplements; and
- vitamin and mineral supplements.

These are designed to 'supplement' an individual's intake of ordinary food and their use should be reviewed regularly, both in terms of quantity and variety consumed. It is important to change the flavour and type of supplement in response to changing preferences to ensure that the prescribed dose is consumed.

Drinks that are sipped are most frequently used, and some of their practical advantages and disadvantages are listed in Table 13.8.

Some individuals prefer to drink the supplement from the carton using a straw, but they may need assistance opening the packaging and inserting the straw. Shake the carton thoroughly prior to opening. Other people prefer savoury or sweet supplements to be warmed and served in a cup or bowl, or poured over other foods. If a supplement is to be taken cold, it is more palatable when chilled. Sweet supplements can be frozen if the individual wishes to suck them as 'ice cubes' or an 'ice lolly'.

Other forms of supplement are designed to be added to normal food to increase energy or nutrient intake. Details, including recipe suggestions, are provided on the packaging and from the various company websites.

If someone is not able to consume sufficient energy and nutrients via the oral route to meet their nutritional requirements,

Table 13.8 Practical advantages and disadvantages of sip feeds

Advantages of sip feeds	Disadvantages of sip feeds
Source of balanced nutrition when someone is unable to eat an adequate diet Can be easy to take Little preparation needed Consumption can be monitored Variety of sweet and savoury flavours Can stimulate the appetite Can be seen as medicine and therefore consumed Can be taken hot or cold Less effort to drink than eat a meal	The importance of ordinary foods is sometimes forgotten May affect appetite for ordinary food Packaging difficult to open Over-reliance on special 'medicine' products Expensive Waste, because any cartoons must be discarded on same day as opened Taste fatigue Staff may spend less time with the individual encouraging them to eat and drink foods May encourage social isolation

then artificial feeding, such as nasogastric or gastrostomy feeding, may be required.

A systematic review of oral nutritional supplements in clinical practice found that there are consistent clinical benefits—particularly with older people who are acutely ill, for example following orthopaedic surgery or with pressure ulcers (Stratton and Elia, 2007).

Changing texture in food and fluids

People with dysphagia (that is, swallowing difficulties) and physical obstructions (see Box 13.5 for causes), or a problem with chewing (due to ill-fitting dentures or cancer of the mouth), may need a diet that has a modified consistency.

Specialist dietitians, and speech and language therapists, collaborated to produce the *National Descriptors for Texture Modification in Adults* (BDA/RCSLT, 2002), with detailed descriptions of the various textures in food and fluids. Fluids are grouped into 'thin', 'naturally thick', and 'artificially thickened' using one of the commercial thickeners to be drunk via a straw, from a cup, or using a spoon. Foods are classified A–F according to smoothness and uniformity of consistency, with A, B, and C textures all being pureed and sieved to remove any lumps.

All companies that produce commercial artificial thickeners have literature about their products that includes recipes and handy hints.

Box 13.5 Causes of dysphagia

Obstructions

- Cancer of head, neck, and oesophagus—particularly those affecting the pharynx, oesophagus, and tongue
- Severe inflammation
- Severe oedema
- Oesophageal spasm
- Oesophageal strictures

Neurogenic

- Stroke
- Dementia
- Cerebral tumours
- Motor neurone disease
- Multiple sclerosis

This means that, once a swallow assessment has been undertaken, appropriately textured food and fluid can be offered. Many people who have experienced choking are fearful to eat or drink, so need to be supported by being seated comfortably and offered suitable foods using appropriate cutlery. Eating will require considerable concentration and effort, causing fatigue, so it is important not to overwhelm someone with large quantities of food at one point in time.

Certain foods are especially high risk, because of the structure, and should be avoided when someone has an impaired swallow reflex. These foods include vegetable skins (such as beans), fruit skins (such as grapes), stringy fibrous textures (such as pineapples and runner beans), floppy textures (such as lettuce), and crunchy items (such as bread crust, pie crust, crumble, and dry biscuits). Similarly, mixed-consistency foods—for example, muesli with milk, mince with thin gravy, soup with lumps—should be eaten with care

Why eating can be difficult for older people

As the previous section on dysphagia highlights, eating can be very difficult for older people. However, it can be for a wide variety of reasons, including social, economic, environmental, and social, as well as health, and this further emphasizes the need for good assessment and screening in order to address the issues and barriers.

The following section highlights reasons why older people have problems and the appropriate interventions.

NURSING PRACTICE INSIGHT: NURSING ACTIONS—LINDA DITCHBURN, COMMUNITY NUTRITION NURSE SPECIALIST

Actions linked to physical assessment of capabilities

- Dexterity—consider the need for adapted utensils or referral to occupational therapy.
- Position—ensure the patient's position is conducive for eating and consider the seating, etc.
- Cognitive impairment—see below.
- Mouth problems—address dry mouth, thrush, altered taste, poorly fitting dentures, etc. Consider referral to dental service.
- Sight problems—can the person with sight loss see their food and fluids? For example, consider a coloured beaker rather than a glass beaker.
- Nutritional intake assessment—obtain information from family, carers, and friends regarding intake, weight loss, reasons for poor appetite, etc.
- Nutritional screening using appropriate tool—ensure that an action plan is put in place and followed with ongoing monitoring. Referral to dietitian as appropriate.
- Ensure that weighing equipment is available and in good working order.
- Access training for other measurements—for example, mid-upper-arm circumference (MUAC)—especially if the majority of your patients cannot be weighed.

It is also important for the nurse to beware of the older patient's illness and how this relates to their appetite—for example, whether they are nauseous or are awaiting gastrointestinal surgery, whether their medications are impacting on appetite/nausea, and whether the type, dose, or timing of medications be changed to alleviate this. Consider a GP or pharmacy review of medications.

Actions linked to psychological and environmental assessment of barriers to eating

- Social isolation/low income/poor local shopping facilities/reliance on others/unable to make own food choices—consider social service or voluntary sector interventions, such as Age UK.
- Unfamiliar surroundings and people
- Change in routine
- Apathy/depression—ascertain and discuss reasons before making a referral.
- Lack of encouragement/interaction
- Staff time restraints
- Different food/presentation

Other practical actions

- Reduce distractions at mealtimes—for example, medical investigations—and enforce protected mealtimes. Save food or offer snacks if a meal missed.
- Give timely prescribed analgesia or anti-emetics, so as to reduce pain or nausea at mealtimes.
- Ensure adequate staffing at mealtimes to assist those who require help with feeding.
- Use red trays (Essence of Care initiative) to identify those who require assistance.
- Develop a care plan for nutritional needs and use as a communication aid between staff.
- Ensure that all staff work consistently in their approach to older patients who need help with nutrition and fluids.
- Maintain eye contact and adopt a calm, unhurried approach.
- Encourage the patient to feed self—ensuring that they have the right utensils, seating, etc. Refer to occupational therapist if necessary.
- Ensure the patient is in a good position for feeding—Sit out/at table or sit up in bed. Ensure bed table is at the right height and in reach. Ensure clear of clutter—especially vomit bowl/urinal!
- Encourage social interaction—eating together is important: using a dining room in an acute elderly medical ward has been found to increase energy intake (Wright et al., 2006).
- Try to give the older patient some choice with food offered and honour food choices. Enlist help from family and friends regarding preferences, etc.
- Ensure that portion sizes are appropriate.
- Ensure that food is at the right temperature and given at right time—liaise with kitchen/catering staff.
- Look at times between meals Too long? Too short? Are snacks and drinks available at other times?
- Liaise with dietitian if weight loss evident.

See Chapter 3 for more on sight loss.

Dementia and cognitive impairment

A loss of appetite is a normal progression of dementia, and thus careful attention and support are required. People with dementia often require verbal prompting, reassurance, and encouragement to eat. The nurse needs to ensure that sufficient time is provided for the person to finish their meal—particularly in cases in which there is a slow eating pace. Other interventions include sitting with others around a table (social interaction) and reducing environmental distractions—particularly noise from radios and televisions, or ward rounds.

Carers and family should always be involved in assessment, and for ascertaining normal routines and requirements with dementia patients. When two or more meals have been refused or not eaten, it is important to ensure that a nutritional assessment is carried out.

Where there is no diagnosis, but a dementia condition is suspected, a referral to a doctor is required for identification or exclusion of other medical reasons for confusion, such as an infection. Following a physical screening, a referral to a memory assessment service or input from the mental health team may be required.

See Chapter 11 for more on dementia.

Organizational initiatives to improve nutrition

There have been many initiatives to tackle malnutrition among older people, with varying degrees of success, in care homes and hospitals.

Initiatives to tackle problems of malnutrition among older people can be grouped into four broad areas:

- regular monitoring by staff to detect signs of malnutrition;
- better nutritional knowledge and heightened nutrition awareness;
- adequate appetizing food served and eaten; and
- access to and use of specialists.

Care homes

Davies and Holdsworth (1979), as a consequence of assessing the nutritional status of residents in care homes in London, developed the 'A–Z' checklist to enable home managers to identify and change their practice as needed. Recommendations included varying the menu cycle, always offering choice of food and portion size, improving the presentation and timing of meals, assisting frail residents to eat and drink, and investigating further any regular observation of weight changes in residents.

The Caroline Walker Trust (1995; 2004) developed these points further, making additional recommendations focusing on the nutritional adequacy of the food provided.

- Nutritional guidelines should be a minimum standard for food prepared for older people.
- Cost should not override the need for adequate nutritional content in planning and preparing meals.
- Regular monitoring of the nutritional standard of meals should be part of the registration process.

The *Care Homes for Older People National Minimum Standards* (DH, 2001a) restated these recommendations, stressing the importance of initial assessment (Standard 3) and regular nutrition screening with appropriate interventions (Standard 8).

The environment has an impact on an older person being encouraged and motivated to eat and drink—for example, the dining area must be clean and tidy. Ullman (2009) also states that the following factors are important and conducive to encouraging older people to participate in mealtimes within care homes:

- personal tastes should be considered (residents should be consulted on preferences);
- food should look good;
- food should be served by caring staff, assisting where necessary; and
- the meal should meet the residents' expectations.

See also the section on 'Fluid' above and the Water UK's *Hydration Best Practice Toolkit for Care Homes* (2005).

Hospitals

Nutrition Guidelines for Hospital Catering (DH National Task Force, 1995), *Not Because They Are Old* (HAS, 1998), and the more recent exploration of patients' experience in hospitals (Savage and Scott, 2005; Age Concern, 2006) all show that there is a wide variation in nutritional care in hospitals. The Age Concern campaign still reported inappropriate food being offered, no assistance being given with cutting meat, and food trays being placed out of reach.

The *Better Hospital Food* programme was launched in 2001, as part of the NHS plan to revitalize NHS food services. Key steps for *Better Hospital Food* included the NHS menu, a 24-hour catering service, and ward housekeeping, so that specified nutritional requirements would be delivered through the menu to all patients, utilizing protected mealtimes and flexible menus.

In 2003, the Council of Europe issued a Resolution including '*ten key characteristics of good nutritional care*' (Council of Europe, 2003), and recommending nutrition screening on admission, the identification of nutritional needs in patient care plans, protected mealtimes, guidance on food services and nutritional care in clinical governance arrangements, and appropriate staff with skills to ensure that patient's nutritional needs are met.

This was reiterated in one of the patient-focused benchmarks for food and nutrition identified in the *Essence of Care* (NHS Modernization Agency, 2003), which stated that '*patients* [should be] *enabled to consume food (orally) which meets their individual need*'.

In 2009, the National Reporting and Learning Service of the National Patient Safety Agency undertook a review of the 'protected mealtime' initiative to identify barriers and critical success factors. It found inconsistencies around which mealtimes were protected, and barriers, such as ward and drug rounds, diagnostic tests, and healthcare professional activities (National Patient Safety Agency, 2009).

In 2007, *Improving Nutritional Care: A Nutrition Action Plan* (DH, 2007) outlined a range of actions to tackle malnutrition, aiming to ensure that health and social care staff and managers are well informed, equipped, and supported to provide good nutrition and effective nutritional care.

BAPEN (2009) reinforced the importance of 'screening' and 'risk' assessment for all patients on admission to hospital, and further recommended that this should extend to ongoing monitoring and rescreening.

Conclusion

Screening and assessing nutritional needs is paramount to identifying the nutritional requirements of the older person. And should be embedded in person-centred care.

The need to ensure that older people receive the assistance that they require with eating and drinking is a key component of dignity in care (DH, 2006). In busy, dynamic care environments, providing assistance can be demanding and difficult, but it is essential to nursing care, a core skill, and a fundamental human right for those older people who require assistance whether they have a physical disability, a medical condition, and/or a communication or cognitive impairment.

Case studies

Miss Alice Sutton, who is 80 years old, has limited mobility and relies on a Zimmer frame to move around her ground-floor warden-controlled flat. She is fearful of having an 'accident' before she can reach the toilet and regularly complains of being constipated. You notice that Miss Sutton rarely finishes her cup of tea and other drinks.

- **How could you encourage her to increase her fluid consumption?**
- **How might you adapt the information in the Eat Well Plate to her needs?**

Mr Boyd Hobson, who is 68 years old, has recently retired from working on the railways. He fell off a ladder while painting the outside of his house and is now in hospital recovering from surgery, having fractured his femur. You notice that he does not appear interested in anything, including eating. His wife is very worried about this and thinks that he has lost weight.

- **What measures should be in place for you to respond to Mrs Hobson's concerns?**
- **What obstacles might have occurred to prevent the procedures from being followed?**
- **How would you find out what Mr Hobson was eating?**
- **What practical suggestions could you implement?**

Mrs Elaine Morgan, a widow aged 85, had a stroke four weeks ago, which has left her with left-sided weakness and a delayed swallow. She has made steady progress and is now going to be transferred to intermediate care for further rehabiliation. As part of the discharge process, you have been asked to itemize what steps have been taken on the ward to support Mrs Morgan with her eating and drinking.

- **List the probable support that Mrs Morgan has been offerred on the ward.**
- **How could you communicate this information in an effective written format?**

Questions and self-assessment

- Next time you visit a supermarket, apply Webb's food selection framework to your food choice.
- How closely does your own food intake adhere to the proportions in the Eat Well Plate?
- Identify someone you know who has recently retired and ask them about their eating habits. How closely do they follow the recommendations of the Eat Well Plate? In what ways, does their food intake differ from yours?
- Write a list of what you ate in the last 24 hours, noting the times, portion size, types, and combinations of food eaten.
- Count the type and number of cups of fluid (excluding alcohol) that you consume during a day and compare your fluid intake to that of someone who has restricted mobility due to ill health.
- What practical measures could be put into place on a busy ward to ensure that every older person is offered and drinks sufficient fluid to meet their requirements?
- Use the nutrition screening tool within a health organization on three patients. What difficulties did you encounter?
- Think of an older person with whom you have been involved in nursing who had a poor appetite. Consider the potential reasons and offer practical suggestions that you could implement.
- The Council of Europe (2003) stressed the value of protected mealtimes in hospitals. List the obstacles that may prevent these from being fully implemented.

Self-assessment

- Having read the chapter, how will you change your practice?
- Identify up to three areas relating to nutrition in which you need to develop your knowledge and understanding further.
- Identify how you are going to develop this knowledge and understanding, and set deadlines for achieving this.

References

Age UK (2006) *Hungry to be Heard*, available online at http://www.scie.org.uk/publications/guides/guide15/files/hungrytobeheard.pdf.

Bond, S. (ed) (1997) *Eating Matters: A Resource for Improving Dietary Care in Hospital*, Newcastle-upon-Tyne: Centre for Health Services Research, University of Newcastle.

British Association for Parenteral and Enteral Nutrition (2009) *Improving Nutritional Care and Treatment: Perspectives and Recommendations from Population Groups, Patients and Carers*, Redditch: BAPEN.

British Dietetic Association/Royal College of Speech and Language Therapists (2002) *The National Descriptors for Texture Modification in Adults*, Birmingham: BDA.

Caroline Walker Trust (1995) *Eating Well for Older People*, London: Caroline Walker Trust.

Caroline Walker Trust (2004) *Eating Well for Older People*, 2nd edn, London: Caroline Walker Trust.

Charney, P. (2008) 'Nutrition screening vs nutrition assessment: How do they differ?', *Nutrition in Clinical Practice*, 23(4): 366–72.

Copeman, J. and Hyland, K. (1999) 'Nutrition Issues in Older People', in G. Corley (ed.) *Older People and Their Needs: A Multidisciplinary Perspective*, London: Whurr.

Council of Europe (2003) *Food and Nutritional Care in Hospitals*, Resolution 12/11/2003, Strasbourg: Council of Europe Publishing.

Davies, L. and Holdsworth, D. (1979) 'A-Z checklist: A technique for assessing nutritional "at risk" factors in residential homes for the elderly', *Journal of Human Nutrition*, 33: 165–9.

Denny, A. (2008) 'An overview of the role of diet during the ageing process', *British Journal of Community Nursing*, 13(2): 58–67.

Department of Health (1991) *Dietary References Values for Food Energy and Nutrients for the UK: Report of the Panel on DRV of the Committee on Medical Aspects of Food Policy*, Report on Health and Social Subjects No. 41. London: HMSO.

Department of Health (1992) *The Nutrition of Elderly People: Report of the Panel on Nutrition of Elderly People of the Committee on Medical Aspects of Food Policy*, Report on Health and Social Subjects No. 43, London: HMSO.

Department of Health (2000) *The NHS Plan: A Plan for Investment, a Plan for Reform*, London: HMSO.

Department of Health (2001a) *Care Homes for Older People National Minimum Standards*, London: HMSO.

Department of Health (2001b) *Essence of Care*, London: HMSO.

Department of Health (2001c) *National Service Framework for Older People*, London: HMSO.

Department of Health (2004) *At Least Five a Week: Evidence of the Impact of Physical Activity and Its Relationship to Health—A Report from the Chief Medical Officer*, London: DH.

Department of Health (2006) *A New Ambition for Old Age*, London: DH.

Department of Health (2007) *Improving Nutritional Care: A Nutrition Action Plan*, London: HMSO.

Department of Health National Task Force (1995) *Nutritional Guidelines for Hospital Catering*, London: HMSO.

Edington, J. Kon, P., and Martyn, C.N. (1996) 'Prevalence of malnutrition in patients in general practice', *Clinical Nutrition*, 15: 60–3.

Elia, M. (ed.) (2003) *Screening for Malnutrition: A Multidisplinary Responsibility—Development and Use of the Malnutrition Universal Screening Tool (MUST) for Adults*, Redditch: BAPEN.

Finch, S., Doyle, W., Lowe, C., Bates, C.J., Prentice, A., Smithers, G., and Clarke, P.C. (1998) *National Diet and Nutrition Survey: People Aged 65 years and Over—Report of the Diet and Nutrition Survey*, London: HMSO.

Food Standards Agency (2008) *Eat Well Plate*, available online at http://www.eatwell.gov.uk/healthydiet/eatwellplate/.

Green, S.M. and Watson, R. (2006) 'Nutritional screening and assessment tools for older adults: Literature review', *Journal of Advanced Nursing*, 54(4): 477–90.

Health Advisory Service (1998) *Not Because They Are Old: An Independent Inquiry into the Care of Older People on Acute Wards in General Hospital*, London: Health Advisory Service.

Health and Social Care Information Centre, The (2009) *Statistics on Obesity Physical Activity and Diet England: February 2009*, available online at http://www.ic.nhs.uk/webfiles/publications/opan09/OPAD%20Feb%202009%20final.pdf.

Hodgkinson, B., Evans, D., and Wood, J. (2003) 'Maintaining oral hydration in older people: A systematic review', *International Journal of Nursing Practice*, 9: S19–28.

Hubley, J. and Copeman, J. (2008) *Practical Health Promotion*, Cambridge: Polity.

King, D.E., Mainous, A.G., and Geesey, M.E. (2007) 'Turning back the clock: Adopting a healthy lifestyle in middle age', *American Journal of Medicine*, 120(7): 598–603.

Lennard-Jones, J.E. (1992) *A Positive Approach to Nutrition as Treatment: Report of a Working Party on the Role of Enteral and Parenteral Feeding in Hospital and Homes*, London: King's Fund.

Lochs, H., Allison, S.P., Meier, R., Pirlich, M., Kondrup, J., Schneider, S., van den Berghe, G., and Pichard, C. (2006) 'Introductory to the ESPEN Guidelines on enteral nutrition: Terminology, definitions and general topics', *Clinical Nutrition*, 25: 180–6.

Malnutrition Advisory Group Standing Committee of BAPEN (2003) *Malnutrition Universal Screening Tool*, Redditch: BAPEN, available online at http://www.bapen.org.uk/must_tool.html.

McWhirter, J.P. and Pennington, C.R. (1994) 'Incidence and recognition of malnutrition in hospital', *British Medical Journal*, 308: 945–8.

National Health Service Modernization Agency (2003) *Essence of Care Patient-Focused Benchmarks for Food and Nutrition*, London: NHS.

National Institute for Health and Clinical Excellence (2006a) *Nutrition Support in Adults*, London: NICE, available online at http://www.nice.org.uk.

National Institute for Health and Clinical Excellence (2006b) *Obesity: The Prevention, Identification, Assessment and Management of Overweight and Obesity in Adults and Children*, London: NICE, available online at http://www.nice.org.uk.

National Patient Safety Agency (2009) available online at http://www.nrls.npsa.nhs.uk/.

Rogers, P.J., Kainth, A., and Smit, H.J. (2001) 'A drink of water can improve or impair mental performance depending on small differences in thirst', *Appetite*, 36: 57–8.

Royal College of Nursing (RCN) (2008) *Nutrition Now*, available online at http://www.rcn.org.uk/newsevents/campaigns/nutritionnow.

Savage, J. and Scott, C. (2005) *Patients' Nutritional Care in Hospital: An Ethnographic Study of Nurses' Roles and Patients' Experience*, A Report to the NHS Estates, London: RCN.

Shepherd, A. (2009) 'The role of nutrition in maintaining good health in later life', *Nursing and Residential Care*, 11(7): 337–45.

Sofi, F., Cesari, F., Abbate, R., Gensini, G.F., and Casini, A. (2008) 'Adherence to Mediterranean diet and health status: Meta-analysis', *British Medical Journal*, 337: a1344.

Steele, J.G., Sheiham, A., Marcenes, W., and Walls, A.W.G. (1998) *National Diet and Nutrition Survey: People Aged 65 Years and Over, Vol 2: Report of the Oral Health Survey*, London: HMSO.

Stratton, R.J. and Elia, M. (2007) 'A review of the reviews: A new look at the evidence for oral nutritional supplements in clinical practice', *Clinical Nutritional Supplements*, 2(1): 5–23.

Stratton, R.J., Hackston, A., Longmore, D., Dixon, R., Price, S., Stroud, M., King, C., and Elia, M. (2004) 'Malnutrition in hospital outpatients and inpatients: Prevalence, concurrent validity and ease of use of the malnutrition universal screening tool (MUST) for adults', *British Journal of Nutrition*, 92(5): 799–808.

Teitelbaum, D., Guenter, P., Howell, W.H., Kochevar, M.E., Roth, J., and Seidner, D.L. (ASPEN Board of Directors and Standards Committee) (2005) 'Definitions of terms, style and conventions in ASPEN guidelines and standards', *Nutritional Clinical Practice*, 20: 281–5.

Ullman, S. (2009) 'The contribution of care homes staff to nutrition and hydration', *Nursing and Residential Care*, 11(3): 128–34.

Vanderkroft, D., Collins, C.E., Fitzgerald, M., Lewis, S., Neve, M., and Capra, S. (2007) 'Minimizing undernutrition in the older inpatients', *International Journal of Evidence-Based Healthcare*, 5: 110–81.

Water UK (2005) *Water for Health: Hydration Best Practice Toolkit for Care Homes*, available online at http://www.water.org.uk/home/water-for-health/older-people.

Webb, G. (2002) *Nutrition: A Health Promotion Approach*, 2nd edn, London: Arnold.

Webb, G. and Copeman, J. (1996) *The Nutrition of Older Adults*, London: Arnold.

Webster, J., Healy, J., and Maud, R. (2009) 'Nutrition in hospitalized patients', *Nursing Older People*, 21(10): 31–7.

Wilson, M.-M.G. and Morley, J.E. (2003) 'Impaired cognitive function and mental performance in mild dehydration', *European Journal of Clinical Nutrition*, 57(Suppl2): 524–9.

Wright, L., Hickson, M., and Frost, G. (2006) 'Eating together is important: Using a dining room in an acute elderly medical ward increases energy intake', *Journal of Human Nutrition and Dietetics*, 19: 23–6.

For further reading and information

Department of Health (2007) *Improving Nutritional Care: A Nutrition Action Plan*, London: DH.

Elia, M. (ed.) (2003) *Screening for Malnutrition: A Multidisplinary Responsibility—Development and Use of the Malnutrition Universal Screening Tool (MUST) for Adults*, Redditch: BAPEN.

Food Standard Agency (2008) *Manual of Nutrition*, 11th edn, London: TSO

http://www.bapen.org.uk/

http://www.cwt.org.uk/

Online Resource Centre

You can learn more about nutrition, fluids, and older people at the Online Resource Centre that accompanies this book:
http://www.oxfordtextbooks.co.uk/orc/hindle/

Elimination and continence and the older adult

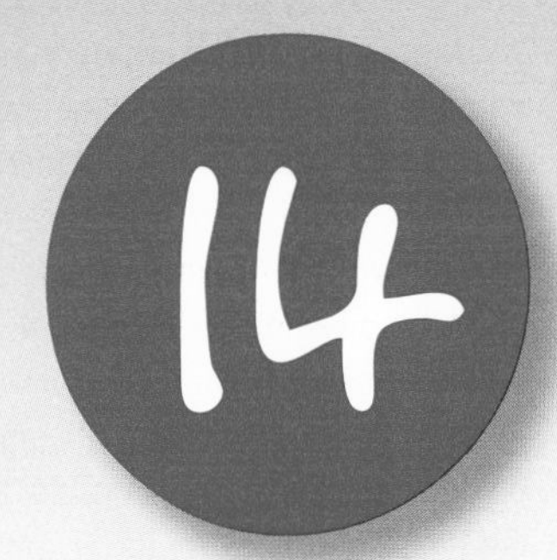

Alison Coates and Gill Davey

Learning outcomes

By the end of the chapter, you will be able to:

- identify the extent and impact of incontinence on older people's lives;
- identify the causes of incontinence;
- identify normal elimination;
- explain the assessment process, tools, and skills needed by the nurse when working with people who are incontinent;
- discuss treatment strategies for incontinence; and
- recognize the importance of maintaining the patient's dignity.

Introduction

This chapter will provide the reader with an understanding of the causes, assessment, and treatment options for incontinence that older adults may experience.

Incontinence is not part of the normal ageing process and, for the most part, the causes of incontinence are the same for older adults as they are for younger people. Incontinence is not a diagnosis, but rather a symptom of an underlying disorder. The precise number of people who are affected by incontinence is not known, but worldwide the World Health Organization (1998) estimates some 200 million adults are affected. The difficulty in determining the precise numbers who suffer from incontinence arises because many people do not seek help due to embarrassment. The perceived stigma associated with incontinence means that many older people who do seek health advice often do so only after they have had incontinence problems for some time and may be put off by negative experiences with health professionals (Royal College of Physicians, 2009). Thus, ensuring that patient dignity is maintained is an important part of providing health care for continence issues.

Whilst ageing is not the direct cause of incontinence, older people are more likely to experience incontinence, because they have a greater likelihood of having a health problem that increases the risk of incontinence. The Department of Health (2000) identified that between one in 14 and one in 10 men living at home, and between one in 10 and one in 5 women living at home, may be incontinent. This figure rises to 2 in every 3 in nursing homes.

The need to develop integrated (that is, across health and social care systems) continence services has been identified by the *National Service Framework for Older People* (NSFOP) (DH, 2001). Continence services employ nurses who offer specialist advice and support; referral can be made directly by the patient or by the healthcare professional. The services are also a source of information and support for health professionals.

Normal urinary elimination and the ageing process

This section will provide a brief overview of normal elimination and the effects of ageing, before explaining why incontinence occurs.

Urine is produced when the kidneys filter the blood to remove waste products. Urine passes from the kidneys, down the ureters, and into the bladder. The bladder lies behind the symphysis pubis and, in males, it lies in front of the rectum and above the prostrate; in females, it lies in front of the uterus and vagina (see Figure 14.1). The urethra is the duct by which urine is discharged from the bladder. In women, it is about 4 cm long; in men, it is about 20 cm long. Behind the bladder are a group of muscles known as the 'pelvic floor', which support the bladder, bowels, and, in females, the womb. (To develop your knowledge and understanding further, you should refer to an anatomy and physiology book.)

As urine collects in the bladder, sensory nerve endings called 'stretch receptors' send messages to the brain that result in the contraction of the detrusor muscle (the smooth muscle that comprises the bladder wall) and relaxation of the internal sphincter muscle. Urine is then released from the bladder. However, in order for this to happen, the conscious relaxation of the external sphincter muscle needs to occur; for most people, this occurs when and where they choose to go to the lavatory. This requires complex nervous system input from the higher centres. The process of messages being sent and the patient consciously relaxing the external sphincter muscle may be compromised by neurological disorders, and incontinence may occur (see below). For other people, damage to the pelvic floor may be the cause of incontinence (see below).

The amount of urine passed will depend on fluid input; older people should have a daily fluid intake of 1.5–2 litres, including that contained in foodstuffs, but this will depend upon the patient's weight. The physiological requirement is for 28 mL/kg body mass each 24 hours (Abrams and Klevemark, 1996). Due to physiological changes, urine production at night often increases in older people, and this can lead to disturbed sleep, and the frequent need to get out of bed and go to the lavatory.

As the body ages, kidney function declines and loses some of the ability to remove waste from the blood. The muscles of the ureters, bladder, and urethra also weaken, and this may result in the bladder not fully emptying each time the patient goes to the lavatory, leaving behind a 'residual volume'. This might result in an increase in urinary infections or urinary frequency.

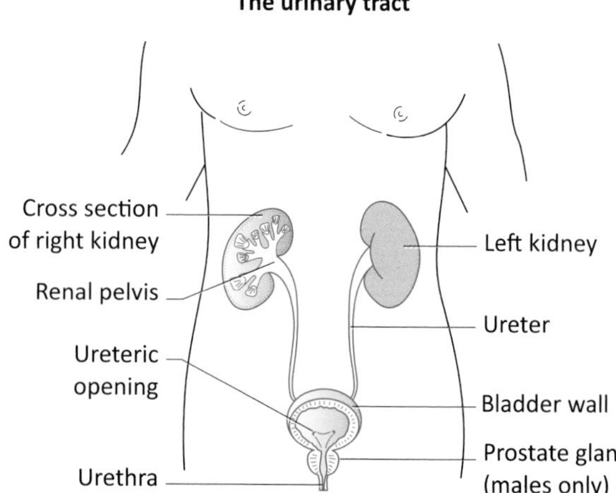

Figure 14.1 The urinary tract

Common causes and types of urinary incontinence

Stress incontinence

'Stress incontinence' refers to involuntary leakage occurring when people laugh, cough, sneeze, or exercise. It is more common in women than in men due to pregnancy and childbirth, when damage can occur to the pelvic floor muscles and the urethral sphincter; this problem may have developed several years before the woman seeks help. Women may also be affected by low oestrogen levels after the menopause, causing thinning and decreased vascularity in the submucosal urethral tissues, which reduces urethral closure.

For men, stress incontinence may occur following prostate surgery if accidental damage occurs to the bladder neck or internal sphincter. Other causes of stress incontinence may include repeated heavy lifting, a chronic cough that strains the pelvic floor, and obesity leading to a decrease in pelvic floor strength.

Urgency incontinence (or overactive bladder)

'Urgency incontinence' occurs when there is a sudden desire to empty the bladder and the patient is not able to get to the lavatory in time. The symptom of urinary urgency is defined as a sudden, compelling desire to void that is difficult to overcome (Abrams et al., 2002).

Also known as 'overactive bladder' (OAB), urgency incontinence is sometimes referred to as 'OAB wet'. Urgency without urgency incontinence is sometimes referred to as 'OAB dry'. Overall, of people with OAB, a third are incontinent. Causes of urge incontinence include urinary tract infections.

Functional incontinence

'Functional incontinence' occurs when the lower urinary tract and bowel function is, to all intents, normal, but the person is still incontinent. This may be because of physical impairments causing, for example, poor mobility and difficulties in getting out of a chair to visit the lavatory. A new environment may cause functional incontinence if the patient is not aware of whom to ask for help, or of the location of the lavatory. Other factors might include poor eyesight or not wearing the correct strength glasses, and poor foot care, which can make walking painful.

Overflow incontinence

'Overflow incontinence' occurs when the bladder remains full and does not empty completely (that is, chronic retention). This can be accompanied by poor flow of urine and continual dribbling. This is more prevalent in older adults than younger adults, due to progressive bladder muscle failure, coupled with the effect of outflow tract obstruction in men.

Overflow incontinence can occur in medical conditions such as diabetes, multiple sclerosis, and motor neurone disease, in which neurological damage has occurred. Severe constipation can also cause overflow incontinence.

Mixed urinary continence

Many people report symptoms of both urgency incontinence and stress incontinence. This is referred to as 'mixed symptoms'. About 50 per cent of women report mixed symptoms (Sykes et al., 2005).

Investigations to determine the cause of urinary incontinence

Student and newly qualified nurses will usually undertake fluid balance charts and urinalysis. However, it is important to be aware of other investigations, for which you will probably need to refer your patients to a more senior member of staff who has been specifically trained to carry these out.

Fluid balance charts

A fluid balance chart may also be called a 'fluid diary', 'bladder diary', 'frequency–volume chart', or 'fluid chart'. Fluid balance charts are necessary to establish the fluid input and output of the patient. The chart should contain information concerning volume, type of fluids, frequency of input, and volume and frequency of output. If incontinence occurs, then the patient keeping the chart should record whether the fluid lost was large, medium, or small.

It is recommended that these charts are kept over three days to allow for changes in the patient's normal day. Normal fluid output is proportional to input, but input (and therefore output) should be proportional to the patient's weight (Abrams and Klevmark, 1996). Advice to the patient should be that about six to eight cups of fluid a day should be drunk, but if the patient says that caffeine-containing drinks worsen their symptoms, then a trial of withdrawal should be recommended.

A fluid balance chart can be completed by the patient, nurse, or carer, whoever is most appropriate.

An example of a fluid balance chart can be found later in this chapter.

Urine testing

The nurse should collect a sample of urine for a urinalysis to be carried out using a medical urine test strip (multistick/dip stick). A good clinical skills book will show you how to undertake this. If the stick indicates that protein, blood, glucose, leucocytes, or nitrates are present, then a specimen should be sent for culture and analysis.

When collecting a sample from an older person, the nurse should recognize that they may have difficulty providing a clean catch sample due to restrictions in mobility or dexterity, and assistance may be required or consideration given to the how the specimen is to be collected. A receptacle placed in the toilet may make collection easier than giving the person a small bottle. Make sure that your instructions are clear and properly understood—for example, if you require a midstream specimen of urine (MSSU), explain exactly what that is and how they must first pass urine into the toilet, then, without stopping the flow of urine, catch some urine in a sterile bottle, then pass the rest of the urine in the toilet. The nurse should ensure that privacy and dignity are maintained.

Bladder scans

Bladder scans assist in detecting any residual urine following urination.

Digital rectal examination

A digital rectal examination (DRE) will establish if the patient's bowel is impacted with faeces, which can be a factor in urinary incontinence. Rectal examination will also allow for an assessment of the prostate in men. However, such procedures should only be carried out by someone competent and trained (NMC, 2008). (See 'Digital rectal examination' below.)

Abdominal examination

Abdominal examination allows for an assessment of retention of urine in the bladder, but will only detect a fairly large bladder (that is, more than 500 mL), which is why, if you suspect that there might be a residual volume, a bladder scan or in-and-out catheter should be done. The examination is usually done by a specialist doctor or a nurse competent to carry out the examination (NMC, 2008).

Vaginal examination

An urogential prolapse may be the cause of voiding problems and if a mass protruding from the vagina is seen, then a specialist opinion should be sought.

Pelvic floor muscle assessment

Digital assessment of the pelvic floor should be carried out by a specialist nurse or physiotherapist before pelvic floor muscle training. The Oxford grading system can be used to grade the strength of the pelvic floor muscles (NICE, 2006) (see Box 14.1).

Other assessments

Mobility, dexterity, and environment

A patient who is experiencing mobility or dexterity problems may need assessment to determine how easily they are able to access a lavatory and remove clothing. The environment should also be assessed. For example, are the access routes to the lavatory clear? Hand rails, adapted clothing, raised lavatory seats, good lighting, and other environmental adaptations may be useful.

Referral to an occupational therapist may be made for a full assessment.

Box 14.1 Oxford grading system (for assessing pelvic floor strength)

0 Nil
1 Flicker
2 Weak
3 Moderate
4 Good
5 Strong

Mental health

It may be appropriate to assess the patient's mental health and degree of cognitive impairment in order to assess the patient's ability to comply with any treatment programme. The mini-mental state examination (Folstein et al., 1975) and the six-item cognitive impairment test (Katzman et al., 1983) may be used. However, it should not be assumed that cognitive impairment is the cause of the incontinence and patients should be assessed to determine if other factors are responsible.

Treatment for stress incontinence

Each treatment option should be discussed with the patient in order to find the most suitable option.

Pelvic floor muscle exercises

The National Institute of Health and Clinical Excellence (2006) recommends a minimum of 32 pelvic floor muscle contractions a day, although it provides no specific guidelines for older people and there is not much evidence of effect in older people. The aim of these exercises is to increase pelvic muscle strength and successful performance can not only cure stress incontinence, but also allow the older person to 'hang on' long enough to reach the lavatory in time.

NURSING PRACTICE INSIGHT: HOW TO TEACH PELVIC FLOOR EXERCISES

Ask the patient to try the following steps.

- Sit comfortably, without moving your abdomen muscles or bottom, and without holding your breath.
- Try to squeeze the muscle around your back passage, as if you are trying to stop wind from escaping.
- Next, try to do the same squeeze around the front and breathe.
- After tightening, try to lift the muscle—for example, by imagining being in a lift and going up. Aim to pull as hard and hold as long as you are able, then relax.
- Repeat this eight times, with a rest in between each contraction.
- Then, squeeze the muscles quickly for one second and repeat five times.

To see an improvement in incontinence symptoms requires motivation and commitment, because the exercises need to be carried out regularly and over a long period of time. Progress is reviewed at regular intervals by the specialist nurse or physiotherapist.

Medication

There is only one medication licensed for stress incontinence. It is called duloxetine. It is not recommended by NICE for this condition. Although it may be helpful, its main side effect, nausea, severely limits its use.

Urethral bulking agents

Bulking agents can be injected into the submucosal tissue of the urethra or bladder neck and these prevent stress incontinence. This improves the closure mechanism (sphincter) of the bladder neck. The effectiveness of these agents is short-term (months), so the procedure may need to be repeated.

Surgery

Several surgical options aim to prevent the leakage of urine for women. The commonest operation for this involves the insertion of a plastic mesh tape underneath the middle of the urethra. The tension-free vaginal tape is the best known of these options. They are effective in older women.

Vaginal cones

Vaginal cones are a device for weight training of the pelvic floor. They can assist the patient in improving muscle strength and can have positive feedback if utilized properly. There is no evidence that these are effective in older women.

Electrical stimulation

Electrical stimulation treatment is usually carried out by physiotherapists or a continence nurse. A small probe is placed in the rectum for men and the vagina for women, and this stimulates the pelvic floor muscles. This treatment is useful for people who cannot do normal pelvic floor muscle exercises.

Treatment for urgency incontinence

Treatment options for both overactive wet or dry urge incontinence include those listed below. Each should be discussed with the patient in order to find the most suitable option.

Bladder training (behavioural therapies)

Bladder training is a process of establishing patterns of toileting and behaviour. The aim is to increase the interval between the desire to void and the actual void. Different regimes emphasize either a strict schedule in which times are set for or by the patient. Most specialists advise that a chart recording frequency and volume is kept for a minimum of three days, and up to seven days if possible, to establish a baseline. Once a baseline is obtained, then the patient is asked to increase the time between visits to the lavatory. Commitment from the patient is important, because improvement can take between three and six months, or even longer (NICE, 2006).

Bladder training can be used with people who have neurological changes, such as dementia, and should be initiated every two hours when toileting (Getliff and Doleman, 2007).

Pharmacological treatment

NICE (2006) recommends the use of immediate-release non-proprietary oxbutynim if bladder training has not been successful for women with overactive bladder or mixed urinary incontinence. Other drugs may be prescribed, but women should be counselled about the adverse effects of antimuscarinic drugs. Medication may be used alongside bladder training.

Forthcoming recommendations for men suggest that an alpha blocker (for example, tamsulosin) should be given initially, and then an antimuscarinic medication (for example egg oxybutynin) after four weeks should symptoms not resolve.

The patient pathway illustrated in Figure 14.2 demonstrates the use of medication in continence management.

Surgical treatment

For detrusor overactivity that does not respond to pharmacological measures, there are surgical procedures that can help. Injection of botulinum toxin A into the bladder is rapidly becoming the commonest procedure. Alternatives, recommended by NICE after appropriate counseling, are neuromodulation, using an implantable stimulator of the sacral nerve roots (see anatomy), which control the bladder, and a clam ileocystoplasty, whereby the bladder is opened and a patch of bowel patched into the hole. This controls the urgency and frequency, but means that patients often cannot empty their bladder properly and have to self-catheterize to achieve this.

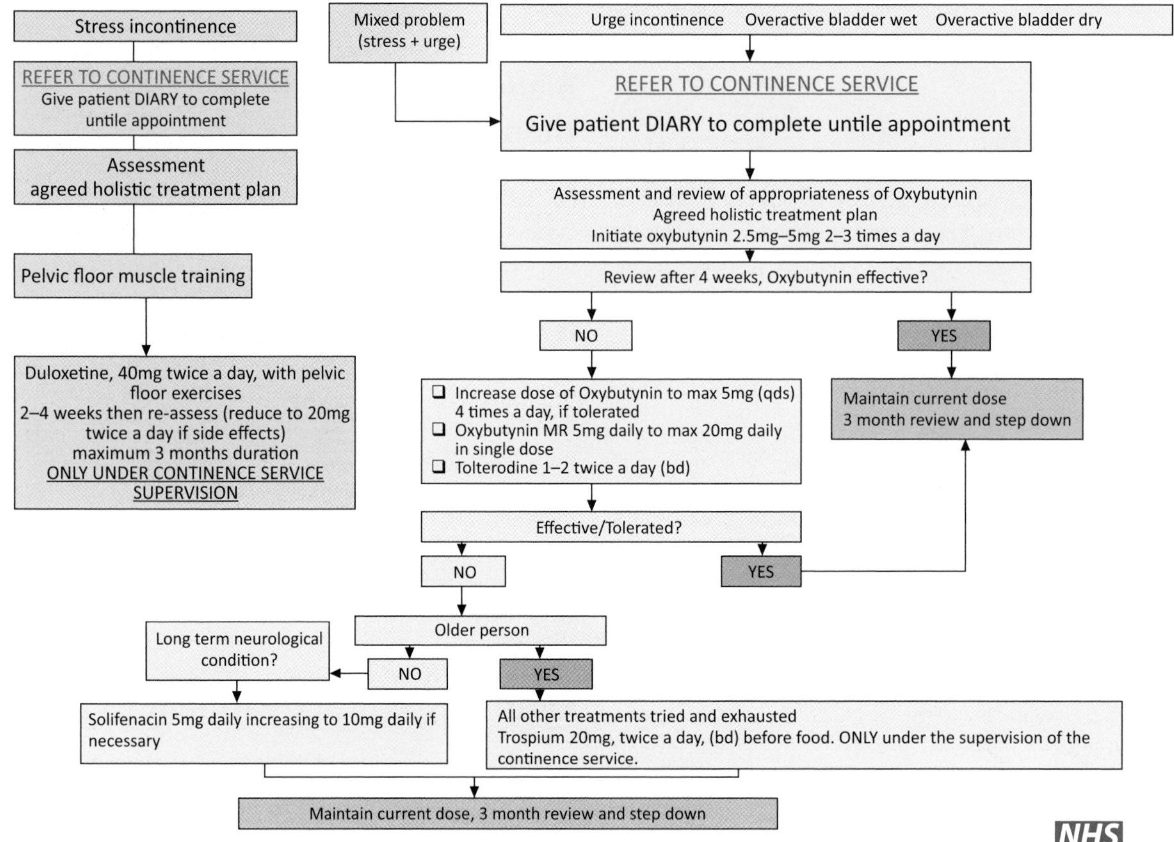

Figure 14.2 The use of medication in continence management
Source: © Dudley Continence Service.

Non-pharmacological treatment

Pads

Pads may be necessary, but should not be a first choice of management. Consideration should be given to the size of the pads and whether the patient can change the pad on their own. The quality and quantity of pads needed, and how the patient can dispose of used pads, also needs consideration. In the UK, pads are available through local continence services, presently free of charge, and this includes delivery and collection. Many types are available and some recognition of patient choice should be made in selection of the most appropriate product.

Sheaths

Penile sheaths (that is, a soft rubber sleeve that fits over the penis) may be used with men as a means of collecting urine in a bag attached to the leg. Measurement for the correct size of sheath needs to be carried out. Some men may prefer sheaths to wearing a pad. Evidence shows that they can be more acceptable and less costly.

Catheters

If the incontinence is intractable and pads would be insufficient, a urinary urethral catheter (a permanent indwelling catheter) may be a solution. Catheters may also be used temporarily if the patient has pressure ulcers and skin healing is being hampered by maceration of the skin. Catheters should not be used because of nursing convenience and should be avoided if at all possible. Infection can be introduced by poor aseptic technique and the Department of Health (2007) identifies urinary tract infections as the second largest single group of healthcare-associated infections in the UK, amounting to 19.7 per cent of all hospital-acquired infections.

Intermittent catheterization (self-catheterization) is an option when a patient is unable to void, has voiding difficulties, or retains large quantities of residual urine. This skill is taught by a nurse specialist and the patient's dexterity has to be considered as part of the assessment process.

The use of catheters are also indicated where there is urinary retention—for example, either before or following surgery—or where there are other medical conditions, such as deteriorating renal function.

Skin care and incontinence

As people age, the epidermis of the skin thins, and there is a reduction in the contact between the dermis and the epidermis, which leads to a reduction in the exchange of nutrients and metabolites between these two layers. Because of these changes, the skin is more liable to damage, so the nurse needs to be particularly vigilant when moving older adults and in keeping the skin clean if incontinence occurs.

Reflection point

Incontinence—either urinary, faecal, or both—can lead to skin breakdown caused by faecal enzymes and wet skin.

This damage can lead to excoriation and dermitus, in which case the skin becomes red, inflamed, and sore. When incontinence does occur, nurses should make sure that the patient's skin is cleaned properly using a product that contains a moisturizing agent (silicone, titanium, or zinc-based) (Nazarko, 2007). Good hygiene will prevent skin breakdown and is essential in helping to maintain dignity.

Assessment process

Whilst some assessments should be part of the standard nurse baseline assessment, a more in-depth assessment might be required by a nurse specialist from a continence service. If the non-specialist nurse identifies that the patient has a continence problem, they should maintain a fluid balance chart and carry out a 'multistick' urine test. If a problem is identified and a referral is made to a nurse specialist, then the following example of an assessment might be used in determining the cause of incontinence and identifying an appropriate treatment strategy.

Before starting a continence assessment, it is important to remember that this is an embarrassing topic for most people. In order to minimize embarrassment and maintain dignity, you should:

- ensure privacy and prevent interruptions;
- ensure that there is plenty of time, so that the patient does not feel rushed; and
- offer reassurance.

The focus of the assessment is on the patient's medical history and the presenting symptoms of incontinence.

Case study: Mrs Nolan

Mrs Nolan, an 65-year-old lady, has an appointment with the practice nurse for a check-up on her asthma. Whilst talking to the nurse, she mentions that she has been experiencing going to the lavatory frequently and occasionally wets herself. She also experiences a sense of urgency and she therefore feels the need to be near lavatory facilities at all times. As a result, she has stopped going out socially—and even going to the local shops is becoming difficult for her.

Mrs Nolan has reduced her fluid intake to try to control the urgency, but this has not helped. She has also been going to the lavatory 'just in case', to try to halt the impact that the bladder problem is having on her life. Mrs Nolan is unhappy, because her quality of life is being affected by her bladder problem, but she does not know who to talk to or if anything can be done to help her.

In relation to Mrs Nolan in the case study above, the nurse would complete an assessment and physical examination, as described in Table 14.1.

Mrs Nolan would have been asked to record her fluid intake and output, along with any incontinence, over a period of three days. Table 14.2 illustrates her fluid balance for one day.

The assessment information would initially suggest that Mrs Nolan may have 'mixed urinary incontinence' (urgency and stress). Her 'urgency' symptoms can be identified because she is going to the lavatory more than 15 times in 24 hours and passing small volumes of urine. Her fluid intake is very restricted and this may have worsened her symptoms. Her 'stress' symptoms are that she is leaking urine on occasions. You will note from the completed assessment form that she might have been offered bladder scanning if she had reported any voiding symptoms or had a prolapse. A urine test was requested, to determine if infection was responsible for the protein and leucocytes in her urine, although she reported no dysuria (pain on micturition) and had no suprapubic tenderness.

Case study continued...

Once the nurse had received the results of the urine test and Mrs Nolan had completed her fluid balance chart, an individual patient care plan was formulated. Mrs Nolan had a urine infection, so antibiotics were prescribed for five days and instructions on the importance of completing the course of tablets was given. The fluid balance chart indicated that Mrs Nolan was overly restricting her fluids, and she was advised to increase her fluid intake and to include non-irritant fluids, such as water. The nurse instructed her on pelvic floor exercises and bladder training.

Table 14.1 Assessment for urinary incontinence

Name/address/postcode:
Mrs Nolan
10 The Meadows
New Town
DOB 14.08.1924
GP: Dr Tyson

Urinary symptoms
Frequency how often?: 15 times
Nocturia how often waking at night?: x 2
Urgency: Yes
Leaking on exercise/coughing: Yes
Passive incontinence (wet without knowing): No
Is the bed ever wet and how often?: No
When did this start?: 45 years, but mild until recently
What were the circumstances?: After menopause
Is the problem worsening/static/improving?: Worsening
How often does the leakage occur?: X 2 daily
Do you use pads and how many?: Yes, 2 pads a day
Where do you get the pads from?: Chemist or uses toilet paper

Bowels: Every 3 days, type 1 stools passing

Do you take laxatives?: No
Have you been constipated how do you treat?: No
Faecal incontinence: No
Psychological: Embarrassed, anxious that she might have an accident or people might smell her

Sexual problems, are there any?: None reported
Social interaction: Limited
Family/relations: Lives on her own, family nearby
Activities: Family events, used to like bowling; finds interacting with others difficult due to incontinence

Signed/date

When seen: 15.8.09
Referred by: Self

Voiding symptoms
Hesitancy: No
Poor stream how often?: No
Any straining: No
Post-micturition dribble: No
Dysuria: No
Haematuria: No

Fluid intake:
Pt asked to keep chart.
Any restriction?: Stops drinking after about 7 p.m. so as to try not to go to the lavatory in the night

Medical history:
Asthma, 1 normal delivery and 1 caesarean
Any neurological problems: No
Medication: Uses inhaler for asthma
Operations: Caesarean, as above

Any treatment for bladder previously?: No
Environment: Own home
Lavatory facilities adequate/or not?: Adequate
Washing/laundry: Twin tub, difficulty in drying in the winter

Physical examination
Skin problems: Sore and red in vulval area
Any prolapse seen(females): No
Retracted penis(males): N/A
MSSU: Protein and leucocytes detected; specimen sent for clarification of micro-organism before treatment (possible antibiotics to be prescribed)
Residual volume/bladder scan: (Possibly on next visit after further information gathered from a bladder diary)
Atrophic changes (females): Yes
Rectal examination: No
Base of work

Table 14.2 Fluid balance chart

Time	Fluid intake	Fluid output	Accidents/ leaks
07:00	250 ml tea	150 ml	
08:00	250 ml tea	350 ml	
08:45		150 ml	
10:00	250 ml coffee	50 ml	Slight leakage
12:00		100 ml	

Table 14.2 *(Continued)* Fluid balance chart

Time	Fluid intake	Fluid output	Accidents/ leaks
14:00	250 ml tea		
15:00		150 ml	
15:45		75 ml	
17:00		100 ml	
18:00		100 ml	

Table 14.2 *(Continued)* Fluid balance chart

Time	Fluid intake	Fluid output	Accidents/ leaks
19:30	100 ml sherry		
19:45		150 ml	
20:00			Slight leakage
22:00	50 ml water	100 ml	
01:00		50 ml	
02:00			
03:00		50 ml	
04:00		150 ml	
05:00			
06:00		200 ml	
Total	1,150 ml	1,925 ml	

At a six-week follow-up appointment, Mrs Nolan reported that her symptoms were improving and that she had recently been out socially. She was advised to continue with the pelvic floor exercises and bladder training. A further appointment was made for her condition to be monitored.

Faecal incontinence

As with urinary incontinence, faecal incontinence is a symptom, not a diagnosis. NICE (2007) estimates that between 1 and 10 per cent of adults are affected by faecal incontinence. Faecal incontinence can be defined as the involuntary passage of faeces in inappropriate circumstances and it should never be considered normal.

Faecal incontinence may be due to a single cause, but it may also be due to several factors leading to incontinence. NICE (2007) notes that certain groups can be identified as at high risk of faecal incontinence, and these groups include frail older people, people with severe cognitive impairment, and people who have urinary incontinence. In addition, specific groups of people are identified as at high risk of developing faecal incontinence, including people with faecal loading or constipation, people with limited mobility, hospitalized patients who are acutely unwell and who develop acute faecal loading and associated incontinence, people with neurological disease/injury, people with learning disabilities, and severely or terminally ill people.

Faecal elimination

Elimination of waste products from the body is necessary for maintaining health; the excreted waste product is called 'faeces', or 'stools'. The digestive system takes in food, removes nutrients, and expels the waste product. On leaving the stomach, peristaltic waves move the waste product through the small intestine into the large intestine, then the rectum, and out of the body through the anus. When faeces enter the rectum, sensory nerves alert the patient that they need to defecate and voluntarily relax the external anal sphincter. The abdominal muscles and the diaphragm assist the process as they increase abdominal pressure, and, with contraction of the muscles of the pelvic floor, faeces moves through the anal canal. The anal sphincter is a circular ring of muscles, located at the opening of the anus. The anal sphincter muscles include the internal and external anal sphincter muscles. These muscles, along with the surrounding pelvic floor muscles, create a barrier that prevents the escape of faeces and flatus. The expulsion of faeces from the anal canal is called 'defecation', or may be called a 'bowel movement' or 'motion' (see Figure 14.3). Some people may have a bowel movement several times a day; others, a few times a week. Ageing alone does not result in a change in bowel frequency; a change in bowel habit in an older person should be investigated, because colonic cancer is common in older people.

To develop your knowledge and understanding further, you should refer to an anatomy and physiology book.

Causes of faecal incontinence

There are many different causes of faecal incontinence and these can be grouped as follows.

Disorders of the anal sphincter and lower rectum

Faecal incontinence can be caused by damage to one or both of the anal sphincter muscles. Typically, damage to the external sphincter will lead to a feeling of urgency, and if the lavatory cannot be reached in time, then incontinence occurs.

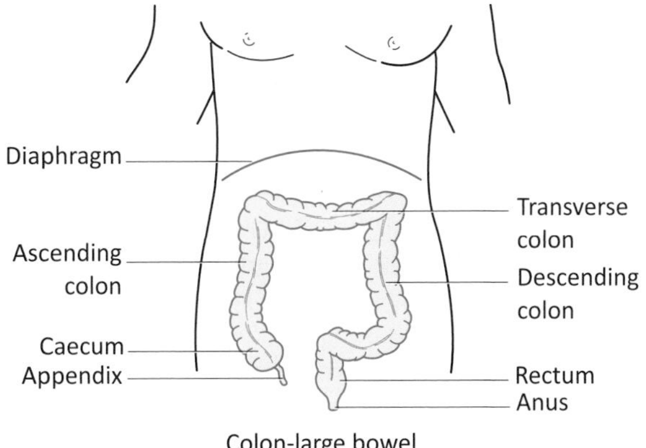

Figure 14.3 The large bowel

Box 14.2 Causes of constipation

- A change in activity levels can affect bowel habit—for example, older people may become less physically active.
- A change in routine or habit, such as an admission to hospital, may change people's lavatory routine.
- People's mental state can have an impact on bowel habit and depression can be associated with constipation.
- Medications may have an impact—for example, some tranquillizers, mineral supplements, and analgesics can cause constipation.
- A low-fibre diet and poor fluid intake is a major cause of constipation.
- Some people have very slow oral–anal transit times (normal is less than five days), which results in constipation.

Damage to the internal sphincter may result in soiling occurring without the patient realizing that it is happening. Damage can occur following giving birth (damage to pelvic floor and perineum), although the symptom of incontinence may occur not at the time, but some years later. Accidental damage may also occur following surgery for piles (haemorrhoidectomy), or an anal fissure or fistula following surgery involving the rectum. Rectal prolapse (often caused by constipation) may also be the cause of faecal incontinence.

Neurological disorders

Neurological disorders with associated nerve injury or disease, such as that caused by multiple sclerosis, stroke, or dementia, may result in the patient suffering from a loss of sensation and not recognizing that they need to go to the lavatory.

Diarrhoea

Diarrhoea can be caused by infection such as food poisoning, some medications such as antibiotics, or medical conditions such as diverticular disease, irritable bowel syndrome (IBS), ulcerative colitis, or Crohn's disease—particularly if accompanied with poor mobility. Diarrhoea may result in incontinence. A common cause of diarrhoea is faecal impaction (constipation). Approximately 50 per cent of cases of faecal incontinence are caused by constipation. This is because a partial blockage caused by hard faeces, which partially stops new waste products from being passed, leads to loose faecal matter passing around the partial blockage.

Investigations to determine the cause of faecal incontinence

Food diary

The nurse may ask the patient to keep a record of the food and fluid intake—usually for a week—in order to gain an understanding of what the patient is eating and drinking. Fibre, fruit, and fluid intake are important to recognize.

Inspection of stool

The nurse should check stools for colour, consistency, amount, shape, and odour. The nurse should also check for any abnormal characteristics, such as the presence of overt blood or foreign bodies. A stool chart helps to clarify the type of stool passed, the frequency and amount, and if the patient experienced any pain. The Bristol stool chart is widely used (Norton and Chelvanayagam, 2000). The chart uses descriptors ranging from 'Type 1' (separate, hard lumps) to 'Type 7' (watery, no solid pieces) and is available online at http://www.bladderandbowelfoundation.org/search/

Physical examination

A physical examination includes listening for bowel sounds and palpitation of the abdomen. This procedure should only be carried out by someone competent and trained to do so (NMC, 2008).

Digital rectal examination

In a digital rectal examination, the patient lies on their left side. If they are unable to lie on the left side, it is acceptable for them to lie on the right side, but because the bowel falls on to the left side, this is the preferred position for the patient to be in. A gloved, lubricated finger is inserted into the rectum to determine if the patient is constipated, and to identify any rectal mass or the presence of blood. In the man, the prostate can be palpated, and its size, consistency, and texture assessed. Hard faeces in the rectum of a Type 1 or Type 2 (see 'Inspection of stool' above) would suggest constipation.

This procedure should be carried out only by a qualified nurse who can demonstrate competence (NMC, 2008).

Stool specimens

If there is diarrhoea or very soft fluffy stool, a specimen may be collected and sent for analysis to detect for bacteria, viruses, parasites, or ova. Occult (hidden) blood may also be detected. Any abnormalities of this type would warrant further investigation and treatments specific to the condition can be implemented.

Other specialist investigations

Specialist X-rays, such as a barium enema or meal and follow-through, plain abdominal X-rays, transit studies, magnetic resonance imaging (MRI), or a defecating proctogram may be undertaken. Visualization examinations include sigmoidoscopy, proctoscopy, and colonoscopy. Anal physiology include colonic manometry and ultrasound may be required if an underlying pathology is suspected (Nicholas, 2004).

Mobility, dexterity, and environment

As with urinary incontinence, the patient's mobility, dexterity, and environment should be assessed.

Table 14.3 Types of laxative and their use

Medication	Purpose
Bulk-forming laxatives	Used with chronic constipation as a maintenance strategy
Osmotic laxatives	Used with chronic constipation May take up to three days to be effective, so not suitable for rapid relief
Stimulant laxatives	Used with acute constipation Effective within 8–12 hours
Faecal softeners	Should be used with patients who need to avoid straining, e.g. people who have had surgery Work within 1–2 days

Treatment options for constipation

Diet and exercise

A diet high in fibre with plenty of fluids is the first-line prevention of constipation and should be combined, where possible, with regular exercise or other activity (DH, 2004).

Oral medication

There are many different types of laxative available: some are suitable for short-term use; others are for longer-term management. These medications are described in Table 14.3.

Rectal medication

Suppositories and enemas may be prescribed, but should not be used as a long-term strategy and should be administered in an acute phase only.

For some people, home rectal irrigation is an acceptable way of achieving control. Kits to do this are available.

Treatment options for disorders of the anal sphincter and lower rectum

Surgery

Surgery may be required, but is generally seen as a last resort for treatment of faecal incontinence.

The Royal College of Nursing (RCN) bowel care guidance for nurses (2008) refers to surgical interventions for faecal incontinence, and includes secondary sphincter repair and stoma.

Surgery for constipation and associated problems includes haemorrhoidectomy, sphincterotomy (a surgical procedure that involves treating mucosal fissures from the anal canal/sphincter), and treatment for prolapse.

Treatment options for disorders of neurological control

Dementia

Depending on the stage of the disease, people with dementia may try to hide the 'evidence' or may go to the lavatory in the wrong places. Nurses can reduce the incidence of incontinence with good care.

Firstly, do not assume that the incontinence is untreatable. It is important that a full assessment is carried out, because the patient may, for example, have a urinary tract infection and neurological changes may not be the cause.

Changes to the environment can be made that minimize the likelihood of incontinence. Make sure that the patient knows where the lavatory is—signs pointing to the lavatory and door or picture signs may help. Leaving the lavatory door open, so that the patient can clearly see the lavatory, may also help, as might changing the colour of the seat to, for example, black to make the lavatory easier to see.

Make sure that people can remove clothing easily and that there are no physical barriers, such as tables or chairs, in the way of them reaching the lavatory.

Good observation of behaviour might alert the nurse to the patient's need to go to the lavatory—for example, they may be fidgeting or trying to get out of a chair or bed, because they need to visit the lavatory.

Toileting after breakfast, using the natural gastro-colic reflex, is often useful, but frequent reminders or taking the patient to the lavatory should also be established.

An option for some patients in order to achieve predictable bowel emptying is to use constipating agents and to rely on regular enemas to empty the bowel.

See Chapter 11 for more on dementia.

Other neurological conditions

People who have neurological conditions such as multiple sclerosis or Parkinson's disease may become incontinent. This can be caused by nerve damage and loss of sensation or constipation. As discussed, an adapted exercise regime and a healthy diet, high in fibre and plenty of fluids, may help to resolve or alleviate the issues.

Referral to a continence service and specialist neurological services is recommended in more complex cases.

Treatment options for diarrhoea

Treatment for diarrhoea will depend upon the cause, and diarrhoea that is persistent for more than a few days will require a sample for culture and sensitivity analysis to identify appropriate antibiotics.

Food poisoning will frequently settle with rest and plenty of fluids. Anti-diarrhoeal medications may also be required.

Patients with ulcerative colitis, which commonly result in diarrhoea, are usually under the care of a specialist clinician.

Pelvic floor muscle exercises

These are essential not only for urinary incontinence, but also for faecal incontinence. (See 'Pelvic floor muscle exercises' above.)

Pads

As with urinary incontinence pads, there needs to be a comprehensive assessment, and pads should be correctly fitted and not used for nursing convenience. Most pads that are used for urinary continence can be used for faecal incontinence and patient preference for design type should be sought (Fader et al., 2008).

NURSING PRACTICE INSIGHT: DISCUSSING OPTIONS WITH PATIENTS

It is important that, when discussing the application of pads, the patient's carer is invited to be included in the discussion—particularly where the carer is the person who will be assisting the patient. The nurse should always be reassuring and sensitive, and the patient and carer need to be given time to pose questions and enable discussion.

Skin care

See 'Skin care and incontinence' above.

Nursing care

The impact that incontinence has on the patient is likely to be extremely upsetting and people who are incontinent are likely to be highly embarrassed by their condition. Incontinence can lead to isolation, as people withdraw from social situations due to embarrassment.

The nurse has an important role to play in ensuring that incontinence does not occur because of poor care or because of the environment in which the older person is living. Nurses must ensure that older people in their care receive a healthy diet, including plenty of fluids, and ensure that older adults are kept mobile, because exercise will help bowel movement and help to maintain independence in accessing lavatory facilities. The environment needs to be suitable, and issues such as accessibility, providing clean and private lavatory facilities, and ensuring access with good lighting will all help to maintain continence.

When incontinence has been identified, the nurse must ensure that the patient's dignity is maintained by ensuring privacy and dealing sensitively with the issues.

Assessment

As with urinary incontinence, a full assessment needs to be carried out, including relevant medical history (any medication being taken, prescribed or non-prescribed), dietary habits including fluid intake, cognitive assessment, and an environmental assessment, before focusing specifically on the assessment of bowel habits.

Assessment may include self-assessment questionnaires recording:

- how frequently the patient passes stools;
- the consistency of stools;
- any pain before, during, or after defecating;
- any blood loss; and
- any unintended weight loss.

Case study

During his 'Well Man' check-up with the practice nurse, Mr Jones mentions problems going to the lavatory. He has, at times, been incontinent of faeces and is extremely embarrassed about it. Since his wife died last year, he has not been eating or drinking properly. He generally sits at home, rarely going out, and has become quite isolated.

In relation to Mr Jones in the case study above, the nurse would complete an assessment, as illustrated in Table 14.4.

Table 14.4 Assessment for bowel dysfunction

Name: Mr Jones
Address: 89 Haycroft Road
Little Riding
HY 1 2BG

Telephone no.: 01456 27890
GP: Dr Blud
NHS no.: 4547484940
Medical history
Hypertension (controlled by medication)
Hip replacement 9 years ago

Bowel symptoms:
Was daily; now every 4–5 days

Is there urgency?
Occasionally

How long can you delay?
5 mins maximum

What are your stools like?
Hard/little drops

Do you have 'accidents'?
Yes, but no set pattern when they occur

Do you have bowel leakage?
Yes, soiling of underwear and can occur after he has emptied his bowels; has also had diarrhoea

When does the leakage occur?
Twice a week, but no set pattern

What is the loss like?
Diarrhoea

Do you wear pads?
Yes

Do you get flatus?
More now

Do you leak on passing flatus?
No

Do you have pain on defecating?
Yes, very uncomfortable; can sometimes sit on lavatory for 20 mins

DOB: 21/01/29
Referrer: Self
Weight
Has not lost weight, feels bloated

What size pad used?
Small pant liner; uses some that he found in his wife's cupboards

Is it restricting what you are able to do?
Yes, finding that he needs to know where the toilets are when he goes out

Do you have trouble emptying your bowels?
Yes, does not feel fully empty

How much fluid do you have per day?
About 3 cups of tea

How much fruit/vegetables per day?
Limited; finds he is not eating properly since wife died

Medication
Over-the-counter laxative; milk of magnesium
A couple of spoonfuls when feeling bloated
Ramipril 5 mg
Bendroflumethiazide 2.5 mg

Environment
Lavatory is downstairs
Stairs are quite steep and is finding them difficult to climb

Washing/drying facilities
Has a washing machine; drying is by putting clothes on a line

Social
Use to go the Legion Club every Friday
Family live nearby (1 son and 1 daughter plus family)
Lives on his own since wife died

Investigations
Abdomen: swollen and hard faeces felt on transverse colon
Anus: haemorrhoids—red and have been bleeding
Skin: generally is intact and hydrated
Digital rectal examination: This would normally be mandatory, but Mr Jones declined, agreeing that it might be necessary at a later date

Action to be taken
Food diary for 1 week
Bowel diary for 1 week
Sign/Date

Table 14.5 Food diary

Day	Breakfast	Lunch	Dinner
Monday	Tea/toast white bread x 1	Biscuit/tea	Pot noodles/tea
Tuesday	Tea	Soup/tea	Sandwich cheese/crisps/tea
Wednesday	Tea/toast x 2 white bread	Sandwich ham/tea/juice	Microwave roast dinner/tea
Thursday	Tea/toast x 2 white bread	Sandwich cheese/water/apple	Tin spaghetti on toast (white bread)/tea
Friday	Tea/toast x 2 white bread	Sandwich ham and cheese/tea	Meat pie and potatoes/tinned peas/tea
Saturday	Tea/toast x 2 white bread	Juice/soup /tea	Chicken roll/mashed potatoes/tinned peas
Sunday	Tea/toast x 2 white bread	Microwave beef and potato dinner/tinned peaches	Sandwich with meat paste/tea

Table 14.6 Bowel chart

Day	Time	Type of stool (Bristol Stool Chart)	How long to defecate?	Pain Yes/No
Monday	07:00	1 (hard lumps)	20 minutes	Yes
Wednesday	10:00	1 (hard lumps)	30 minutes	Yes
Thursday	No bowel movement 'mess on pants', with liquid and staining	Loose		
Friday	08:00	1 (hard lumps)	5 minutes	No
Saturday	07:30	1 (hard lumps)	20 minutes	No
Sunday	No bowel movement			

Having completed the assessment, the nurse would ask Mr Jones to keep a food diary (see Table 14.5) and a bowel chart (see Table 14.6) for seven days to establish the type of bowel dysfunction that he has. Mr Jones would be given a copy of the Bristol stool chart in order to record his stools using this scale.

The food diary above suggests that Mr Jones does not eat enough fibre. The Department of Health (2004) recommends five portions of fruit and vegetables a day, and on some days, Mr Jones eats none.

The bowel chart indicates that he is passing small, hard, dry lumps, which suggests constipation. The 'accident' of liquid stool suggests overflow (faecal incontinence). A diet so low in fibre is likely to be the cause of constipation, and the diarrhoea and incontinence is 'overflow'.

Case study continued...

The practice nurse developed an individual care plan and, in consultation with Mr Jones, a laxative was prescribed with advice on taking the medication. Dietetic advice and a recommendation to drink more fluids were given. The patient was advised to take up exercise, such as walking, on a daily basis, to aid bowel movement/peristalsis.

At a two-month follow-up appointment, Mr Jones reported feeling better and having no further 'accidents'. He also reported getting a dog that keeps him company and which he takes for a walk each day. He is following the dietary advice by ensuring that he sticks to the five recommended portions of fruit and vegetables, and is drinking more water.

The practice nurse advised Mr Jones to discontinue the laxative medication, because his bowels were now functioning normally, but to ensure that he continues with his plan. He was advised to return or contact the nurse at any time if he experienced incontinence problems in future.

Conclusion

Dealing with patient elimination issues is part of many nurses' working days, but it is important to remember that, for most patients, receiving care or giving information on their toileting habits can be deeply embarrassing and distressing. In order for the nurse to develop the skills required to assess incontinence issues, it is equally important that there is recognition of the taboos surrounding the sharing of information on this topic and steps must be taken to ensure the patient's dignity is maintained. The nurse should also recognize that incontinence is not an inevitable part of growing older, and older people should receive a full assessment and care based on need; their problems should not be dismissed as an inevitable part of ageing. Promoting good bowel and bladder health is an important part of any nurse's role, and good care can make a huge and positive impact on patient's lives—surely the goal of every nurse.

Questions and self-assessment

Now that you have worked through the chapter, answer the following questions.

- How would you demonstrate respect when assessing and managing continence with an older adult?
- What impact might incontinence have on the patient's social and physical well-being?
- What are the main causes of urinary and faecal incontinence?
- Describe normal urinary and faecal elimination.
- List the key areas of assessment that are important in the assessment of incontinence.
- What treatment strategies are available for the treatment of urinary incontinence?
- What treatment strategies are available for the treatment of faecal incontinence?

Self-assessment

- Having read the chapter, how will you change your practice?
- Identify up to three areas relating to continence in which you need to develop your knowledge and understanding further.
- Identify how you are going to develop this knowledge and understanding, and set deadlines for achieving this.

References

Abrams, P. and Klevemark, B. (1996) 'Frequency volume charts: An indispensible part of lower urinary tract assessment', *Scandinavian Journal of Neurology*, 179: 47–53.

Abrams, P. Cardozo, L. Fall, M., et al. (2002) 'The standardisation of terminology in lower tract function: Report from the Standardisation Subcommittee of the International continence Society', *Neurourology and Urodynamics*, 21(2): 167–78.

Bladder and Bowel Foundation (2010) *Bladder Problems*, available online at http://www.bladderandbowelfoundation.org/bladder/bladder-problems/.

Department of Health (2000) *Good Practice in Continence Services*, London: DH, available online at http://www.dh.gov.uk/prod_consum_dh/groups/dh_digitalassets/@dh/@en/documents/digitalasset/dh_4057529.pdf.

Department of Health (2001) *National Service Framework for Older People*, London: DH, available online at http://www.dh.gov.uk/prod_consum_dh/groups/dh_digitalassets/@dh/@en/documents/digitalasset/dh_4071283.pdf.

Department of Health (2004) *Choosing Health: Making Healthy Choices Easier*, available online at http://www.dh.gov.uk/en/Publicationsandstatistics/Publications/Publications PolicyAndGuidance/Browsable/DH_4097491.

Department of Health (2007) *Saving Lives: Reducing Infection—Delivering Clean and Safe Care*, available online at http://www.dh.gov.uk/en/Publicationsandstatistics/Publications/PublicationsPolicyAndGuidance/DH_078134.

Fader, M., Cottenden, A.M., and Getliffe, K. (2008) 'Absorbent products for moderate-heavy urinary and/or faecal incontinence in women and men', *Cochrane Database of Systematic Reviews*, 4, Art. No. CD007408, DOI 10.1002/14651858.CD007408, available online at http://www2.cochrane.org/reviews/en/ab007408.html.

Folstein, M.F., Folstein, S.E., and McHugh, P.R. (1975) 'Mini-mental state: A practical method for grading the cognitive state of patients for the clinician', *Journal of Psychiatric Research*, 12: 189–98.

Getliffe, K., and Dolman, M. (2007) *Promoting Continence: A Clinical and Reseach Resource*, Edinburgh: Balliere Tindall.

Katzman, R., Brown, T., Fuld, P., Peck, A., Schechter, R., and Schimmel, H. (1983) 'Validation of a short orientation-memory-concentration test of cognitive impairment', *American Journal of Psychiatry*, 140: 6.

National Institute for Health and Clinical Excellence (2006) *Urinary Incontinence: The Management of Urinary Incontinence in Women*, available online at http://www.nice.org.uk/nicemedia/live/10996/30281/30281.pdf.

National Institute for Health and Clinical Excellence (2007) *Faecal Incontinence*, available online at http://www.nice.org.uk/guidance/index.jsp?action=download&o=36582.

Nazarko, L. (2007) 'Skin Care: ID', *Nursing and Residential Care*, 97: 310–13.

Nicholas, T. (2004) 'Ano-rectal Physiology: Investigation Techniques', in C. Norton and S. Chelvanayagam (eds) *Bowel Continence Nursing*, London: Beaconsfield Publishers Ltd, ch. 8.

Norton, C. and Chelvanayagam, S. (2000) 'A nursing assessment for adults with faecal incontinence', *Journal of Wound, Ostomy and Continence Nursing*, 27: 279–91.

Nursing and Midwifery Council (2007) *Chaperoning*, London: NMC, available online at http://www.nmc-uk.org.

Nursing and Midwifery Council (2008) *The Code*, London: NMC, available online at http://www.nmc-uk.org.

Royal College of Nursing (2008) *Bowel Care Including Digital Rectal Examination and Digital Removal of Faeces: RCN Guidance for Nurses*, London: RCN.

Royal College of Physicians (2009) *Privacy and Dignity in Continence Care Project*, available online at http://www.rcplondon.ac.uk/clinical-standards/ceeu/Current-work/Documents/Privacy-and-Dignity-in-Continence-Care-Phase-1-Report-Nov-2009.pdf.

Sykes, D.C., Castro, R., Pons, M.E., Hampel, C., Hunskaar, S., Papanicolaou, S., Quail, D., Samsioe, G., Voss, S., Wagg, A., and Monz, B.U. (2005) 'Characteristics of female outpatients with urinary incontinence participating in a six-month observational study in 14 European Countries', *Maturitas*, 52(Supp2):13–23.

Wagg, A., Andersson, K.E., Cardazo, L., Chapple, C., Kirby, M., Kelleher, C., Lose, G., and Milsom, I. (2005) 'Nocturia in adults', *Journal of Clinical Practice*, 59(8): 938–45.

Wagg, A.S., Cardozo, L., Chapple, C., De Ridder, D., Kelleher, C., Kirby, M., Milsom, I., and Vierhout, M. (2007) 'Overactive bladder syndrome in older people', *British Journal of Urology International*, 99(3): 502–9.

World Health Organization (1998) 'World Health Organization calls First International Conference on Incontinence', Press release, 1 July, available online at http://www.who.int/inf-pr-1998/en/pr98-49.html.

For further reading and information

http://bladderandbowelfoundation.org/

http://www.ageuk.org.uk/

http://www.promocon.co.uk/

PromoCon provides a national service—working as part of Disabled Living, Manchester—to improve the life for all people with bladder or bowel problems by offering product information, advice, and practical solutions to both professionals and the general public.

Online Resource Centre

You can learn more about continence, elimination, and older people at the Online Resource Centre that accompanies this book:
http://www.oxfordtextbooks.co.uk/orc/hindle/

Hygiene, infection control, and the older adult

Debbie Weston

Learning outcomes

By the end of this chapter, you will be able to:

- explain what is meant by the term 'healthcare-associated infection' (HCAI);
- discuss the implications of HCAIs, both to patients and the healthcare economy;
- discuss the specific risk factors for the development of HCAIs in older people;
- describe the various components that facilitate the spread of infection; and
- analyse the importance of hand decontamination, the correct use of gloves and aprons, and isolating/cohort nursing in breaking the links in the chain of infection.

Introduction

With more than 18 per cent of the UK population over retirement age, and 1.3 million people in the UK aged 85 years or older (NOS, 2009), older people are amongst the biggest users of the National Health Service (NHS), with 65 per cent of hospital beds occupied by people over the age of 65 (DH, 2007a). They are, therefore, one of the most vulnerable 'at risk' groups with regard to healthcare-associated infections (HCAIs).

In 2004, the Department of Health estimated that there were some 300,000 cases of HCAI in the UK each year, which cost the NHS in excess of £1 bn, caused the deaths of at least 5,000 people annually, and were also considered to be a contributing factor in 15,000 other deaths each year (NAO, 2004; 2009).

Older people are at more risk from potentially life-threatening infections than ever before due to advances in medical care, which enable major surgery and invasive diagnostic procedures to be undertaken on a patient group with weakened immunity and increased susceptibility to infections, as a result of underlying illness and disease, and the ageing process.

As we age, the body's ability to fight infection naturally declines. Natural barriers, such as the skin, weaken as the collagen content of the dermis, responsible for the skin's elasticity, decreases, leaving the skin more susceptible to trauma and facilitating the entry of microorganisms into the soft tissues or into the blood stream, and delaying wound healing (Candore et al., 2006; de la Fuente, 2007; Bianchi and Cameron, 2008). In the respiratory tract, lung capacity diminishes by up to 40 per cent by the age of 70 and the effectiveness of the cough reflex is reduced, leaving older people vulnerable to serious respiratory tract infections such as pneumonia (Knight and Nigam, 2008a). In the digestive tract, the protective mucosa lining the stomach becomes weakened and damage from gastric acid secretion can lead to the development of gastric ulcers (Knight and Nigam, 2008b). These commonly require treatment with proton-pump inhibitors, which reduce gastric acid secretion, such as Omeprazole, but their use has been implicated as a possible contributing factor in cases of infection with *Clostridium difficile* (Dial et al., 2004).

Anorexia and weight loss are common problems in older people, and 40–60 per cent of older people admitted to hospital are found to be malnourished (Morse and High, 2004). Poor nutritional intake compromises the immune system (High, 1999) and low concentrations of serum albumin, as a result of malnutrition, can be a poor prognostic indicator when treating serious infections. Loss of mobility can lead to skin damage, which increases the risk of pressure sore formation; these sores may become infected, requiring admission to hospital for surgical debridement. It may also adversely affect the older person's ability to remain continent. In addition to this, oral intake in older patients is often reduced, and this can lead to dehydration and the need for admission to hospital. The use of an indwelling urethral catheter to manage urinary incontinence or to monitor urine output substantially increases the risk of a urinary tract infection developing.

Much of the focus on the prevention and control of HCAIs generally is within the acute hospital setting, because this is where the risk to patients is the greatest. For example, with regard to the risk of infection in an older person on an acute hospital ward, there are often high bed occupancy rates, rapid patient turnaround times, and the mixing of different patient populations. Invasive clinical interventions, such as open surgery, laparoscopic surgery, and the insertion of invasive indwelling devices, increase the risk of microorganisms entering 'sterile' areas of the body, such as the bloodstream. Exposure to microorganisms from other patients can result in cross-infection. *Clostridium difficile* (*C. difficile*) may be acquired through exposure to a symptomatic patient and inadequate cleaning/decontamination standards. However, the basic principles of infection prevention and control, and the requirement to implement evidence-based guidelines that inform best practice, must be applied to *all* healthcare settings.

Guidelines that are specific to the community setting are available in the Department of Health document *Infection Control Guidance for Care Homes* (DH, 2006a); the National Institute for Health and Clinical Excellence (NICE) Clinical Guideline *Infection Control: Prevention of Healthcare-associated Infections in Primary and Community Care* (NICE, 2003), and the recently published document by the Care Quality Commission (2009) *Working Together to Prevent and Control Infections: A Study of the Arrangements for Infection Prevention and Control between Hospitals and Care Homes*. Primary care trusts (PCTs) will also have their own local infection control policies and best practice guidelines based on *Essential Steps to Safe, Clean Care* (DH, 2007b).

This chapter begins with some background information on the problem of HCAIs in general. The chain of infection is then discussed in detail, enabling the reader to understand how infections can be transmitted in the healthcare setting and the particular risk factors associated with older people. This is then followed by an explanation of the principles of infection control, which, if applied consistently, can break the chain of infection. The chapter concludes with 12 important points on the prevention of HCAIs in the older person. National guidance and Department of Health policies, drives, and initiatives are referred to throughout the chapter, and provide the evidence base for best practice.

It is important to note that, in spite of the physiological effects of the aging process and the general risk factors associated with health care, which may predispose patients to the development of HCAIs, the most important risk factors for the development of a healthcare-associated infection in the older person—or indeed any individual—are not, in fact, age related; rather, they are the presence of invasive indwelling devices and the degree of underlying illness.

See the Online Resource Centre that accompanies this book for more detail on the common HCAIs, such as Meticillin-resistant Staphylococcus aureus (MRSA) and C. difficile.

The problem of healthcare-associated infections

Healthcare-associated infections are defined as infections caused by any infectious agent acquired as a consequence of a person's treatment/intervention within a healthcare setting, which may be community or hospital-based (NAO, 2004; DH, 2006b). As well as being a major patient safety concern, and causing high levels of anxiety and distress to affected patients, their families, and the public in general, which cannot be underestimated, HCAIs also impact on the wider health economy and on all aspects of NHS performance. Each HCAI costs between £4,000 and £10,000 to treat, and extends the patient's stay in hospital on average by 11 days (Plowman et al., 2000). Delayed discharges from hospital equate to lost bed days and subsequent loss of revenue, with money spent on litigation, empirical therapy, personal protective equipment, medical equipment, and cleaning services. High-profile outbreaks of infection such as *C. difficile* at South Buckinghamshire NHS Trust in 2006, and Maidstone and Tunbridge Wells NHS Trust in 2007, attract adverse publicity and severely damage the public's confidence in the NHS (HCC, 2006; 2007) Failure to meet government targets for Methicillin-resistant staphylococcus aureus (MRSA) and *C. difficile* reduction can also result in hefty financial penalties.

In 2006, the Department of Health introduced the *Health Act 2006: Code of Practice for the Prevention and Control of Healthcare Associated Infections* (the 'Hygiene Code') (DH, 2006b), which was superseded in January 2009 by the *Health and Social Care Act 2008: Code of Practice for the NHS on the Prevention and Control of Healthcare-associated Infections and Related Guidance*. As of April 2009, NHS trusts are *legally* required to prevent and control HCAIs under the Health Act 2006, and must register with the regulators of health and adult social care services in England—that is, the Care Quality Commission (CQC). By registering with the CQC, trusts are self-declaring their implementation of, and compliance with, the Hygiene Code, therefore demonstrating their absolute commitment to the prevention and control of HCAIs. The CQC undertakes unannounced annual spot checks, and in the event of an NHS organization breaching the Hygiene Code, it can take enforcement action, such as issuing the organization with a warning notice, issuing a financial penalty notice in lieu of prosecution, suspending or cancelling the organization's registration with the CQC, or prosecuting for specified offences.

In spite of these challenges, the reader must be aware of their own responsibility for the prevention and control of HCAIs, and while not all infections can be avoided, 15–30 per cent (and perhaps as much as 50 per cent) can (DH, 1995). The culture within the NHS is rapidly moving to one of 'no avoidable infections' and 'zero tolerance' in respect of avoidable infections and non-compliance or poor infection control practice. The Hygiene Code clearly states that the '*effective prevention and control of HCAI has to be embedded into every-day practice and applied consistently by everyone* [...] *all staff should demonstrate good infection control and hygiene practice*' (DH, 2006b: 2). In other words, the prevention and control of HCAIs are everybody's business, because it is fundamental and integral part of patient care.

Box 15.1 summarizes the general risk factors that can increase the risk of infection in older people in community and hospital settings.

> ***Reflection point***
>
> What do you think are the most common types of HCAI, in order of prevalence?

> **Box 15.1** General risk factors that can increase the risk of infection in older people in community and hospital settings
>
> - Undergoing surgery/invasive procedures
> - The presence of invasive, indwelling devices
> - Underlying illness/disease
> - Exposure to colonized/infected patients
> - Medication, including antibiotics
> - The growth of antibiotic-resistant organisms and the emergence of hypervirulent strains of bacteria
> - Lack of isolation/cohort nursing facilities
> - Poor standards of environmental hygiene/cleanliness
> - Patient movement between wards/departments and care facilities
> - High bed occupancy rates
> - Patient turnaround times
> - Poor staff to patient ratios
> - Inadequate supplies of equipment—equipment may be shared between multiple patients
> - Lack of adequate resources for decontamination

The chain of infection

A thorough understanding of the 'chain of infection'—that is, the process through which infections can spread from one individual to another—is essential in order to prevent or reduce the risk of infections occurring. There are several interacting links in the chain and for an infection, or an outbreak of infection, to occur, all of the links have to be present and in the correct order.

The organism

Bacteria, viruses, and fungi (microorganisms) can all cause infections, but the extent to which a microorganism is 'problematic' for the patient depends upon a number of factors. The organisms discussed here all cause infections in older people.

Firstly, an organism needs to demonstrate pathogenicity and/or virulence. 'Pathogenicity' refers to its ability to cause infection, and 'virulence' is its ability to overwhelm the host's immune responses and cause severe infection/disease. There are at least 50 species of bacteria that are considered to be pathogenic, but the spectrum of illness and disease that they can cause is diverse, ranging from asymptomatic colonization (the adherence of the organism to the skin or mucosal surfaces without any adverse effect to the host), to infection that may be mild, severe, or potentially life-threatening (Burton and Engelkirk, 2004). For example, MRSA can harmlessly colonize the skin and the anterior nasal nares, but it can also cause boils and abscesses, deep-seated wound and soft tissue infections, and bloodstream infections. Long-term care facilities, such as nursing and residential homes, are widely recognized to be reservoirs for MRSA, predisposing residents to colonization and potentially seeding the spread into acute care facilities (Eveillard and Joly-Guillou, 2009). Group A beta-haemolytic streptococcus (*Streptococcus pyogenes*) is a normal inhabitant of the upper respiratory tract and the commonest bacterial cause of throat infections, but it is also one of the most prevalent and lethal human pathogens, responsible for devastatingly invasive skin/soft tissue and bloodstream infections, such as necrotizing fasciitis and streptococcal toxic shock syndrome (Bisno and Rouff, 2004; HPA, 2004a). Some bacteria are opportunistic pathogens, meaning that they only cause infection when the patient's immune defences are impaired (that is, as a result of underlying illness) or breached (that is, as a result of surgery or the insertion of an invasive, indwelling device).

Many bacteria produce toxins, which are either shed from the living organism or released in large quantities when the organism is dead or dying, having been destroyed by the host's immune response or the bactericidal (killing) action of antibiotics (Gladwin and Trattler, 2004). Some bacterial toxins, known as 'super-antigens', can overstimulate the immune system, causing an aggressive immune response that can actually damage the host (Torres et al., 2001). Some strains of *Staphylococcus aureus* (including MRSA) produce an extremely potent toxin called 'panton valentine leukocidin' (PVL) and these strains cause extremely invasive infections (HPA, 2008). The emergence of a hypervirulent strain of *C. difficile*, ribotype 027, has resulted in a more acute illness in affected patients, with reduced response to treatment with antibiotics and greater rate of progression to serious complications, such as pseudomembranous colitis, toxic megacolon, and risk of death (Bartlett and Perl, 2005; Brierly, 2005).

Bacteria may secrete 'slime', which enables them to slide along solid services, or possess capsules, which help to protect the organism from some of the defensive actions of the immune response, such as phagocytosis, and from the effects of certain antibiotics. Spore-forming organisms such as *C. difficile* are able to survive in the situations in which the nutrient or moisture supply is low, and they are resistant to the killing effects of heat, cold, drying, and chemicals, including some disinfectants. Other bacterial cell structures, dependent upon the type of organism, include flagella ('tails'), which enable them to move—for example, towards a source of nutrients or to evade the host's immune response—and pilli (fimbriae), which enable them to adhere to host cells (Petri et al., 2004).

Reservoir/source of infection

Nutrients and moisture are necessary for an organism's survival, and these can be found in its site or reservoir, which may be animal, human, or environmental. In terms of preventing HCAIs, human and environmental reservoirs are obviously the most important and the most problematic reservoirs to control, because the human body is the reservoir for organisms that colonize the skin, and the respiratory and gastrointestinal tract, some of which may be shed from the patient into the environment. On a square centimetre of skin, there may be as many as 10 million aerobic bacteria, such as *Staphylococcus aureus* and *Staphylococcus epidermidis*, and 80 per cent of resident skin flora may be found in the top five cell layers of the epidermis. Therefore, infected skin lesions, such as venous leg ulcers in the older person, and various secretions and excretions, can contaminate the patient's general environment, medical/patient equipment (that is, commodes, mattresses, bed frames, patient monitoring equipment, and soft furnishings), and the hands of healthcare staff. They can also be transferred on the patient's hands from one body site to another, giving rise to endogenous infections (that is, infections arising from the patient's own resident bacteria). Faecal bacteria, which normally colonize the gastrointestinal tract, such as antibiotic-resistant *Enterococus faecalis*, are a common cause of wound, urinary tract, and bloodstream infections (Cookson et al., 2001; HPA, 2004b). *Clostridium difficile* is part of the normal bowel flora in 2–5 per cent of the population, but carriage rates of 13–50 per cent have been reported in hospitalized patients, and 7 per cent in community settings, such as nursing and residential homes, where a heavily contaminated environment can result in the ingestion of bacterial spores (Chang and Nelson, 2000; Poutanen and Simor, 2004).

Outbreaks of viral gastroenteritis, such as Norovirus infection, in which older people are often severely affected (Goller et al., 2004), can result in widespread environmental contamination, because the virus can survive in the environment for up to 12 days (Cheesebrough et al., 1997). Therefore, contact with frequently touched surfaces, such as door handles, patient call bells, equipment, and furnishings in toilets and bathrooms, can result in transmission of Norovirus via the faecal–oral route.

Route of exit

The routes that enable the microorganism to leave the reservoir are varied. They can be secreted via the skin, mucous membranes, and the respiratory and gastrointestinal tracts in secretions, excretions, respiratory droplets, blood, and body fluids, and carried on the hands of healthcare staff.

Mode of transmission

The way in which microorganisms can spread is also varied.

- **Direct/indirect contact**—Direct contact with infected/colonized patients can result in the spread of microorganisms from infected skin lesions, secretions, blood, and body fluids. They can also be transferred to other patients from equipment that has become contaminated and on the hands of healthcare staff.
- **Airborne**—Particles containing microorganisms, such as dust, water, and respiratory droplets, can be inhaled, or can settle on equipment, furniture and bedding, and wounds. Pathogens can also be expelled from the respiratory tract through coughing and sneezing.
- **Ingestion**—Contaminated food and water can be consumed, or ingestion can occur via the faecal–oral route if hands become contaminated and are then moved to the mouth.
- **Inoculation**—Blood-borne viruses can be transmitted through needlestick injury, human bites that break the skin, splashes of blood/body fluids into the mucosa, and the contamination of non-intact skin with infected blood/body fluids.

Route of entry

The route that the microorganism uses to enter the host may be the same as the route of exit or different. For example, tuberculosis is spread and acquired via the respiratory tract, whereas *C. difficile* and Salmonella are excreted via the gastrointestinal tract in faeces, but have to be ingested in order for the individual to become infected. In 1984, an outbreak of food poisoning caused by *Salmonella typhimurium* at the Stanley Royd Hospital in Yorkshire killed 19 elderly patients (DHSS, 1984).

Susceptible host/patient

There are numerous patient factors that substantially increase the risk of infection in patients including the following.

- **Age**—While any patient in hospital will be susceptible to developing an infection, older people are particularly vulnerable, because the immune system declines with age (Loebenstein-Grubeck, 1997; Castle, 2002; Scheinfeld, 2005). The adaptive/acquired immune response, which is targeted against specific antigens (that is, microorganisms) and is responsible for immunological memory, weakens. The innate/natural immune response, which consists of natural defence mechanisms such as the skin, defence mechanisms of the respiratory, gastrointestinal, and genito-urinary tracts, white blood cells, macrophage production, and phagocytosis, also declines. In 2006, the National Prevalence Survey found that the risk of acquiring an infection substantially increases with age: 3.2 per cent in patients under the age of 35; increasing to 8.3 per cent in those aged 65–84; and 9.8 per cent in those aged 85 and over (Hospital Infection Society/Infection Control Nurses Association, 2006). Infections can be difficult to identify in older people, because the normal clinical manifestations such as fever may be absent due to a weakened immune response and they may instead present with relatively non-specific complaints, such as lack of appetite, confusion, and malaise (Rajagopalan and Yoshikawa, 2001; Destarac and Ely, 2002)
- **Non-intact skin**—Wounds, including small breaks in the skin, breach the body's first line of defence. Poor skin integrity is a common problem in the older patient.
- **The presence of invasive indwelling devices, such as vascular access devices (that is, peripheral intravenous cannulae and central venous catheters) and urinary catheters**—Urinary tract infections (UTIs) accounted for 19.7 per cent of all HCAIs in the 2006 National Prevalence Survey, with 80 per cent of all UTIs associated with urinary catheters. The risk of infection is strongly associated with the method and duration of catherization, and the susceptibility of the patient (Pratt et al., 2001).
- **Surgical intervention**—Open wounds/non-intact skin, intubation and mechanical ventilation, the insertion of 'foreign' material, such as prosthetic implants and sutures, all increase the risk of infection (National Collaborating Centre for Women's and Children's Health, 2008).
- **Duration of stay in hospital**—The 'average' length of stay in hospital varies from 10.9 days to 44.5 days, during which time patients may be exposed to infected/colonized patients. Delayed discharges, due to 'social' problems such as securing placements in long-term care facilities, increase the risk of exposure to microorganisms causing HCAIs.
- **Immunocompromization**—This may arise as a result of underlying illness or disease and its treatment: for example, chemotherapy/radiotherapy for malignant disease depresses the immune response.
- **Medication**—For example, steroids (which may be used in the treatment of asthma or rheumatoid arthritis) alter the immune response, antibiotics disrupt the normal body flora, and the use of ciprofloxacin for the treatment of UTIs and chest infections can predispose patients to MRSA infection (Coia et al., 2004; Weber et al., 2004).

● *Reflection point*

Think of a patient in your clinical area who has an infection. Work your way in the chain of infection to identify why or how the infection occurred.

Did the patient have any specific risk factors besides their age?

The principles of infection control

Introduction to standard precautions

The chain of infection can easily be interrupted or broken through the application of the principles of infection control. The principles of infection control are essentially the set of basic standard precautions that healthcare workers need to apply to all patients in all healthcare settings all of the time, such as: hand hygiene; the correct use of personal protective equipment and clothing; the safe handling and disposal of sharps; the management of spillages (blood/body fluids); the management of waste and linen; the decontamination of equipment and the environment; the decontamination of reusable medical devices; and patient isolation/cohort nursing. If healthcare workers apply these principles consistently, there will be fewer opportunities for infections to occur.

The Department of Health commissioned the development of national evidence-based guidance on the prevention of HCAIs in NHS hospitals in England, which were published in 2001 and revised and updated in 2006. The 2006 version is known as EPIC2 ('evidence-based practice in infection control') (Pratt et al., 2001; 2006), and provides the evidence-based best practice recommendations for:

- hospital environmental hygiene;
- hand hygiene;

- the use of personal protective equipment (gloves, aprons, masks, and face/eye protection);
- the safe use and disposal of sharps;
- prevention of infections associated with the use of short-term, indwelling, urethral catheters; and
- the prevention of infections associated with the use of central venous catheters (the principles of which are applicable to the use of peripherally inserted vascular devices).

This section looks at the importance of hand hygiene, the correct use of gloves and aprons, and the isolation/cohort nursing of infected or colonized patients.

Hand hygiene

Without a doubt, the transmission of microorganisms via the hands of healthcare staff is a huge factor in the spread of HCAIs and effective hand hygiene is simply *the* most important intervention that can be undertaken. The hands of healthcare staff can transmit both resident and transient bacteria. Deep-seated resident skin flora, which reside in skin crevices, hair follicles, sweat glands, and beneath the finger nails, may be of lower pathogenicity than transient bacteria, but they can act as pathogens if they are transferred to wounds, intravascular devices, or urinary catheters. Transient microorganisms are associated with HCAIs and are acquired from contact with other people (that is, skin, body sites, blood/body fluids, secretions, and excretions), and surfaces and equipment that may look visibly clean, but are highly likely to be heavily contaminated. MRSA and *C. difficile* are obvious examples of transient microorganisms. Fortunately, they are easily removed from the hands through the simple application of liquid soap and water. However, washing hands only renders hands socially clean and, given the vulnerability of patients in healthcare settings, the nature of the medical interventions that they undergo, and the amount of interaction that takes place between patients and healthcare staff, 'socially clean' hands do not always suffice.

The introduction of alcohol-based hand rubs at the point of care were first recommended in 2001 in the first version of the EPIC guidelines (Pratt et al., 2001) Their use in clinical practice has become a best practice recommendation. However, the placement of alcohol hand rubs in healthcare settings—that is, at the patient's bedside and at the entrance to wards/departments—must be subject to a clinical risk assessment. In 2008, the National Patient Safety Agency (NPSA) reissued an alert bulletin advocating that the need to prevent HCAIs and to ensure that alcohol hand rub was provided at the point of care was balanced against the risks of accidental ingestion (that is, by older confused patients or children) and deliberate ingestion (that is, by individuals with alcohol use disorder).

The advantages and disadvantages of alcohol hand rubs are listed in Box 15.2.

Student activity

Read the hand hygiene policy in the infection control manual for your area to ensure that you are compliant with its recommendations.

You can watch a video on the importance of hand hygiene online at http://www.npsa.nhs.uk/cleanyourhands. You can also download a poster that demonstrates the correct techniques for hand washing and for applying alcohol hand rub.

Watch the video, study the poster, and then look at your own hand decontamination technique. How thorough is it? Ask if you can have your technique assessed in the workplace.

'Five Moments for Hand Hygiene'

The World Health Organization (WHO) has developed an initiative known as the 'Five Moments for Hand Hygiene', in order to improve hand hygiene compliance by enabling staff

Box 15.2 Advantages and disadvantages of alcohol hand rubs

Advantages

- Rapid action (15–30 seconds) and effective against a wide range of microorganisms
- Do not require the use of water, soap, and towels, therefore more practical, easy to use, and more likely to achieve compliance
- Added emollients, so kinder to the skin than soap and water
- Rapid hand decontamination between patients and procedures
- Portable—can be taken/placed at the point of care and packaged into pocket-sized containers, so useful for situations in which access to hand basins are limited

Disadvantages

- Alcohol is not a cleansing agent and will not work on visibly soiled hands
- Alcohol is not effective against *C. difficile* spores and should not be used for hand decontamination after contact with patients with diarrhoea (hand washing is indicated in these instances to wash bacterial spores physically off of the skin's surface)
- They are astringent and can sting if they come into contact with non-intact skin (that is, minor cuts/abrasions)

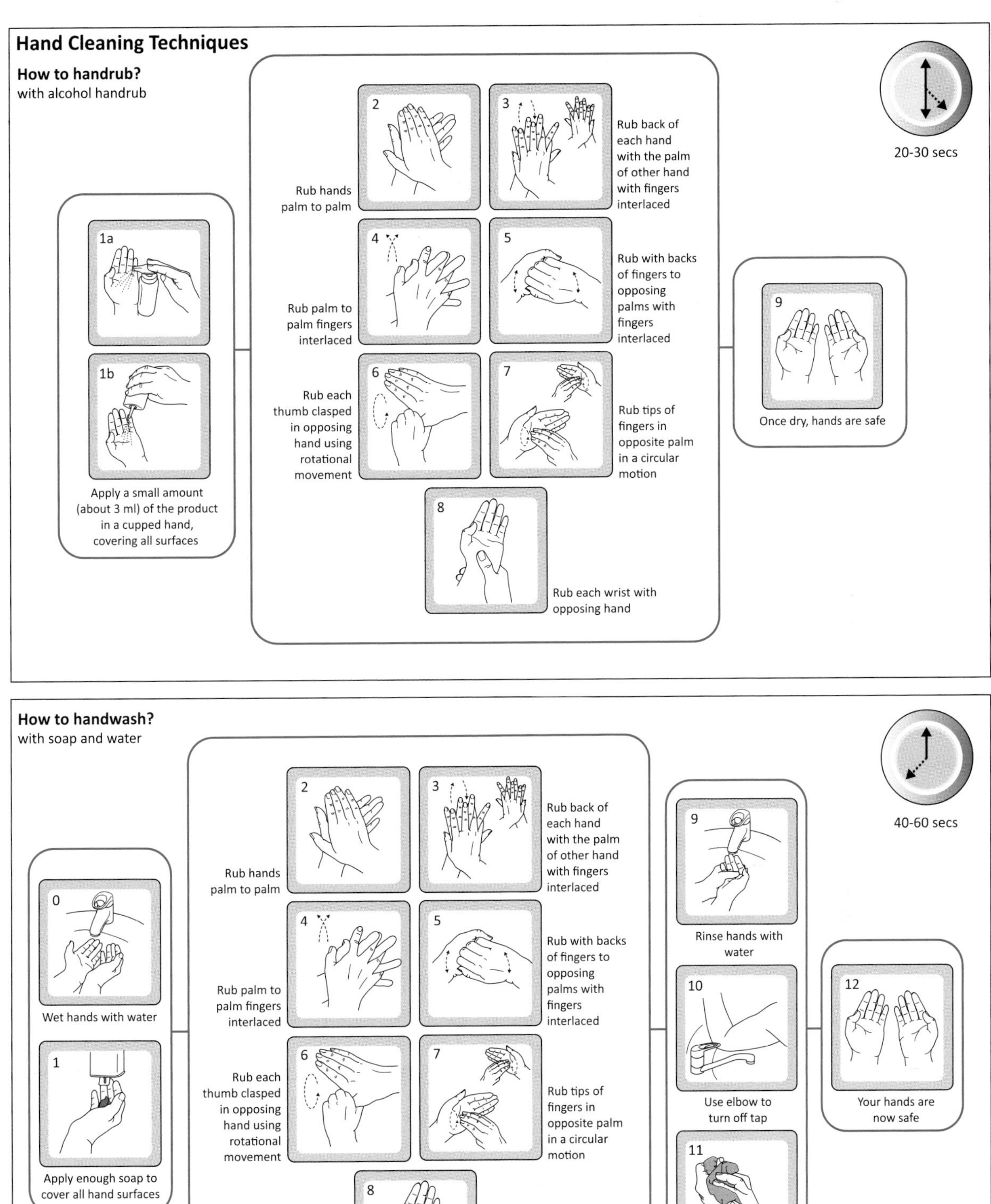

Figure 15.1 Hand-cleaning techniques
Source: © 2009 National Patient Safety Agency.

to better understand how microorganisms can be transmitted in clinical practice. This is now being widely implemented in most healthcare settings and Sax et al. (2007) offers further exploration of the background to the development of the 'Five Moments' and its rationale and implementation.

The healthcare setting (whether community, home, ambulance, or hospital) is viewed as consisting of two zones.

- The **patient zone** is the vicinity in which immediate patient care is provided and is likely to be heavily colonized or contaminated with the patient's microbial flora. It includes the patient's intact skin, inanimate objects, and surfaces touched by, or in direct contact with, the patient (that is, bed rails, bedside locker/table, patient/medical equipment), and surfaces frequently touched by healthcare staff.
- The **healthcare zone** is the rest of the environment, made up of other patients and their own patient zones, and is also likely to be heavily contaminated with microorganisms, some of which may be antibiotic-resistant.

The 'Five Moments' for hand hygiene can be described as follows.

1. Moment One occurs *before* patient contact and takes place within the patient zone as near to the patient as possible. The purpose of hand decontamination at this point is to prevent the spread of microorganisms on the hands of healthcare staff to the patient and any equipment within the patient zone.
2. Moment Two must take place before any clean or aseptic procedure, so as to prevent the introduction of microorganisms from the environment, and also from the patient's own microbial flora, into susceptible sites such as wounds and the sites of invasive indwelling devices.
3. Moment Three is after body fluid exposure and should include hand decontamination following the removal of gloves, in order to prevent contamination of the area outside of the patient zone.
4. Moment Four is after patient contact and takes place on leaving the point of care. The aim of hand decontamination here is to prevent the transfer of microorganisms between the patient zone and the healthcare zone.
5. Moment Five takes place following contact with any object (including furniture) or piece of equipment in the patient zone, because it will be colonized with the patient's microbial flora.

For more information on the 'Five Moments', and their application in hospital and community settings, visit http://www.npsa.nhs.uk/cleanyourhands

The use of personal protective equipment: Gloves and aprons

The purpose of wearing of gloves and aprons is twofold: they protect the healthcare worker; and they prevent the transmission of pathogens/microorganisms. EPIC2 makes it very clear that the use of any form of personal protective equipment (PPE) must be based on a risk assessment. However, healthcare staff are often unsure as to what item of PPE to wear and when, and this uncertainty—together with a general lack of understanding as to how infections are spread—can lead to practices that are haphazard, inconsistent, and increase the risk of the spread of infection to vulnerable patients.

The requirements can be summarized as follows.

- Aprons must be worn for close contact with patients, equipment, or materials, and where there is a risk of clothing becoming contaminated with pathogenic microorganisms or blood, body fluids, secretions, or excretions (with the exception of perspiration).
- Aprons must be single-use items, worn for one procedure or episode of direct patient care, and then discarded as clinical waste.
- They must be worn where there is risk of extensive splashing of uniform, clothing, or skin of healthcare workers with blood, body fluids, secretions, or excretions (except perspiration). Disposable, fluid-repellent, full-body gowns may be required.
- Aprons must be put on immediately before contact/treatment, and removed and disposed of immediately afterwards.
- They must be changed between different care activities on the same patient to prevent the spread of microorganisms from one body site to another.
- They must be changed in between patients, to prevent the transmission of microorganisms from one patient/the patient's immediate environment to another patient.
- Gloves must be worn for invasive procedures, contact with sterile sites, contact with non-intact skin and mucous membranes, where there is a risk of exposure to blood, body fluids, secretions, or excretions, and when handling sharp or contaminated instruments.
- They must be put on immediately before contact/treatment, and removed and disposed of immediately afterwards.
- They must be changed between different care activities on the same patient to prevent the transfer of microorganisms from one body site to another.
- Gloves must be changed in between each patient to prevent the transfer of microorganisms from one patient to another.
- Polythene gloves can leak and must not be used for contact with blood/body fluids.
- Gloves are classified as medical devices and must not be reused (DH, 1998).
- Gloves must not be worn all of the time, or for *routine* activities such as bed-making, assistance with mobility, recording

vital signs, or taking items into a patient's isolation room. This is because these activities are less likely to cause extensive contamination of the healthcare workers hands, and hand washing or the use of alcohol hand rub will effectively remove transient microorganisms from the skin.

- Gloves are not a substitute for handwashing. They will become heavily contaminated when in contact with dirty/contaminated equipment and blood/body fluids, and some of this contamination will be invisible. Healthcare workers who routinely wear gloves and fail to remove them in between patients, or who fail to wash/decontaminate their hands following the removal of gloves, are simply seeding the spread of microorganisms to other patients and equipment.

> ***Reflection point***
>
> Look at the use of gloves and aprons in the area in which you are working (the infection control manual for your area should also contain guidance on when they should be worn).
>
> - Are they being used correctly, according to best practice guidelines, or can you identify any inappropriate practices?
> - If so, what might be the most appropriate way in which to address these issues?

The isolation/cohort nursing of infected or colonized patients

Because infected or colonized patients can act as a source of infection for other patients and healthcare staff, 'source isolation' in a single room is often necessary. Enforced isolation can have a serious detrimental effect on older people, giving rise to feelings of social isolation, sensory deprivation, acute anxiety, psychological distress, and depression (Newton, 2001; Madeo, 2003), and healthcare workers must acknowledge this and take steps to reduce the impact that it may have. In spite of this, however, source isolation is an important component in the spread of HCAIs, and can reduce the microbial bio-burden in the environment and prevent other patients from becoming infected or colonized. While the use of single rooms is the most effective form of isolation, there are occasions on which demand outweighs capacity, and a risk assessment has to be undertaken that takes into account the patient, the organism, its mode of transmission, the risk of cross-infection that it poses to other patients and staff, and the facilities available.

In 2007, best practice guidance was published by the Department of Health on *Isolating Patients with a Healthcare-associated Infection: A Summary of Best Practice* (DH, 2007c). Where isolation facilities are not available, cohort nursing (that is, the grouping together of patients with the same infection or who are colonized with the same organism, such as MRSA or *C. difficile*) is an acceptable and practical alternative.

Box 15.3 summarizes the infection control precautions that must be in place when patients are source isolated/cohort nursed.

Conclusion

Twelve important points for the prevention of healthcare-associated infections in the older person

1. Know where the infection control manual is located within your area of practice, and familiarize yourself with the key policies and clinical practice guidelines.
2. Consider the chain of infection at all times.
3. Do not insert invasive devices, such as intravascular devices or urinary catheters, unless the indication for their use can be justified on clinical grounds.

> **Box 15.3** Infection control precautions that must be in place when patients are source isolated/cohort nursed
>
> - Hand washing facilities must be available within the single room/cohort bay and alcohol hand rub must be available at the point of care.
> - Gloves and aprons must be available at the entrance to the room/cohort bay.
> - Waste bins must be available for the disposal of clinical and domestic waste.
> - 'Dedicated' toilet facilities must be available or patients musts be allocated their own commode.
> - Doors to single rooms/cohort bays should be kept closed (although the safety of the patient isolated in a single room has to be taken into account—that is, in terms of confusion or the risk of falls).
> - Disposable tourniquets, blood pressure cuffs, and medicine pots should be used as standard.
> - Appropriate signage must be used (that is, an isolation sign on the door).
> - The room/bay must be cleaned daily. In the event of *C. difficile* infection, environmental cleaning should take place at least daily using 1,000 ppm available chlorine (DH/HPA, 2008).

4. Where invasive devices are used, ensure that they are managed according to best practice guidelines and that all device-related interventions are clearly documented in the nursing notes, including the indication (justification) for use.
5. Ensure that you change your gloves and aprons in between each episode of care on the same patient, and in between each patient contact.
6. Decontaminate your hands with alcohol hand rub at the point of care in accordance with the 'Five Moments for Hand Hygiene'.
7. Wash your hands with liquid soap and water if they are visibly soiled or contaminated with dirt, blood, or body fluids, and after contact with patients with diarrhoea.
8. Decontaminate equipment in between each patient contact.
9. Allocate equipment to patients in isolation/cohort bays and use disposable equipment where possible (that is, tourniquets, blood pressure cuffs, etc.).
10. Ensure that patients are isolated/cohort nursed where required in accordance with local policy and following a risk assessment.
11. Ensure that the patient environment is kept tidy and free from clutter in order to facilitate cleaning.
12. Remember: infection prevention and control is the responsibility of all healthcare staff.

Questions and self-assessment

Now that you have worked through the chapter, answer the following questions.

- Explain what is meant by the term 'healthcare-associated infection' (HCAI) and describe the various components that facilitate the spread of infection.
- What are the implications of HCAIs, both to patients and the healthcare economy?
- What are the specific risk factors for the development of HCAIs in older people?
- Discuss the importance of hand decontamination, the correct use of gloves and aprons, and isolating/cohort nursing in breaking the links in the chain of infection.

Self-assessment

- Having read the chapter, how will you change your practice?
- Identify up to three areas relating to infection control in which you need to develop your knowledge and understanding further.
- If you were to identify a member of staff putting a patient at risk by not following infection control procedures, how might you deal with this situation?

References

Bartlett, J.G. and Perl, T. (2005) 'The new *Clostridium difficile*: What does it mean?', *New England Journal of Medicine*, 353(23): 2503–5.

Bianchi, J. and Cameron, J. (2008) 'Assessment of skin integrity in the elderly 1', *British Journal of Community Nursing*, 13(3): S26–S32.

Bisno, A.L. and Rouff, K.L. (2004) 'Classification of Streptococci', in G.L. Mandell, J.E. Bennett, and R.D. Dolin (eds) *Mandell, Bennett and Dolin's Principles and Practices of Infectious Diseases*, 6th edn, London: Churchill Livingstone.

Brierly, R. (2005) '*Clostridium difficile*: A new threat to public health?', *The Lancet*, 5: 535.

Burton, G.R.W. and Engelkirk, P.G. (2004) 'Microbiology: The Science', in *Microbiology for Health Sciences*, Philadelphia, PA: Lippincott, Williams, and Wilkins Health, pp.1–4.

Candore, G., Bailistreri, C.R., Listi, F., Grimaldi, M.P., Vasto, S., Colonna-Romoulo, G., Franceschi, C., Lio, D., Caselli, G., and Caroliso, C. (2006) 'Immungenetics, gender and longevity', *Annals of the New York Academy of Sciences*, 1089: 516–37.

Care Quality Commission (2009) *Working Together to Prevent and Control Infections: A Study of the Arrangements for Infection Prevention and Control between Hospitals and Care Homes*, available online at http://www.cqc.org.uk/_db/_documents/Working_together_to_prevent_and_control_infections.pdf.

Castle, S.C. (2002) 'Clinical relevance of age-related immune dysfunction', *Clinical Infectious Diseases*, 31: 578–85.

Chang, V.T. and Nelson, K. (2000) 'The role of physical proximity in nosocomial diarrhoea', *Clinical Infectious Diseases*, 31: 717–22.

Cheesebrough, J.S., Barkess-Jones, L., and Brown, D.W. (1997) 'Possible prolonged environmental contamination survival of small round structured viruses', *Journal of Hospital Infection*, 35(4): 325–6.

Coia, J.E., Duckworth, G.J., Edwards, D.I., Fry, C., Humphreys, H., Mallaghan, C., and Tucker, D.R. for the Joint Working Party of the British Society of Antimicrobial Chemotherapy/Hospital Infection Society/Infection Control Nurses Association (2004) 'Guidelines for the prevention and control of meticillin-resistant Staphylococcus aureus (MRSA) in healthcare facilities', *Journal of Hospital Infection*, 63S: S1–S44.

Cookson, B.D., Macrae, M.B., Barrett, S.P., Brain, D.F.J., Chadwick, C., French, G.L., Hateley, P., Hosein, I.K., and Wade, J.J. (2001) A Report of a Combined Working Party of the HIS/ICNA/BSAC. *Guidelines for the Control of Glycopeptide Resistant Enterococci in Hospitals*, London: Hospital Infection Society.

Department of Health (1995) *Hospital Infection Control: Guidance on the Control of Infections in Hospitals*, HSG(95)10, London: DH

Department of Health (1998) *Medical Devices Directive: CE Marking EL (98)5*, London: HMSO.

Department of Health (2006a) *Infection Control Guidance for Care Homes*, London: DH.

Department of Health (2006b) *The Health Act 2006: Code of Practice for the Prevention and Control of Associated Infections*, London: DH.

Department of Health (2007a) *A Recipe for Care: Not a Single Ingredient—Clinical Case for Change*, Report by Professor Ian Philip, National Director for Older People, London: DH.

Department of Health (2007b) *Essential Steps to Safe, Clean Care: Reducing Healthcare-associated Infections (HCAI) in Primary Care Trusts, Mental Health Trusts, Learning Disability Organizations, Independent Healthcare Facilities, Care Homes, Hospices, GP Practices and Ambulance Services*, London: DH.

Department of Health (2007c) *Isolating Patients with a Healthcare-associated Infection: A Summary of Best Practice*, available online at http://www.clean-safe-care.nhs.uk/toolfiles/116_283198IP_isolating_patients.pdf.

Department of Health and Social Security (1984) *The Report of the Committee of Enquiry into an Outbreak of Food Poisoning at the Stanley Royd Hospital*, London: HMSO.

Department of Health/Health Protection Agency (2008) *Clostridium Difficile Infection: How to Deal with the Problem*, London: DH

Destarac, L.A. and Ely, E.W. (2002) 'Sepsis in older patients: An emerging concern in critical care', *Advances in Sepsis*, 2(1): 15–22.

Dial, S., Airsdsdi, K., Manoukian, C., Huang, A., and Menzies, D. (2004) 'Risk of *Clostridium difficile* diarrhoea among hospital patients prescribed proton pump inhibitors: cohort and case control studies', *Canadian Medical Journal Association*, 171(1): 33–8.

Eveillard, M. and Joly-Guillou, M.L. (2009) 'Meticillin-resistant *Staphylococcus aureus* (MRSA) in the institutionalized older patient', *Reviews in Clinical Gerontology*, 19: 13–23.

Fuente, M. de la (2007) 'Nutrition and immunity in the elderly', *Proceedings of the Nutrition Society*, 67(OCE): 6.

Gladwin, M.T. and Trattler, W. (2004) 'Cell Structure, Virulence Factors and Toxins', in *Clinical Microbiology Made Ridiculously Simple*, 3rd edn, Miami, FL: MedMaster Inc., pp. 8–15.

Goller, J.L., Dimitriadias, A., Tan, A., Kelly, H., and Marshall, J.A. (2004) 'Long-term features of *Norovirus gastroenteritis* in the elderly', *Journal Hospital Infection*, 58(4): 286–91.

Healthcare Commission (2006) *Investigation into Outbreaks of Clostridium Difficile at Stoke Mandeville Hospital, Buckinghamshire Hospitals NHS Trust*, London: Commission for Healthcare Audit and Inspection.

Healthcare Commission (2007) *Investigation into Outbreaks of Clostridium Difficile at Maidstone and Tunbridge Wells NHS Trust*, London: Commission for Healthcare Audit and Inspection.

Health Protection Agency (2004a) 'Health Protection Agency Group: A streptococcal working group interim UK guidelines on the management of invasive Group A streptococcal disease', *Communicable Disease Public Health*, 7(4): 354–61.

Health Protection Agency (2004b) *National Glycopeptide Resistant Enterococcal Bacteraemia Surveillance Working Group*, Report to the Department of Health, London: HPA.

Health Protection Agency (2008) *Guidance on the Diagnosis and Management of PVL-associated Staphylococcus Aureus Infections (PVL-SA) in England*, 2nd edn, London: HPA.

High, K.P. (1999) 'Micronutrient supplementation and immune function in the elderly', *Clinical Infectious Diseases*, 28: 717–22.

Hospital Infection Society/Infection Control Nurses Association (2006) *The Third Prevalence Survey of Healthcare-associated Infections in Acute Hospitals*, London: HIS/ICNA.

Knight, J. and Nigam, Y. (2008a) 'Exploring the anatomy and physiology of ageing: Part 2—The respiratory system', *Nursing Times*, 104(32): 24.

Knight, J. and Nigam, Y. (2008b) 'Exploring the anatomy and physiology of ageing: Part 3—The digestive system', *Nursing Times*, 104(43): 22–3.

Loebenstein-Grubeck, B. (1997) 'Changes in the ageing immune system', *Biologicals*, 25(2): 205–8.

Madeo, M. (2003) 'The psychological impact of isolation', *Nursing Times*, 99(7): 54.

Morse, C.G. and High, K.P. (2004) 'Nutrition, Immunity and Infection', in G.L. Mandell, J.E. Bennett, and R.D. Dolin (eds) *Mandell, Bennett and Dolin's Principles and Practice of Infectious Diseases*, 6th edn, London: Churchill Livingstone.

National Audit Office (2004) *Improving Patient Care by Reducing the Risk of Hospital-acquired Infection: A Progress Report*, Report by the Comptroller and Auditor General, HC 876, Session 2003–04, 14 July, London: HMSO.

National Audit Office (2009) *Reducing Healthcare-associated Infections in Hospitals in England*, Report by the Comptroller and Auditor General, HC 560, Session 2008–09, 12 June, London: HMSO.

National Collaborating Centre for Women's and Children's Health (2008) *Surgical Site Infection*, available online at http://www.nice.org.uk/nicemedia/pdf/CG74FullGuideline.pdf.

National Institute for Health and Clinical Effectiveness (2003) *NICE Clinical Guideline CG2: Infection Control—Prevention of Healthcare-associated Infections in Primary and Community Care*, London: NICE.

National Institute for Health and Clinical Effectiveness (2008) *NICE Clinical Guideline 74: Prevention and Treatment of Surgical Site Infection*, London: NICE.

National Office for Statistics (2009) *Older People's Day*, available online at http://www.statistics.gov.uk [accessed 3 July 2010]

National Patient Safety Agency (2008) *Clean Hands Saves Lives*, available online at http://www.nrls.npsa.nhs.uk/resources/?entryid45=59848.

Newton, J.T. (2001) 'Patient's perceptions of methicillin-resistant *Staphylococcus aureus* and source of isolation: A qualitative analysis of source isolation patients', *Journal of Hospital Infection*, 48: 275–80.

Petri, W.A., Mann, B.J., and Huston, C.D. (2004) 'Microbial Adherence', in G.L. Mandell, J.E. Bennett, and R.D. Dolin (eds) *Mandell's Principles and Practices of Infectious Diseases*, 6th edn, London: Churchill Livingstone.

Plowman, R., Graves, N., Griffin, M., Roberts, J., Swan, A.V., Cookson, B., and Taylor, L. (2000) *The Socio-economic Burden of Hospital-acquired Infection*, London: Public Health Laboratory Service.

Poutanen, S.M. and Simor, A.E. (2004) '*Clostridium difficile*-associated diarrhoea in adults', *Canadian Medical Association Journal*, 171(1): 51–8.

Pratt, R.J., Pellowe, C.M., Loveday, H.P., Robinson, M., Smith, G.W., and the Epic Guidelines Development Team (2001) 'The *Epic* Project: Developing national evidence-based guidelines for preventing healthcare-associated infections', *Journal of Hospital Infection*, 47(Suppl): S1–S82.

Pratt, R.J., Pellowe, C.M., Wilson, J.A., Loveday, H.P., Harper, P.J., Jones, S.R.L.K., McDougal, C., and Wilcox, M.H. (2007) 'Epic2: National evidence-based guidelines for preventing healthcare-associated infections in NHS hospitals in England', *Journal of Hospital Infection*, 65(Suppl): S1–S64.

Rajagopalan, S. and Yoshikawa, T.T. (2001) 'Antimicrobial therapy in the elderly', *Medical Clinics of North America*, 85: 133–47; vii

Sax, H., Allegranzi, B., Uckay, I., Larson, E., Boyce, J., and Pittet, D. (2007) '"My five moments for hand hygiene": A user-centred approach to understand, train, monitor and report hand hygiene', *Journal of Hospital Infection*, 67: 9–21.

Scheinfeld, N. (2005) 'Infections in the elderly', *Dermatology Online*, 11(3): 8, available online at http://dermatology.cdlib.org/113/reviews/elderly/scheinfeld.html.

Torres, B.A., Kominsky, S., Perrin, C.Q., Hebeika, A., and Johnson, H.W. (2001) 'Super-antigens: The good, the bad and the ugly', *Experimental Biology and Medicine*, 226: 164–76.

Weber, S.G., Gold, H.S., Hooper, D.C., Karchmer, A.W., and Carmeli, Y. (2004) 'Fluoroquinolines and the risk for methicillin-resistant *Staphylococcus aureus* in hospitalized patients', *Emerging Infectious Diseases*, 9(1): 1415–22.

Online Resource Centre

You can learn more about the prevention and control of infection in older people at the Online Resource Centre that accompanies this book:
http://www.oxfordtextbooks.co.uk/orc/hindle/

Pain and its pharmacological management in older adults

Amelia Williamson-Swift

Learning outcomes

By the end of this chapter, you will be able to:

- recognize different types of pain and appreciate their impact on the older person;
- understand the consequences of poorly managed pain;
- understand pain physiology and key changes associated with ageing;
- assess pain intensity; and
- discuss the pharmacological management of pain in the older adult.

Introduction

Pain is unpleasant sensory and emotional experience associated with actual or potential tissue damage or described in terms of such damage

(Task Force on Taxonomy of the IASP, 1994).

We all suffer from pain from time to time as a result of injury or illness, and these types of pain tend to be no different in nature and frequency in the older adult than in younger members of the population. Some people suffer from pain all of the time—perhaps as the result of an ongoing condition such as osteoarthritis; these pains tend to occur more in older age than in younger age groups.

The consequences of unrelieved acute pain can be serious in older people. Older people are less likely than the young to get prompt or effective treatment (Blomqvist, 2003). Health professionals lack knowledge and skills in assessment of the older adult, knowledge of the specific pharmacological concerns, and have poor attitudes of misconceptions about ageing and older people (Gagliese and Melzack, 1997). The situation is even worse in people with dementia, who are at high risk of suffering undetected severe pain (Husebo et al., 2008).

McCaffrey (1983: 5) defined pain as whatever the patient says it is, occurring whenever they say it does, which reminds us that pain is a subjective experience. Pain affects a person physically, psychologically, socially, and spiritually, and in turn a person's psychological, social, physical, and spiritual well-being affect their perception of pain.

There are a multitude of effective pain treatments and selection should be based on understanding the physiological mechanism of the pain being treated, and also consideration of the person's psychological, social, and spiritual needs. Anatomical, physiological, psychological, and social changes that occur as we age have an influence on the way in which pain can be managed effectively and the support that a person in pain may need.

The 'ABCDE' approach can be a helpful reminder of the important stages of pain management (see Box 16.1).

Effective, individualized care based on sound knowledge of the underlying physiological, psychological, and pharmacological principles can promote recovery or restore quality of life.

Pain physiology and ageing

Pain is evoked when a damaging, or potentially damaging, stimulus activates a specialist nerve receptor (a nociceptor). These stimuli are collectively called 'noxious' and include

> **Box 16.1** The important stages of pain management
>
> A **Assess** the pain by **asking** the person and never make **assumptions**.
>
> B **Believe** the person who is in pain, no matter how challenging that might be.
>
> C **Choose** pain control options that are suitable, based on your assessment of the person and their circumstances.
>
> D **Deliver** your pain management strategy promptly.
>
> E **Empower** the person who is in pain, so that they become knowledgeable and, where possible, in control.
>
> **Evaluate** the effectiveness of the pain management strategy continuously.

things such as strong heat, pinch, or harmful chemicals. If a signal is strong enough to activate the nerve fibre, it creates an 'action potential', which transmits the pain signal to the dorsal horn (the grey matter in the spinal cord) and from there to the brain (see Figure 16.1).

Nociceptors have high 'activation thresholds', which means that it takes a relatively strong stimulus to trigger an action potential (that is, to make them fire). Damaged cells release a 'soup' of chemicals, including prostaglandins, leukotrienes, hydrogen ions, and bradykinin, which lower the activation threshold of the nociceptor (that is, sensitize it), so that other chemicals produced in the injury can activate it.

Anti-inflammatory medications, such as ibuprofen, reduce the amount of prostaglandins formed as a result of tissue damage by blocking the action of cyclooxygenase enzymes. Inhibition of prostaglandin by anti-inflammatory medication makes it more difficult for pain fibres to be activated by the other chemicals released in tissue damage. The result of this will be that fewer fibres will be activated and the patient will feel less pain. Unfortunately, prostaglandins are not only involved in pain signaling, but also in other important processes in the body, such as maintenance of the mucous lining of the stomach. Disruption of this mucous lining because of the use of anti-inflammatory drugs can lead to pain, ulceration, and perforation of the stomach. The downside of these drugs will be considered a little later in the chapter, because it makes these drugs difficult to use by older people.

There are three main types of sensory nerve fibre of interest in pain sensation and management.

- **A-delta** fibres transmit fast sharp pain (for example, a pinprick). They activate nociceptive specific neurons in the superficial layers of the dorsal horn. Nociceptive-specific neurons will always signal pain, no matter what type of incoming fibre synapses with them.
- **C** fibres transmit slow, dull pain (for example, tissue damage or a muscle tear). They activate nociceptive-specific neurons on the superficial layers of the dorsal horn, but also deeper neurons called 'wide dynamic range neurons'. Wide dynamic range neurons send an onward signal that is proportionate to the incoming signal and so can differentiate between a wide range of stimuli, from touch, to pain.
- **A-beta** fibres transmit touch signals, but not pain. They activate wide dynamic range neurons in the deeper layers of the dorsal horn. The wide dynamic range neurons can tell whether they are being activated by a pain fibre or by a touch fibre.

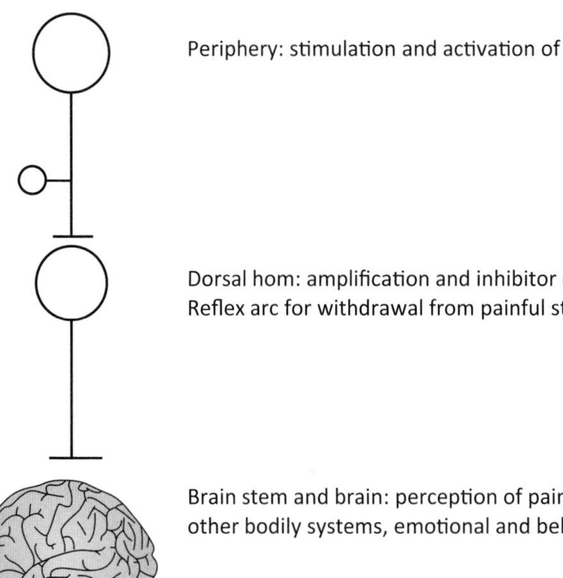

Figure 16.1 Major components of the pain pathway

Ageing leads to degenerative changes in the nervous system, including a loss of density of the fibres that transmit pain signals and degeneration in the dorsal horn of the spinal cord (Gibson and Farrell, 2004). This has been shown in experiments when older people require a stimulus to be more intense before they recognize it as painful (pain threshold). Once the stimulus has activated the nerve, even if this takes a slightly greater intensity to achieve, an older person might rate the pain caused by an intense stimulus to be worse than a younger person, and they might also rate the pain caused by a less intense stimulus as lower than a younger person (Edwards, 2005). What this means in practice is that older people may not recognize a potentially harmful stimulus as quickly as a younger person and this may make them more susceptible to tissue damage. The pain intensity that they experience as a result of a given stimulus might also differ from that experienced by a younger person.

Once a pain signal reaches the dorsal horn, the incoming nerve fibre releases signalling chemicals (neurotransmitters), which cross the gap (synapse) between one nerve cell (neuron) and the next as a means of communicating the signal. One of the most fundamental processes in pain transmission is that an incoming nerve fibre releases neurotransmitters that excite or activate 'projection neurons', which then conduct the pain signal upwards to the brain.

There are many different neurotransmitter molecules. Each fits snugly into a specific receptor on the target cell. Once the neurotransmitter has locked into its receptor, a chemical reaction is initiated within the target cell. This reaction might lead to the release of other neurotransmitters or the generation of an action potential, sending the pain signal further along the pain pathway (towards the brain).

Pain-relieving drugs work by interfering with the process of pain transmission along the pain pathway, often by mimicking naturally occurring neurotransmitters. Morphine and other opioid drugs make it difficult for the incoming pain fibre to release excitatory neurotransmitters (see Box 16.2), such as Substance P. They also make it difficult for the projection neurons to become activated by those excitatory transmitters and they encourage the release of chemicals from the brain that inhibit transmission of the pain signal across the dorsal horn.

Box 16.2 Basic neurotransmitters involved in transmitting or inhibiting the pain signal

Excitatory neurotransmitters (such as Substance P., glutamate, aspartate):

- excite a nerve cell; and
- make it more likely that an action potential will be generated.

Inhibitory neurotransmitters (such as GABA and glycine):

- make it harder for the nerve cell to be excited; and
- make it harder for the nerve cell to produce an action potential.

Tissue damage causes nociceptors to become more sensitive to painful stimuli—a phenomenon known as 'peripheral sensitization' (see above). A similar process happens in the dorsal horn (central sensitization) when the signals reaching it are high frequency or intense. Central sensitization means that less-intense stimuli are needed to activate pain projection neurons. This leads to an increased response to a painful stimulus, called 'hyperalgesia' (that is, something painful hurts more than normal). This makes us more likely to protect the painful area, which allows healing to take place and prevents further injury of vulnerable tissues.

When peripheral nerves are damaged or there is prolonged intense pain, A-beta (touch) fibres activate nociceptive-specific neurons rather than only wide dynamic range neurons. This leads to a situation in which an innocuous (non-painful) stimulus, such as a light touch, produces pain (known as 'allodynia'). This can be caused by something such as sunburn and serves a protective function. However, it can also be caused by nerve damage—for example, in diabetic neuropathy—and then this pain serves no protective function at all, but causes considerable distress to the person, who cannot bear clothing, bedclothes, running water, or a cold breeze on their skin.

When these alterations from straightforward pain processing become long-term, it is usually because of nerve damage (neuropathic pain) and it is not usually a prominent feature of pain caused by damage of other tissues (nociceptive pain).

Pain signals travel from the dorsal horn of the spinal cord in pathways called 'tracts'. There are a number of pathways and tracts that terminate in different brain regions (as illustrated in Table 16.1). Activation of these brain areas by pain signals leads to behavioural responses to pain, such as physiological changes (sweating, increased heart rate, increased blood pressure) and psychological reactions (anxiety and fear).

Pain signals do not only travel in one direction: the dorsal horn sends signals to the brain and it also receives signals back again. The two-way movement of signals between the brain and the spinal cord is managed by the brain stem. In this way, pain can influence behaviour, mood, sleep, even nausea, and in turn the pain intensity that we feel can be influenced by things such as anxiety, fear, or depression.

The brainstem can send signals to the dorsal horn, leading to amplification of pain signaling, and this is called 'descending facilitation' (because it comes down from the brainstem to the spinal cord). Facilitation signals tend to be activated mainly by pain itself—so pain leads to more pain.

The brainstem can also send signals to the dorsal horn to reduce pain signalling and this is called 'descending inhibition'. Pain inhibition tends to be activated by things such as exercise, fear, and relaxation techniques. Importantly, our brainstem tends continually to dampen down pain signalling in the dorsal horn, so that we do not notice much of the

Table 16.1 Destinations in the brain for pain signals

Brain destination	Functional implication of activation
Insular cortex via the thalamus	Integration of sensory information with memory—activation influences our **pain affect** (for example, feeling anxious) Sends signals to the amygdala
Anterior cingulate cortex (ACC) via the thalamus	Modulation of the motor and autonomic responses to pain and pain affect Helps to make the experience of pain feel unpleasant and in pain anticipation and therefore avoidance of, attention to, and escape from pain Also links to the peri-aqueductal gray (PAG) and, in this way, stimulates descending inhibition of pain Crucial area for placebo effect
Primary (S1) and secondary (S2) somatosensory cortex	Location, temporal, and intensity discrimination of pain

stimuli that provoke mild pain all of the time. However, there is some evidence that, in older adults, there is a loss of inhibitory tone—meaning that, in the older person, the ability of the brainstem to damp down pain signals and to ignore relatively minor pain signals will diminish.

Some things cause the brain to produce inhibitory signals and we can incorporate those into pain management strategies. These are things such as relaxation therapy, transcutaneous nerve stimulation (TENS), exercise, and laughter. Other things cause facilitatory signals and we aim to alleviate these as part of the pain management process; this includes pain itself, anxiety, and depression.

Some antidepressants used for pain relief mimic the descending inhibitory system, and increase the amount of norepinephrine and serotonin available to the dorsal horn. These neurotransmitters activate receptors in the dorsal horn that reduce the release of excitatory neurotransmitters, enhance the release of inhibitory neurotransmitters, and can also make it more difficult for the projection neurons to activate. The result of this is a reduction in pain transmission across the dorsal horn.

Pain transmission is a balance between excitation and inhibition. Pain signals excite, while the brainstem both excites and inhibits. This balance was neatly summed up by Ronald Melzack and Patrick Wall (1965), who created a model called the 'gate control theory' (see Figure 16.2). This demonstrates a number of key principles that are still used in pain management today.

The dorsal horn of the spinal cord acts as a gate (or barrier) to the transmission of pain signals through it to the brain. Pain signals must reach the brain in order for us to perceive them. The gate can be opened by events that are excitatory—in other words, things that excite the pain neurons. It can be closed by events that are inhibitory—that is, things that make it more difficult for the pain neurons to respond. Excitation comes in the form of incoming pain signals and events that cause the brain to produce facilitatory neurotransmitters (for example, pain itself and anxiety). Inhibition comes in the form of competing nerve impulses (touch in the form of rubbing, for example) and also from the brain, as descending inhibition stimulated by things such as morphine and relaxation. The amount of pain that we feel depends on the balance of excitation and inhibition—and Melzack and Wall help us to picture this as forces that push open the gate or pull it closed.

Pain signals transmitted via the C fibres are excitatory. If the A-beta fibres are activated at the same time as the C-fibres (for example, by rubbing the skin close to a graze), the pressure and rubbing sensation transmitted via the A-beta fibres will outweigh the dull pain of the graze and, for a short while, the pain sensation can be blocked.

Introduction to acute pain and persistent pain

Acute pain

We can summarize acute pain as pain that:

- warns us about actual or potential tissue damage;
- facilitates healing, because it encourages protection of the injury and rest; and
- usually stops when the injury has healed or the disease has been successfully treated.

Almost everyone experiences short periods of pain associated with injury or interventions, such as surgery (acute pain). This type of pain can be well controlled using pain medication, physical and psychological support, and careful positioning. This type of pain is often nociceptive pain—that is, a type of pain that is caused by injury to the tissues. It includes things such as post-operative pain, a traumatic injury such as a sprain or fracture, and the pain that accompanies infections such as colds and flu.

Some people think that older people experience lower levels of acute pain than younger people (Fecho et al., 2009), while others say that age has no effect (Chou et al., 2008). The important thing for nurses to remember is that all patients, no matter what their age, need good pain assessment, so that we can determine how pain affects them as an individual.

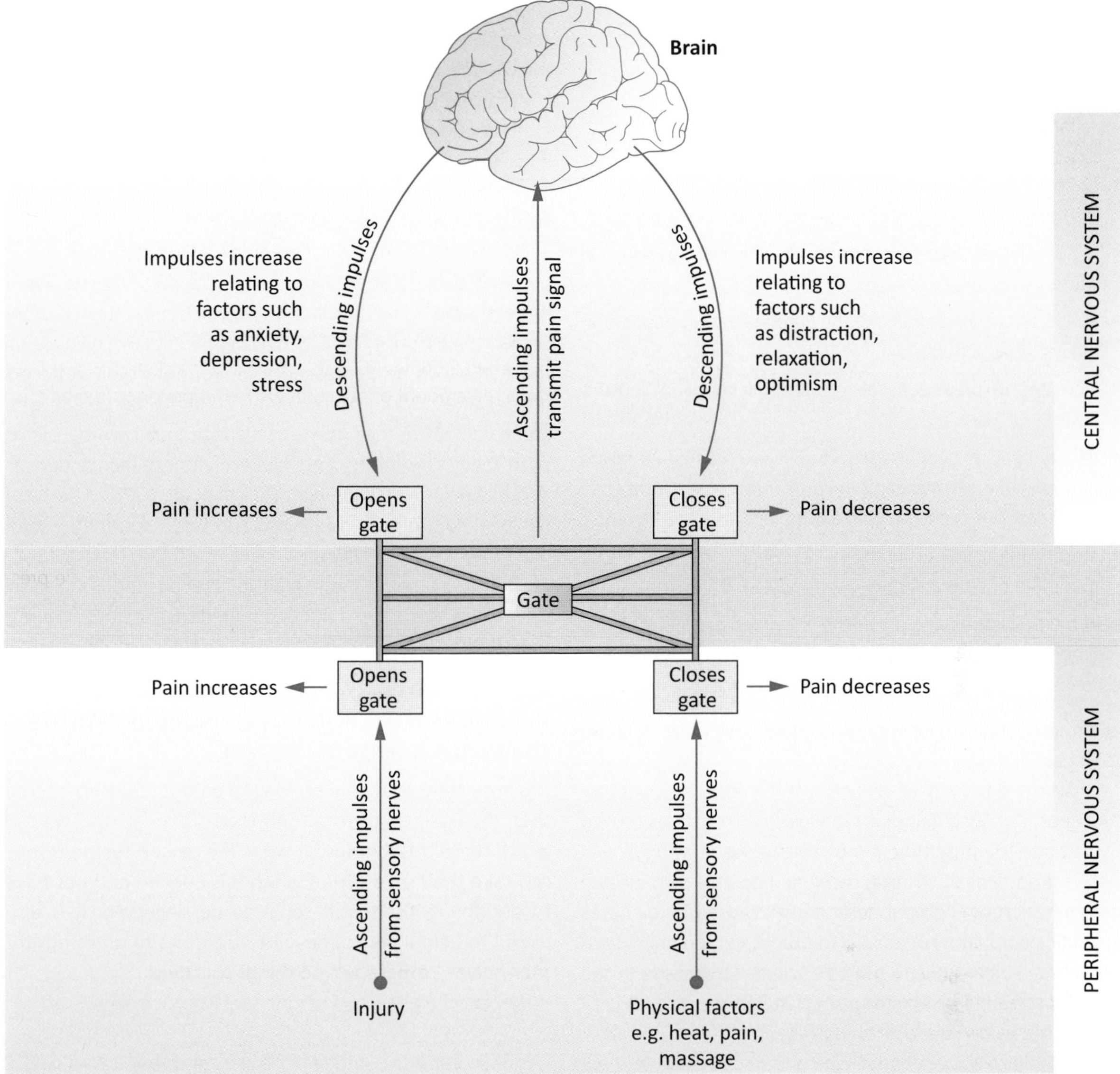

Figure 16.2 Gate control theory

Good pain management can help to prevent acute pain complications, including the following.

- Chest infections can develop when there is difficulty taking deep breaths, coughing, and a reluctance to change position because of pain (Ochroch and Gottschalk, 2005).
- Pain makes people reluctant to move and walk, and this contributes to venous stasis, which increases the risk of deep venous thrombosis (Morrison et al., 2003). Older adults are already at an increased risk of venous stasis due to muscle loss (sarcopenia) and, in some cases, fear of falling.
- The experience of pain increases the incidence of post-operative delirium, a form of confusion, which nurses often fail to appreciate is related to pain (Vaurio et al., 2006).
- Pain causes feelings of anxiety and depression (Carr et al., 2005).

Acute pain leads to a number of short-term physiological changes in the patient, mainly related to autonomic activation—such as:

- increased heart rate;
- nausea and possibly vomiting; and/or
- pale and clammy skin.

Older people may tolerate these changes less well than younger people. Severe pain causes increased heart rate and increased myocardial oxygen demand; in someone who has ischaemic heart disease (which is more prevalent in older age), the coronary circulation may not be good enough to keep up with the extra demand and so acute pain can precipitate angina or even infarction.

The complications of unrelieved acute pain can be life-threatening in older adults who have concurrent medical conditions (Gregory and Haigh, 2008).

Persistent (chronic) pain

Persistent (or chronic) pain can be summarized as pain that:

- is long-term (that is, pain that lasts longer than three months and often even years);
- has minimal protective effect (that is, it is not warning us of anything);
- is sometimes present without an obvious pathological cause;
- affects about 20 per cent of the European adult population (Breivik et al., 2006);
- increases in prevalence as we age (Helme and Gibson, 2001);
- 34 per cent of people aged 75–79 years suffer—a figure that rises in each decade of life until it reaches a prevalence of 50 per cent in people who are more than 90 years old;
- most residents in nursing homes experience frequently to a moderate or severe degree (Cairncross et al., 2007); and
- in medical wards, the prevalence of which in older patients is about 80 per cent (Coker et al., 2008).

The prevalence of persistent pain increases as we get older and frailer people in our society are more likely to be suffering from pain.

Persistent pain may be nociceptive (for example, osteoarthritis) or it may be neuropathic. Neuropathic pain is caused by damage to, or dysfunction of, the nerves or nervous system. The sorts of things that cause neuropathic pain include degeneration of the peripheral nerves caused by diabetes (diabetic neuropathy) or alcohol (alcoholic neuropathy); damage to the myelin sheath (multiple sclerosis), damage to the central processing system for pain (post-stroke pain), or damage caused by disease (post-shingles pain).

The qualities of nociceptive pain and neuropathic pain are different (see Box 16.3). Each type of pain requires a different treatment approach and these differences can help in the assessment of the primary mechanism of the pain.

Box 16.3 The main differences between neuropathic pain and nociceptive pain

Neuropathic pain	Nociceptive pain
Nerve damage	Tissue damage
Burning, shooting, tingling, numbness	Aching, throbbing
No change with movement	Movement often exacerbates
Usually continuous	More likely to vary in intensity over time
Spontaneous shooting pains	Often can identify a cause for changes in pain

Older people are more susceptible to neuropathic pain than younger people, but musculoskeletal pain tends to peak in middle age and tail off as we get older (Gagliese, 2009).

Persistent pain is longer-lasting than acute pain, and often wears patients down physically and emotionally. It can be caused by a variety of mechanisms (see Table 16.2), and is sometimes accompanied by problems such as depression, reduced physical activity, and isolation.

Persistent pain is more commonly associated with mood changes such as depression than acute pain. Depression is more prevalent in all adults with persistent pain than in those without pain (Turk et al., 1995). Older people with pain are no more likely to be depressed than younger pain sufferers (Onder et al., 2005; Arnow et al., 2006). Older people who feel confident of their ability to manage their own pain (that is, of their 'self-efficacy') are less likely to experience depression and pain-related disability (Turner et al., 2005). A sense of personal control over the pain is also very important in mitigating against depression (McIlvane et al., 2007). Older people may also be more prone than younger age groups to social isolation, which is also a significant predictive factor of depression (Rosemann et al., 2007).

NURSING PRACTICE INSIGHT: HELPING YOUR PATIENTS TO DEVELOP A SENSE OF CONTROL

It is important to help people with pain to develop a sense that they are in control. Self-medication is one way in which to do this, because it helps the person feel that they can take their medication when it is needed and not have to ask for it, then wait for it to be delivered. It is also useful to help a person develop strategies to do things for themselves, rather than do things for them.

It is difficult for the sufferer to understand that not all pain is like acute pain, with an obvious cause and a finite lifespan. Poor understanding of persistent pain can be unhelpful, because it often leads to inappropriate self-management. For example, resting to allow healing when there is nothing to heal will lead to muscle weakness. Being less fit physically means that you tire more easily, use your muscles less, and, as a result, experience stiffness and pain when you do try to become more active (see Box 16.4). Risk of injury from unfamiliar levels of physical activity is increased, and poor muscle condition means more rapid fatigue and pain. These physical effects of pain make performing everyday activities more difficult, time-consuming, and energy sapping. Difficulty performing everyday tasks, such as getting out of bed, washing, and dressing, can cause frustration and depression.

Additionally, ageing is associated with sarcopenia (that is, the progressive loss of muscle mass): approximately 25 per cent of older adults suffer from this, which is thought to be a consequence of endocrine and immunological changes (Leveille, 2004).

Table 16.2 Types of persistent pain and their key characteristics

	Nociceptive pain	Neuropathic pain	Mixed pain/idiopathic pain
Cause	From ongoing inflammatory process or disease activity	From damage to or dysfunction of the nerves or nervous system	A mixture of nociceptive and neuropathic (also may have some elements that are not yet fully understood)
Examples	Osteoarthritis Rheumatoid arthritis Spondylitis	Post-herpetic neuralgia (persistent shingles pain) Trigeminal neuralgia Mutliple sclerosis pain Post-stroke pain Post-surgical scar pain Phantom limb pain	Persistent low back pain Fibromyalgia Complex regional pain syndrome (CRPS)
Verbal descriptors	Aching Dull Stiff	Pins and needles Burning Shooting	May have elements of both nociceptive and neuropathic characteristics
Key characteristics	Varies according to activity	Unchanged by activity Often person has allodynia and hyperalgesia	
Useful treatments	Physiotherapy TENS Acupuncture Anti-inflammatory drugs Paracetamol Opioids Acceptance and commitment therapy (ACT), or cognitive behavioural therapy (CBT) Surgery	Opioids Adjuvants (e.g. anticonvulsants and antidepressants) ACT or CBT	Some pains respond to some of the nociceptive and neuropathic treatments

Box 16.4 Poor understanding of pain mechanism can lead to unhelpful management strategies

- John feels pain and thinks 'tissue damage'...
- John rests...
- John's pain persists...
- John's muscles become weaker...
- John's joints become stiff...
- John's pain becomes worse and activity becomes harder...
- John thinks that the tissue damage is becoming worse...
- John rests more...
- John's muscles become weaker...
- John's joints become stiffer...
- John's pain becomes worse and activity becomes harder...

This reduces the functional muscular reserves in the older person and makes it more important to preserve the muscle strength, stamina and suppleness that they already have.

Not all older people experience persistent pain even though it is associated with diseases and pathological processes that are more common in older age, such as osteoarthritis. However, older people are more likely than younger people to attribute their symptoms (including pain) to the ageing process and, as consequence, they tend to under-report symptoms (Prohaska et al., 1987). Nurses also have a tendency to believe that pain is an expected part of ageing and think that the older person should simply 'put up with it' (Brown, 2004: 83). As a consequence, nurses do not always make an effort to assess for pain and older people do not always reveal their pain to healthcare professionals.

Our attitudes towards pain in the older adult are often unhelpful. In one study, nurses described how they felt that some older people exaggerated their pain. These nurses felt frustrated by treatment-related pain or pain that they felt was partly patient's own fault. Most tellingly, patients who endured their pain were admired and it was clear that people who did not complain were favoured above those who did (Blomqvist, 2003). If we add to this the trait of stoicism that some patients in pain exhibit, we have a recipe for failed management. Nurses are not the only healthcare professionals whose attitude to pain in older people is unhelpful. When considering ethical dilemmas associated with caring for older people, many nurses stated that they often felt that medical staff ignored the pain management needs of their patients to the point that some even overrode the doctor's decision to withhold medication (Palviainen et al., 2003).

Our attitudes towards ageing are developed within us from an early age; they are embedded within our culture and perpetuated by the media. We can improve our own attitudes by being aware of them, by working with older people and engaging with them rather than putting up barriers, and by becoming educated. A good start is offered by Lovell (2006), who discusses the realities and the attitudes that we have towards ageing.

Box 16.5 A way of remembering what you need to assess

P	**Provoking factors**	What makes the pain worse?
	Palliating factors	What makes the pain better?
Q	**Quality**	How does the pain feel?
R	**Region/radiation**	Where is the pain and does it radiate elsewhere?
S	**Severity**	How severe or intense is the pain?
T	**Temporal**	How does the pain change during the course of the day? Is it present all of the time, or does it come and go?
	Treatment	What has been tried to help the pain and how well did it work?

Assessment of pain in the older adult

The management of pain must start with its assessment. Pain assessment is a continual activity. Nurses are trained to observe the patient's behaviour and notice signs that further investigation is needed. People often signal their pain by altering their normal behaviour; they may grimace, support the painful area, or move differently. Any sign that a person is in pain, no matter how slight, should be followed up. Whenever any assessment of a patient takes place, a pain assessment should also be done.

NURSING PRACTICE INSIGHT: SPOTTING THE SIGNS

Look for a change from 'normal' in your patients. This often is the first sign that something is wrong. In patients with dementia, it is often the most useful indicator of pain (Bjoro and Herr, 2008).

Pain assessment is used to

- diagnose the problem;
- monitor improvement or deterioration;
- evaluate treatment; and
- help the patient to communicate.

Pain assessment should be a thorough investigation of a person's pain, exploring the cause and history of the pain, and previous attempts to manage it, investigating the person's beliefs about the pain, and establishing how it has affected them physically, socially, psychologically, and spiritually. A useful strategy for making sure that you cover all of the appropriate factors in your pain assessment is to use the reminder 'PQRST' (see Box 16.5).

The British Pain Society (BPS) and the British Geriatrics Society (BGS) (2007) have published a comprehensive guide to pain assessment in the older person, which includes a useful algorithm that can aid decision-making in pain assessment.

If the person in pain demonstrates difficulty coping with a persistent pain, has a complex pain history, or has other complicating factors such as drug dependence, it can be helpful to involve specialist pain practitioners and perhaps to refer the person to a pain team (see Box 16.6). Each member of the team uses their specialist skills to identify the main issues and then the team discusses the case together, before coming up with a comprehensive treatment strategy. It may also be appropriate to consult with other specialist nurses, such as older adult mental health or learning disability nurses.

Box 16.6 Members of the multidisciplinary pain team

Starting with the standard members and including the wider team (indicated by *), the multidisciplinary pain team will include:

- an anaesthetist/pain physician;
- a specialist nurse;
- a psychologist;
- a physiotherapist;
- an occupational therapist;
- a social worker;*
- a family therapist;* and
- an art therapist.*

In acute pain settings—for example, with post-operative pain—the main cause of the pain may be already known and formal pain assessment is often condensed into an intensity rating exercise. However, caution is needed, because it is possible to assume that you know the reason for a patient's pain and so miss an underlying problem—for example, in a patient with long-term low back pain who has come in for a hernia repair, or in a person with cancer who has a headache.

Pain assessment by nurses can be done routinely:

- during drug rounds;
- at the time of other observations;
- prior to nursing interventions such as dressing changes; and/or
- before moving and handling the person.

It can be triggered by the presence of physiological or behavioural cues, such as:

- an increased heart rate;
- pallor;
- grimacing;
- guarding the area;
- a change from usual behaviour; and
- a change in mood.

These signs are often, but not always, present in acute pain and are often absent in persistent pain. Patients might also consciously disguise behavioural signs of pain.

NURSING PRACTICE INSIGHT

An absence of pain behaviour does not indicate an absence of pain.

Stoicism (that is, a reticence to report pain, coupled with a willingness to tolerate it) has been cited as a reason for poor pain control in the older adult. It can lead to the patient suffering needlessly, but it also allows the patient to retain a sense of control over their pain and to cooperate with nursing staff during painful interventions (Spiers, 2006).

Older patients may be fearful of reporting pain in case it leads to an unwanted diagnosis (Gloth, 2000). Nurses need to be sensitive to the implications of admitting pain for the patient. Once a patient does report pain, the nurse's response will have an effect on future assessments. Failure to accept the patient's report and act upon it can make the patient doubt their own appraisal, and make them unwilling to speak up the next time (McAuliffe et al., 2009).

Pain rating scales

The most important function of a pain rating scale is to allow you to determine how a person's pain intensity changes with time or with treatment. Pain intensity ratings should not be used to compare one person's pain with another's. In ward areas and community settings, the verbal descriptor scale (VDS) and numerical rating scale (NRS) (rated 0–10) tend to be the most commonly used intensity rating scales. The BPS provides a numerically based pain rating tool in a number of different languages for those who do not speak English well.

Sometimes, numerical scales are combined with the Wong–Baker FACES pain rating scale (see Figure 16.3). The Wong–Baker FACES scale is popular, but it is not understood by all older people (Herr et al., 1998). However, some studies have found it to be useful, valid, and reliable even in adults with cognitive impairment (Pesonen et al., 2009). A pain rating scale is only useful if the person in pain understands it; finding that out is part of the nurse's role.

The VDS or NRS are recommended for use with older people (BPS/BGS, 2007). They are simple to use, but rely on communication with the person in pain and so they may be less useful in advanced dementia. People who have dementia tend to be less able to describe the quality of their pain or track changes in the intensity of their pain (Kelley et al., 2008), but each person is different and one size does not fit all.

Pain assessment in cognitive impairment

For people with dementia and other cognitive impairments, there are some pain assessment tools that rely on observation of the patient's behaviour (for example, breathing, vocalization, facial expression, and body language). Effective use of these tools often requires additional training and extended periods of observation, and this may limit their usefulness in a general setting. Advice about the most appropriate tool for your patients should be sought from a specialist pain team member. Using a tool without appropriate thought or preparation can lead to you failing to detect pain.

Zwakhalen et al. (2006) systematically reviewed 12 pain assessment tools for use with cognitively impaired older people. They recommended the 'Doloplus-2' pain assessment tool (see Figure 16.4) (Wary and Doloplus, 1999) and the 'pain assessment checklist for seniors with limited ability to communicate' (PACSLAC). However, they concluded that more research was needed to determine whether these tools need any refinement.

Note: This tool should be viewed in conjunction with its lexicon and guidelines, which can be found online at http://www.doloplus.com.

The BPS and BGS discuss these and a number of other tools in their guidance document (2007), and this is strongly recommended as further reading. One of the tools is a relatively brief tool called the 'Abbey pain scale' (see Figure 16.5).

Verbal descriptor scale (VDS)

0 No pain

1 Mild pain

2 Moderate pain

3 Severe pain

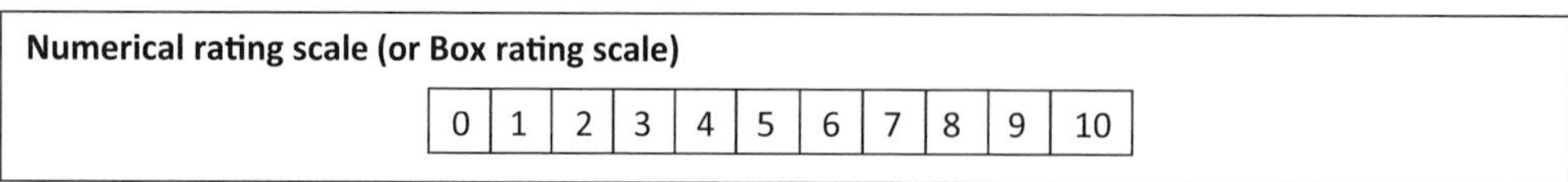

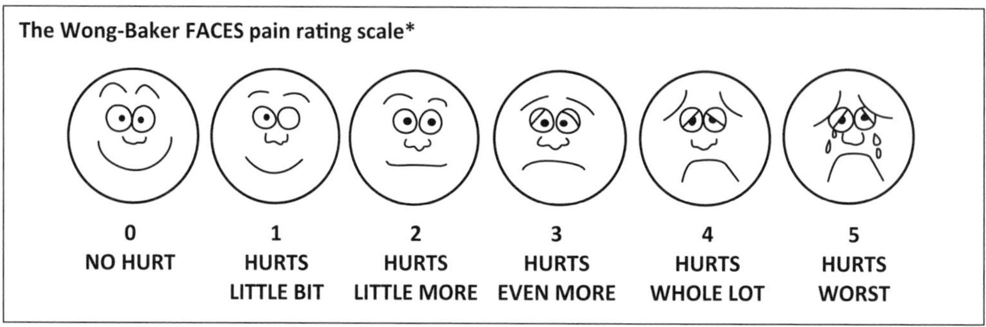

Figure 16.3 Three types of pain rating scale
* Wong–Baker FACES pain rating scale reproduced with permission from Hockenberry et al. (2005: 1259).

Like the other behavioural pain tools mentioned here, it requires further testing and perhaps revision, but it illustrates the principle of observation of behaviour to detect pain.

Changes in a patient's behaviour often indicate pain (whether there is cognitive impairment or not). Pain can make a person aggressive or withdrawn. Listen to people who know the person best—for example, their main carer or close family—who will be more familiar and better able to spot subtle changes in behaviour. It is difficult to assess pain in a person who has a cognitive impairment if you do not have a good understanding of what their normal behaviour is.

Case study: Pain assessment in cognitive impairment

Julian, aged 83, is a retired professor of music. He has been admitted to your medical ward with a chest infection. He has been suffering from Alzheimer's disease for three years and, in the past year, has deteriorated rapidly. His wife Anna, aged 79, is his main carer and, although she is tired, she says that she copes well at home. Usually, Julian is content to sit and listen to his favourite music, and enjoys his wife's company.

Julian's chest infection is improving slowly, although he is still pyrexic; his temperature is 38.5. He has been quiet on the ward, spending most of his time conducting music that he listens to via headphones. Today, he has been a little restless and has begun to wander out of his bay into the corridor. He allows himself to be guided back to his bed space, but then wanders off again. Attempts to get him to eat lunch, which he usually enjoys, have been resisted.

When Julian's wife comes to see him at visiting time, he becomes very agitated Upset, Anna leaves the ward in tears. She returns some time later and Julian tries to hit her. You sit with her for a time and talk about Julian's behaviour during the day. She tells you that this is very out of character. In order to rule pain out as a cause of the change of behaviour, you make an assess-ment of Julian using the Abbey scale. You and Anna think that the cause of his behavioural change is pain. After discussion with the doctor, an analgesic is administered.

Later that day, Julian is back to normal, sitting with Anna.

Reflection point

If you were to have no opportunity to get to know what normal behaviour was for Julian, how would you know to do a pain assessment?

DOLOPLUS-2 SCALE	BEHAVIOURAL PAIN ASSESSMENT IN THE ELDERLY	DATES			
NAME :	Christian Name : Unit :				
Behavioural Records					
SOMATIC REACTIONS					
1• Somatic complaints	• No complaints	0	0	0	0
	• Complaints expressed upon inquiry only	1	1	1	1
	• Occasionnal involuntary complaints	2	2	2	2
	• Continuous involontary complaints	3	3	3	3
2• Protective body postures adopted at rest	• No protective body posture	0	0	0	0
	• The patient occasionally avoids certain positions	1	1	1	1
	• Protective postures continuously and effectively sought	2	2	2	2
	• Protective postures continuously sought, without success	3	3	3	3
3• Protection of sore areas	• No protective action taken	0	0	0	0
	• Protective actions attempted without interfering against any investigation or nursing	1	1	1	1
	• Protective actions against any investigation or nursing	2	2	2	2
	• Protective actions taken at rest, even when not approached	3	3	3	3
4• Expression	• Usual expression	0	0	0	0
	• Expression showing pain when approached	1	1	1	1
	• Expression showing pain even without being approached	2	2	2	2
	• Permanent and unusually blank look (voiceless, staring, looking blank)	3	3	3	3
5• Sleep pattern	• Normal sleep	0	0	0	0
	• Difficult to go to sleep	1	1	1	1
	• Frequent waking (restlessness)	2	2	2	2
	• Insomnia affecting waking times	3	3	3	3
PSYCHOMOTOR REACTIONS					
6• Washing &/or dressing	• Usual abilities unaffected	0	0	0	0
	• Usual abilities slightly affected (careful but thorough)	1	1	1	1
	• Usual abilities highly impaired, washing &/or dressing is laborious and incomplete	2	2	2	2
	• Washing &/or dressing rendered impossible as the patient resists any attempt	3	3	3	3
7• Mobility	• Usual abilities & activities remain unaffected	0	0	0	0
	• Usual activities are reduced (the patient avoids certain movements and reduces his/her walking distance)	1	1	1	1
	• Usual activities and abilities reduced (even with help, the patient cuts down on his/her movements)	2	2	2	2
	• Any movement is impossible, the patient resists all persuasion	3	3	3	3
PSYCHOSOCIAL REACTIONS					
8• Communication	• Unchanged	0	0	0	0
	• Heightened (the patient demands attention in an unusual manner)	1	1	1	1
	• Lessened (the patient cuts him/herself off)	2	2	2	2
	• Absence or refusal of any form of communication	3	3	3	3
9• Social life	• Participates normally in every activity (meals, entertainment, therapy workshop)	0	0	0	0
	• Participates in activities when asked to do so only	1	1	1	1
	• Sometimes refuses to participate in any activity	2	2	2	2
	• Refuses to participate in anything	3	3	3	3
10• Problems of behaviour	• Normal behaviour	0	0	0	0
	• Problems of repetitive reactive behaviour	1	1	1	1
	• Problems of permenent reactive behaviour	2	2	2	2
	• Permenent behaviour problem (without any external stimulus)	3	3	3	3
COPYRIGHT	SCORE				

Figure 16.4 The Doloplus-2 pain assessment tool
Note: This tool should be viewed in conjunction with its lexicon and guidelines, which can be found online at http://www.doloplus.com.

Pharmacological management of pain in the older adult

Pain-relieving drugs are often the first thing to which healthcare professionals turn when thinking about pain management. They should, however, be used in conjunction with other strategies, including ensuring that the patient is positioned comfortably, well nourished and hydrated, and is being cared for respectfully and in a way that promotes dignity. Non-pharmacological pain management strategies are equally important and should be used as adjuncts to pain medications.

See Chapter 7 for more on medication management.

Abbey Pain Scale

For measurement of pain in people with dementia who cannot verbalise.

How to use scale : While observing the resident score questions 1 to 6.

Name of resident : ....

Name and designation of person completing the scale : ....

Date : .... **Time :** ....

Latest pain relief given was..**at**.........**hrs.**

Q1. Vocalisation
e.g. whimpering, groaning, crying
Absent 0 Mild 1 Moderate 2 Severe 3
Q1 ☐

Q2. Facial expression
e.g. looking tense, frowning, grimacing, looking frightened
Absent 0 Mild 1 Moderate 2 Severe 3
Q2 ☐

Q3. Change in body language
e.g. fidgeting, rocking, guarding part of body, withdrawn
Absent 0 Mild 1 Moderate 2 Severe 3
Q3 ☐

Q4. Behavioural Change
e.g. increased confusion, refusing to eat, alteration in usual patterns
Absent 0 Mild 1 Moderate 2 Severe 3
Q4 ☐

Q5. Physiological change
e.g. temperature, pulse or blood pressure outside normal limits, perspiring, flushing or pallor
Absent 0 Mild 1 Moderate 2 Severe 3
Q5 ☐

Q6. Physical changes
e.g. skin tears, pressure areas, arthritis, contractures, previous injuries
Absent 0 Mild 1 Moderate 2 Severe 3
Q6 ☐

Add scores for 1–6 and record here ⇨ Total Pain Score ☐

Now tick the box that matches the Total Pain Score ⇨

0–2 No pain	3–7 Mild	8–13 Moderate	14 + Severe

Finally, tick the box which matches the type of pain ⇨

Chronic	Acute	Acute on Chronic

Abbey, Jp De Bellis, A: Piller, N: Esterman, A: Giles, L: Parker, D and Lowcay, B.
Funded by the JH & JD Gunn Medical Research Foundation 1998–2002

Figure 16.5 The Abbey pain scale
Source: Abbey et al. (2004).

People must consent to be given medicines, including pain-relieving drugs. In some cases, it may be desirable to give an older person pain medication, but they may lack the capacity to consent (for example, due to a significant learning disability or cognitive impairment). In these cases, the nurse needs to understand the Mental Capacity Act 2005, how to assess the capacity to refuse or consent to medication, and how to act in the person's best interest.

See Chapter 4 for more on the law relating to consent.

There are numerous anatomical and physiological changes that alter the way in which we absorb, metabolize, and excrete drugs as we age. A number of these are extremely relevant to the use of pain-relieving drugs, but not all can be covered in sufficient detail within this chapter and the reader is referred to a textbook on the subject such as Banning (2007).

Some of the major considerations for use of medications in older adults concern anatomical changes, such as a reduction in lean body mass and total body water, which mean that lower doses of some drugs may be needed to achieve therapeutic levels. Alterations in the liver and renal systems will affect the time taken for drugs to be eliminated from the body, and also the likelihood and intensity of side effects. Older people are three times more likely to suffer an adverse reaction to a drug than someone in their 30s (Banning, 2007).

Different types of medication

Pain medications can be divided into a number of different categories according to the way in which they work. In addition to having different mechanisms of action, these drugs also work at different places in the pain pathway.

- **Paracetamol**—This inhibits prostaglandin synthesis in the central nervous system. It has many similarities with NSAIDs (below), and for some people, will produce the same side effects and have the same risks of use.
- **Non-steroidal anti-inflammatories (NSAIDs)**—This group includes drugs such as aspirin, ibuprofen, and naproxen. These drugs inhibit prostaglandin synthesis in the periphery (at the site of injury) and also within the dorsal horn of the spinal cord. Prostaglandins enhance the pain-producing effect of other chemicals released during tissue injury, or released within the dorsal horn as part of the pain-signalling process. NSAIDs reduce sensitization of the peripheral and central components of the pain pathway.

  CAUTION: Anti-inflammatory medications have a number of side effects, including gastric irritation, renal failure, and development of thrombosis, potentially leading to stroke or myocardial infarction. These are more likely to happen in older age and, as a result, NSAIDs are not recommended for long-term use in the older adult. In fact, many practitioners prefer not to use them at all in older adults. Although paracetamol is currently not included in the NSAID group, many experts are encouraging cautious use of this drug too, and would not recommend that more than 3 grams a day be taken for any length of time (Zhang et al., 2005).
- **Opioids**—This group includes so-called 'weak' opioids such as codeine and tramadol, and more potent drugs such as morphine and fentanyl. The weaker drugs tend to have a maximum useful dose above which little additional pain relief can be gained. The more potent drugs do not have an upper dose limit, except that higher doses are associated with greater side effects.

  CAUTION: Opioids can be used for persistent non-malignant pain such as osteoarthritis, as well as for acute (short-term) pain and cancer-related pain. Long-term use can lead to tolerance to the opioid drug, although this is not a problem for short-term use (Angst et al., 2009). Tolerance means that the longer a drug is used, the greater the dose will be needed to achieve the same pain-relieving affect.

  Opioids have a number of significant side effects, including constipation. Opioid-induced constipation (OIC) does not respond well to laxative therapy, but recently the use of oral naloxone has been tried with some success. This drug better targets the cause of the OIC and can reduce or prevent it (Reimer et al., 2009).

  The use of short-acting opioids for persistent pain is not advised, because it may increase the risk of physical dependence and tolerance (BPS, 2005). Instead, longer-acting preparations should be used wherever possible. The risk of addiction to opioids is very low when they are being used for pain control, but it is still present, and in long-term use, patients are selected carefully and monitored for signs that they are getting into difficulty (Chou et al., 2009).
- **Adjuvant analgesics**—This is a name usually given to drugs that do not belong to the other categories and includes antidepressants (such as nortriptyline) and anticonvulsants (such as gabapentin). These drugs relieve pain by increasing the amount of inhibitory chemicals in the dorsal horn, by blocking the release of excitatory chemicals, or by reducing activity in nerve fibres.

  CAUTION: Adjuvant medications, such as tricyclic antidepressants and anticonvulsants, are known to cause side effects including dizziness, drowsiness, and unsteadiness. These side effects can be particularly difficult in the older person and can contribute to an increased risk of falls (DH, 2001). These are valuable medications because they can alleviate neuropathic pain symptoms, but they need to be used with caution and carefully titrated.

Polypharmacy

It is common to see more than one pain-relieving medication prescribed at one time because the different types of drug target different parts of the pain pathway (see Table 16.3). This is called 'polypharmacy', and although it may be appropriate to use more than one kind of pain medicine, this exposes the person to a greater number of side effects and drug interactions.

The World Health Organization (WHO) analgesic ladder (illustrated, with some modification, at Figure 16.6) illustrates how we increase the potency of our choice of medicine for more severe pain and reduce medication as acute pain resolves. It also shows how different types of drug can be

Table 16.3 Where drugs act (mainly)

Drug	Periphery	Dorsal horn	Brain
Paracetamol	✓	✓✓	
NSAIDS	✓✓	✓	
Opioids	✓	✓✓	✓✓
Anticonvulsants	✓	✓✓	✓
Antidepressants		✓✓	✓✓

Pain increases: move up the ladder

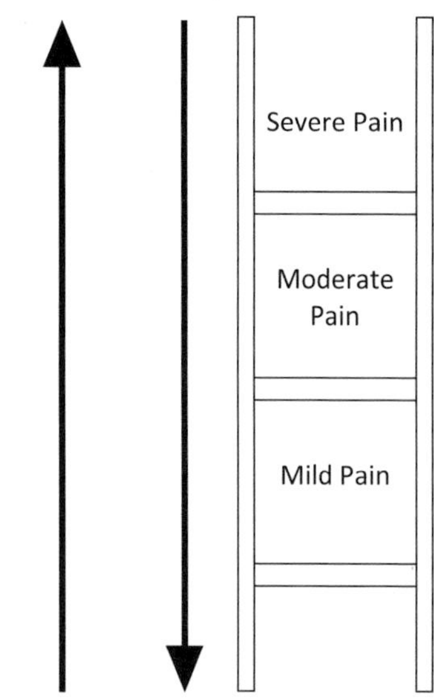

STRONGER OPIOID (e.g. MORPHINE)
plus if needed and appropriate
ANTI-INFLAMMATORIES
ADJUVANTS

MILD OPIOID (e.g. CODEINE)
plus if needed and appropriate
ANTI-INFLAMMATORIES
ADJUVANTS

PARACETAMOL
plus if needed and appropriate

ANTI-INFLAMMATORIES (e.g. Ibuprofen or Diclofenac)
plus is needed and appropriate

ADJUVANTS (e.g. anticonvulstant or antidepressants)

Pain decreases: move down the ladder

Figure 16.6 The analgesic ladder
Source: Adapted from WHO (2010).

combined to improve pain relief. This ladder represents the current practice in many places in the UK and illustrates the combination of paracetamol with anti-inflammatory drugs. This practice is likely to become less common—especially in older adults—because paracetamol may cause the same complications as anti-inflammatories and giving both together will increase the risk to the patient.

The drugs at the top of the ladder include strong opioids, such as morphine and fentanyl. These drugs theoretically have no maximum dose and so can be titrated to the patient's needs. The limiting factor tends to be an increase in side effects with increased dose. Some side effects become less troublesome after a few days or weeks of use, but some, such as constipation, do not and can cause considerable distress.

Polypharmacy also applies to the other drugs that a person is taking to manage coexistent medical conditions. Ageing is associated with increased incidence of many medical conditions affecting all of the major systems and so it is very likely that an older person will be taking a number of medications. Some of these will have an interaction with pain-relieving drugs, and it is important that you look at *all* of the drugs that a person is on and explore these interactions.

One of the examples that illustrates the seriousness of this point is the interaction between warfarin and anti-inflammatory medication. Drugs are carried in the bloodstream in free active form and also bound to protein. The portion of the drug that is bound to protein is inactive. Drugs compete with each other for a limited number of protein-binding sites. Anti-inflammatory drugs displace warfarin from the protein in the blood, thus increasing the amount of warfarin that is active, and this can affect bleeding time (Rang et al., 2007).

The drug(s) chosen to alleviate a person's pain will depend on a number of factors, including:

- type of pain:
  - nociceptive (tissue damage) pain responds well to paracetamol, opioids, and anti-inflammatories;
  - neuropathic (nerve damage) pain responds to opioids, antidepressants, and anticonvulsants used as pain medication;
- previous response:
  - how effective the drug was at relieving the same or a similar pain;
  - how troubling any side effects that the person experienced were;
- concurrent conditions and medicines:
  - conditions that the person has that might prevent them taking the suggested pain medicine—for example, a gastric ulcer or asthma prohibits the use of anti-inflammatories;
  - medicines that the person is taking that might interact—for example, warfarin, monoamine oxidase inhibitor (MAOI) antidepressants, and other antidepressants;
- known sensitivity—for example, the development of a rash with paracetamol or bronchoconstriction with NSAIDs;
- the ageing process:
  - most doses will need to be reduced for the older person because of the effect of the ageing process on drug metabolism and clearance (gradual liver and renal function decline is normal as we age);

– older people are more likely to experience side effects of medications;

- **cognitive and/or physical impairments**:
  – taking medications requires organizations skills, good memory, and dexterity;
  – concurrent medical conditions that may affect ability to take drugs—for example, swallowing problems relating to Parkinson's or stroke;
- **beliefs and preferences**—such as concerns that a person may have about the reason a drug is being prescribed, a desire to avoid being 'labelled' by drug use, or worries about side effects.

Pain medication should be taken regularly because it takes time for the amount of drug to build up in the bloodstream to a useful therapeutic level (about five doses, but this can be more in the older person). 'By-the-clock' dosing is encouraged, as opposed to taking it intermittently or when the pain is bad. The latter option will mean that the level of drug in the bloodstream will be lower than the therapeutic level and will have less chance of controlling the pain well.

It may take some time to build up to a therapeutic dose of a drug. When nortriptyline is used as a neuropathic pain reliever, it may be started at a dose as low as 5 mg at night to reduce the risk of side effects. It would then take two or three weeks to reach a therapeutic dose of between 25 mg and 75 mg. The person who is taking it will need to understand that they may not feel any benefit from it straight away and that it is hoped that any side effects will abate or become tolerable.

> ***Reflection point***
>
> If a patient tells you that they have tried a pain medication and did not find it helpful, what questions can you ask to find out whether they used it appropriately?

Side effects

All drugs have side effects and the following factors must be taken into account.

- The benefit to the patient needs to outweigh the harm.
- Older people may suffer more and worse side effects than younger people (McGeeney, 2009).
- Side effects can sometime be prevented.
- Side effects will stop a patient from taking potentially helpful medication.

It is also important that the right amount of the drug is taken, although the amount required may vary from person to person. The appropriate dosage in the older person is sometimes lower than in younger people. These issues, and others relevant to medications management in the older adult, are covered in useful depth in *Medicines and Older People: Implementing Medicines-related Aspects of the National Service Framework for Older People* (DH, 2001).

Routes of administration and formulation

There are a number of different routes of administration of pain medication (see Table 16.4). It is important to choose one that is appropriate to the person who is in pain.

Concordance

The nurse must investigate when the offer of pain medications are rejected. Try to make time for this, because the person may need an unhurried discussion about their pain and its treatment.

There are many ways in which to improve concordance with pain medication, including:

- helping the pain sufferer to understand the risks of pain and the benefits of pain relief;
- helping the pain sufferer to make an informed choice, which means that they need to know about the side effects as well as the benefits of good pain relief;
- respecting what the sufferer tells you and respecting their choice;
- considering other factors that might be causing concern—for example, whether the person is worried about their diagnosis; and
- exploring fears and concerns that the person has about the suggested medication.

See Chapter 7 for more on medicines management and concordance.

Case study: Medication

Mary, who is aged 78, has osteoarthritis and osteoporosis. She has pain in her back, hips, and wrists, and has not been walking much for the past few months. Mary has been seeing a pain consultant and a pain specialist nurse on a regular basis. She has been experiencing moderate to severe pain (described as 7–8 on a ten-point scale) for the past several months. She has been unable to leave the house without help, and is beginning to feel depressed—and fearful that her pain and quality of life will get worse still.

The following is a summary of the meetings between Mary and the pain management nurse. This nurse is a prescriber, but will be discussing her management plan with the rest of the pain management team, including the consultant.

Table 16.4 Routes of drug administration with advantages and disadvantages

Route	Advantages	Disadvantages
Oral	Easy storage Portable Cheap Non-invasive Minimal training	Variable **bioavailability** Patient needs to be able to swallow Interference between drugs and food Some drugs unsuitable, because gastric degradation inactivates them (e.g. diamorphine) Much of the drug lost in **first-pass metabolism**
Rectal	Can be used when gastric function is poor and if person has nausea or vomiting episodes Avoids first-pass metabolism for some of the drug	The amount of drug entering first-pass metabolism is variable and so amount reaching circulation from each dose can vary People may have an aversion to rectal administration
Sublingual or buccal	Rapid onset Avoids first-pass metabolism No need to be able to swallow	Few drugs available via this route (other than Fentanyl and Buprenorphine) Not good for nauseous people Local irritation may develop—need to vary the placement of the lollipop or lozenge Some people have an aversion to some styles of administration (e.g. the obviousness of the lollipop)
Pulmonary (inhaler)	Rapid onset Easy to titrate required dose	Needs good coordination Not appropriate in significant lung disease
Topical (creams), e.g. topical anti-inflammatory or capsaicin	Drug is required to be applied close to site	Requires frequent application Some people find them messy and difficult to apply
Transdermal, e.g. Fentanyl	Sustained release—up to 72 hours from one patch Some side effects may be reduced Continuous level of analgesia for duration	Allergic reaction/sensitivity to the adhesive Friable skin may be damaged by adhesive Thinned skin and poor circulation can affect adsorption Takes 6–8 hours to reach therapeutic levels Not ideal for use in acute pain (because skin depot forms and can interact with short-acting drugs given via other routes in unpredictable ways)
Intranasal	Rapid onset	Frequent application required Small volumes only
Subcutaneous	Most usually via an infusion Good when patient unable to swallow Good adsorption	Suitable only for small volumes Adsorption not always at same rate from different sites
Intravenous	Rapid onset	Rapid onset of side effects Needs cannula Needs additional training Needs monitoring
Intramuscular	Can be used to administer drugs that are carried in oily solutions (e.g. depot injections) Accessible without cannula Can give greater volumes than subcutaneous	Pain at injection site (patients may avoid injection and so get poor pain relief) Variable speed of onset Variable bioavailability
Epidural/spinal (intrathecal)	Smaller doses needed because administered close to dorsal horn Some drugs more effective via this route (e.g. opioids for neuropathic pain) Can be used in most settings providing user and supporters are trained	Risk of infection Requires specialist skills/training and monitoring

Reflection point

Look at the WHO ladder and relate the different drugs that Mary was prescribed to the appropriate levels.

- What side effects did Mary experience as a result of trying the different drugs to control her pain?
- How do you feel about opioid medication being used for the management of persistent non-cancer pain?

Conclusion

Pain is poorly managed in older people and the situation is even worse in those with a learning disability and/or dementia. Many problems stem from the prejudices, attitudes, and beliefs that we develop as we grow up, which are often a reflection of our culture and can be intensified by the portrayal of older people in the media. Being aware of these issues can help us, as nurses, to overcome them, gain knowledge, and improve pain management in the older adult.

Pain affects quality of life and independence. It can cause depression, isolation, and physical disability. Nurses are fundamentally important in the detection of pain, the support of people with pain, and the management of pain. The key to good pain management is good observation, good communication, and knowledge. Understanding pain physiology and the way in which pain treatments work can help nurses to work with patients in finding the best treatment for them. Pain assessment and management need to be tailored to the individual, taking into account their abilities and their preferences. The older adult with cognitive impairment requires an appropriate assessment tool to identify pain, but nothing replaces getting to know the person, so that a change from normal can be quickly noticed and followed up.

Table 16.A

Treatment plan	Rationale
Update medical history.	Be aware of current medication use, concurrent medical problems, and any issues that imply a higher risk for certain drugs (e.g. previous history of drug abuse, renal failure, liver failure). Ascertain Mary's understanding of her current conditions. Explore Mary's feelings about her medication, including her expectations, any problems that she has encountered, and whether Mary uses her medication optimally.
Prescription: Paracetamol 1 g, three times per day and then review in two weeks.	Step 1 of the WHO ladder. Paracetamol is good for mild or moderate pain, but can also be useful in severe pain—people often underestimate its potential. Careful counselling will be needed to make sure that Mary understands the rationale and does not think that she is being misled. Side effects are rare. It works in the dorsal horn, targeting the pain centrally. Taking medicines regularly gives them the best chance of achieving therapeutic levels and being effective. Time is needed for Mary to evaluate whether the drug is helping, allowing for normal variation in pain levels.
Review appointment: no side effects, pain level now between 5 and 8. Would like better pain relief Teach Mary how to use a TENS machine and follow this up at the next appointment. Consider the use of an anti-inflammatory as needed.	TENS helps to increase the power of descending inhibition on the dorsal horn of the spinal cord. It can be as effective as pain medication when used correctly, but some people struggle with the application of pads. An anti-inflammatory such as ibuprofen is an NSAID and will target the inflammatory component of the pain in the periphery. It has less risk of causing thrombotic events than some NSAIDs, especially when the dose is kept below 1,200 mg per day. The nurse is following recent guidelines (Zhang et al., 2008; EMA, 2006). However, there are risks with these drugs and they are not recommended for long-term use in older people. Using a TENS machine may help without adding a second drug, but Mary could take ibuprofen from time to time to help her to improve her pain management. Taking drugs ad hoc is not advised, but in this case this may be helpful because regular use is contra-indicated.

Treatment plan	Rationale
Review appointment: no side effects. Pain level still 5–8, but activity level has increased. TENS machine is helpful, but she is only using it once or twice per day. Would like better pain relief. Add Tramadol 50 mg per day, increasing gradually as needed to 100 mg twice per day. Review in 2 weeks.	An increased activity level, when combined with static pain intensity, suggests that the treatment plan is partially effective and that perhaps Mary's confidence is increasing. Step 2 of the WHO ladder. Tramadol is a mild opioid when used at this dose. It can cause drowsiness, unsteadiness, nausea, and diarrhoea. The risk of side effects increases with dose and starting slowly, and building up helps some people to escape them. Mary can increase the use of the TENS machine, but needs to develop confidence with this over time. Mary needs to consider whether she wants to continue with the paracetamol as well at this time: the number of drugs that she is taking may put her off adding another to her list.
Review appointment: pain level 7–8 Tramadol making her feel sick and unsteady, stopped taking it after 4 days on 50 mg per day. Had stopped Paracetamol at the same time, because she was fed up of the number of tablets and their lack of effect. Prescription: oxycodone 5 mg twice per day instead and review in 2 weeks.	Tramadol does not suit Mary well. It is important to note that the side effects were a problem and stayed a problem even on the lowest dose. A different opioid may suit her better. The number of tablets per day is important to Mary.
Review appointment: pain level 3–5. Activity level increasing gradually, but some fear of falling is restricting her ability to go out. Refer to the physiotherapist for assessment and advice. The nurse takes this opportunity to check how Mary is using the TENS machine: she is using it properly, but not very often. Continue present regime and review in 3 months.	Step 3 of the WHO ladder. Caution is needed when using opioids for persistent pain, and the nurse and doctor are aware the British Pain Society recommendations (2005). Exercise is important and Mary may also benefit from the knowledge that the physiotherapist can give her, as well as general non-pharmacological pain management strategies. The physiotherapist can also continue with the training that Mary needs to get the most from her TENS machine.
Review appointment: pain level 3–5, sleeping better, constipation problematic. Physiotherapy helpful to boost confidence and knowledge. Now walking outside each day. Advised to monitor fluid intake and start a stimulant laxative (e.g. senna) and keep under review.	Exercise will help improve Mary's constipation. It does not respond well to laxatives, and the nurse and doctor may consider changing Mary's opioid to transdermal Fentanyl, which has a reduced incidence of constipation, or using one of the new opioid–naloxone combination drugs, which have been reported to be very effective in preventing opioid-induced constipation (Reimer et al., 2009).

Older age is associated with an increased incidence of persistent pain—but that does not make it something that must be endured. Age increases susceptibility to side effects from pharmacological treatments and alters drug metabolism and excretion. Ageing makes it more likely that a person will have more than one medical problem and this makes it vital that we take a holistic view of each person whom we treat, taking into consideration what other therapies or treatments are being used, being watchful for interactions, and being mindful of the burden that we might place on an individual by asking them to add more treatment to their list.

Helping to relieve a patient's pain is a rewarding role that can make an enormous difference to a person's quality of life.

Questions and self-assessment

Now that you have worked through the chapter, answer the following questions.

- How is acute pain distinguished from persistent pain?
- What impact does pain have on an older person's life?
- What are the consequences of poorly managed pain to the older person?
- How is pain physiology associated with ageing?
- What assessment tools are available for the assessment of pain?
- Discuss the pharmacological management of pain in the older adult.

Self-assessment

- Having read the chapter, how will you change your practice?
- Identify up to three areas relating to pain management and older people in which you need to develop your knowledge and understanding further.
- Identify how you are going to develop this knowledge and understanding, and set deadlines for achieving this.

References

Abbey, J., Piller, N., De Bellis, A. et al. (2004) 'The Abbey pain scale: A 1-minute numerical indicator for people with end-stage dementia', *International Journal of Palliative Nursing*, 10: 6–13.

Angst, M.S., Chu, L.F., Tingle, M.S., Shafer, S.L., Clark J.D., and Drover, D.R. (2009) 'No evidence for the development of acute tolerance to analgesic, respiratory depressant and sedative opioid effects in humans', *Pain*, 142: 17–26.

Arnow, B.A., Hunkeler, E.M., Blasey, C.M., Lee, J., Constantino, M.J., Fireman, B., Kraemer, H.C., Dea, R., Robinson, R., and Hayward, C. (2006) 'Comorbid depression, chronic pain, and disability in primary care', *Psychosomatic Medicine*, 68: 262–8.

Banning, M. (2007) *Medication Management in Care of Older People*, Oxford: Blackwell Publishing.

Bjoro, K. and Herr, K. (2008) 'Assessment of pain in the nonverbal or cognitively impaired older adult', *Clinics in Geriatric Medicine*, 24: 237–62; vi.

Blomqvist, K. (2003) 'Older people in persistent pain: Nursing and paramedical staff perceptions and pain management', *Journal of Advanced Nursing*, 41: 575–84.

Breivik, H., Collett, B., Ventafridda, V., Cohen, R., and Gallacher, D. (2006) 'Survey of chronic pain in Europe: Prevalence, impact on daily life, and treatment', *European Journal of Pain*, 10: 287–333.

British Pain Society (2005) *Recommendations for the Appropriate Use of Opioids for Persistent Non-cancer Pain*, London: BPS.

British Pain Society/British Geriatrics Society (2007) *Guidance on the Assessment of Pain in Older People*, London: BPS/BGS.

Brown, D. (2004) 'A literature review exploring how healthcare professionals contribute to the assessment and control of postoperative pain in older people', *Journal of Clinical Nursing*, 13: 74–90.

Cairncross, L., Magee, H., and Askham, J. (2007) *A Hidden Problem: Pain in Older People*, Oxford: Picker Institute Europe.

Carr, E.C., Nicky, T.V., and Wilson-Barnet, J. (2005) 'Patient experiences of anxiety, depression and acute pain after surgery: A longitudinal perspective', *International Journal of Nursing Studies*, 42: 521–30.

Chou, L.B., Wagner, D., Witten, D.M., Martinez-Diaz, G.J., Brook, N.S., Toussaint, M., and Carroll, I.R. (2008) 'Postoperative pain following foot and ankle surgery: A prospective study', *Foot and Ankle International*, 29: 1063–8.

Chou, R., Fanciullo, G.J., Fine, P.G., Adler, J.A., Ballantyne, J.C., Davies, P., Donovan, M.I., Fishbain, D.A., Foley, K.M., Fudin, J., Gilson, A.M., Kelter, A., Mauskop, A., O'Connor, P.G., Passik, S.D., Pasternak, G.W., Portenoy, R.K., Rich, B.A., Roberts, R.G., Todd, K.H., and Miaskowski, C. (2009) 'Clinical guidelines for the use of chronic opioid therapy in chronic non-cancer pain', *Journal of Pain*, 10: 113–30.

Coker, E., Papaioannou, A., Turpie, I., Dolovich, L., Kaasalainen, S., Taniguchi, A., and Burns, S. (2008) 'Pain management practices with older adults on acute medical units', *Perspectives*, 32: 5–12.

Department of Health (2001) *Medicines in Older People: Implementing Medicines-related Aspects of the National Service Framework for Older People*, London: DH.

Edwards, R.R. (2005) 'Age-associated Differences in Pain Perception and Processing', in S.J. Gibson and D.K. Weiner (eds.) *Pain in Older Persons*, Seattle, WA: IASP Press, 45–65.

European Medicines Agency (2006) *Opinion of the Committee for Medicinal Products for Human Use Pursuant to Article 5(3) of Regulation (EC) No. 726/2004, for Non-selective Non-steroidal Anti-inflammatory Drugs (NSAIDs)*, EMEA/CHMP/410051/2006, EMEA/H/A-5.3/800, available online at http://www.ema.europa.eu/pdfs/human/opiniongen/nsaids.pdf.

Fecho, K., Miller, N.R., Merritt, S.A., Klauber-Demore, N., Hultman, C.S., and Blau, W.S. (2009) 'Acute and persistent postoperative pain after breast surgery', *Pain Medicine*, 10(4): 708–15.

Gagliese, L. (2009) 'Pain and aging: The emergence of a new subfield of pain research', *Journal of Pain*, 10: 343–53.

Gagliese, L. and Melzack, R. (1997) 'Chronic pain in elderly people', *Pain*, 70: 3–14.

Gibson, S.J. and Farrell, M. (2004) 'A review of age differences in the neurophysiology of nociception and the perceptual experience of pain', *Clinical Journal of Pain*, 20: 227–39.

Gloth, F.M.I. (2000) 'Geriatric pain: Factors that limit pain relief and increase complications', *Geriatrics*, 55: 46–54.

Gregory, J. and Haigh, C. (2008) 'Multi-disciplinary interpretations of pain in older patients on medical units', *Nurse Education in Practice*, 8: 249–57.

Helme, R.D. and Gibson, S.J. (2001) 'The epidemiology of pain in elderly people', *Clinics in Geriatric Medicine*, 17: 417–31.

Herr, K.A., Mobily, P.R., Kohout, F.J., and Wagenaar, D. (1998) 'Evaluation of the Faces pain scale for use with the elderly', *Clinical Journal of Pain*, 14: 29–38.

Hockenberry, M.J., Wilson, D., and Winklestein, M.L. (2005) *Wong's Essentials of Pediatric Nursing*, 7th edn., St Louis, MI: Mosby.

Husebo, B.S., Strand, L.I., Moe-Nilssen, R., Borgehusebo, S., Aarsland, D., and Ljunggren, A.E. (2008) 'Who suffers most? Dementia and pain in nursing home patients: A cross-sectional study', *Journal of the American Medical Directors Association*, 9: 427–33.

Kelley, A.S., Siegler, E.L., and Reid, M.C. (2008) 'Pitfalls and recommendations regarding the management of acute pain among hospitalized patients with dementia', *Pain Medicine*, 9: 581–6.

Leveille, S.G. (2004) 'Musculoskeletal aging', *Current Opinion in Rheumatology*, 16: 114–18.

Lovell, M. (2006) 'Caring for the elderly: Changing perceptions and attitudes', *Journal of Vascular Nursing*, 24: 22–6.

McAuliffe, L., Nay, R., O'Donnell, M., and Fetherstonhaugh, D. (2009) 'Pain assessment in older people with dementia: Literature review', *Journal of Advanced Nursing*, 65: 2–10.

McCaffrey, M. (1983) *Nursing the Patient in Pain*, 2nd edn., London: Longman Higher Education.

McGeeney, B.E. (2009) 'Pharmacological management of neuropathic pain in older adults: An update on peripherally and centrally acting agents', *Journal of Pain and Symptom Management*, 38: S15–S27.

McIlvane, J.M., Schiaffino, K.M., and Paget, S.A. (2007) 'Age differences in the pain-depression link for women with osteoarthritis: Functional impairment and personal control as mediators', *Women's Health Issues*, 17: 44–51.

Melzack, R. and Wall, P.D. (1965) 'Pain mechanisms: A new theory', *Science*, 150: 971–9.

Morrison, R.S., Magaziner, J., McLaughlin, M.A., Orosz, G., Silberzweig, S.B., Koval, K.J., and Siu, A.L. (2003) 'The impact of post-operative pain on outcomes following hip fracture', *Pain*, 103: 303–11.

Ochroch, E.A. and Gottschalk, A. (2005) 'Impact of acute pain and its management for thoracic surgical patients', *Thoracic Surgery Clinics*, 15: 105–21.

Onder, G., Landi, F., Gambassi, G., Liperoti, R., Soldato, M., Catananti, C., Finne-Soveri, H., Katona, C., Carpenter, I., and Bernabei, R. (2005) 'Association between pain and depression among older adults in Europe: Results from the Aged in Home Care (AdHOC) project—A cross-sectional study', *Journal of Clinical Psychiatry*, 66: 982–8.

Palviainen, P., Hietala, M., Routasalo, P., Suominen, T., and Hupli, M. (2003) 'Do nurses exercise power in basic care situations?', *Nursing Ethics*, 10: 269–80.

Pesonen, A., Kauppila, T., Tarkkila, P., Sutela, A., Niinisto, L., and Rosenberg, P.H. (2009) 'Evaluation of easily applicable pain measurement tools for the assessment of pain in demented patients', *Acta Anaesthesiologica Scandinavica*, 53: 657–64.

Prohaska, T.R., Keller, M.L., Leventhal, E.A., and Leventhal, H. (1987) 'Impact of symptoms and aging attribution on emotions and coping', *Journal of Health Psychology*, 6: 495–514.

Rang, H.P., Dale, M.M., Ritter, J.M., and Flower, R.J. (2007) *Pharmacology*, 7th edn, Oxford: Elsevier.

Reimer, K., Hopp, M., Zenz, M., Maier, C., Holzer, P., Mikus, G., Bosse, B., Smith, K., Buschmann-Kramm, C., and Leyendecker, P. (2009) 'Meeting the challenges of opioid-induced constipation in chronic pain management: A novel approach', *Pharmacology*, 83: 10–17.

Rosemann, T., Backenstrass, M., Joest, K., Rosemann, A., Szecsenyi, J., and Laux, G. (2007) 'Predictors of depression in a sample of 1,021 primary care patients with osteoarthritis', *Arthritis & Rheumatism*, 57: 415–22.

Spiers, J. (2006) 'Expressing and responding to pain and stoicism in home-care nurse-patient interactions', *Scandinavian Journal of Caring Sciences*, 20: 293–301.

Task Force on Taxonomy of the IASP (1994) 'Classification of Chronic Pain Syndromes and Definitions of Pain Terms', in H. Merskey and N. Bogduk (eds) *Classification of Chronic Pain*, Seattle, WA: IASP Press.

Turk, D.C., Okifuji, A., and Scharff, L. (1995) 'Chronic pain and depression: Role of perceived impact and perceived control in different age cohorts', *Pain*, 61: 93–101.

Turner, J.A., Ersek, M., and Kemp, C. (2005) 'Self-efficacy for managing pain is associated with disability, depression, and pain coping among retirement community residents with chronic pain', *Journal of Pain*, 6: 471–9.

Vaurio, L.E., Sands, L.P., Wang, Y., Mullen, E.A., and Leung, J.M. (2006) 'Postoperative delirium: the importance of pain and pain management', *Anesthesia & Analgesia*, 102: 1267–73.

Wary, B. and Doloplus, C. (1999) 'Doloplus-2: Une échelle pour évaluer la douleur [Doloplus-2: A scale for pain measurement]', *Soins Gérontologie*, 19: 25–7.

World Health Organization (2010) *WHO's Pain Ladder*, available online at http://www.who.int/cancer/palliative/painladder/en/.

Zhang, W., Doherty, M., Arden, N., Bannwarth, B., Bijlsma, J., Gunther, K.P., Hauselmann, H.J., Herrero-Beaumont, G., Jordan, K., Kaklamanis, P., Leeb, B., Lequesne, M., Lohmander, S., Mazieres, B., Martin-Mola, E., Pavelka, K., Pendleton, A., Punzi, L., Swoboda, B., Varatojo, R., Verbruggen, G., Zimmermann-Gorska, I., and Dougados, M. (2005) 'EULAR evidence-based recommendations for the management of hip osteoarthritis: Report of a task force of the EULAR Standing Committee for International Clinical Studies including Therapeutics (ESCISIT)', *Annals of the Rheumatic Diseases*, 64: 669–81.

Zhang, W., Moskowitz, R.W., Nuki, G., Abramson, S., Altman, R.D., Arden, N., Bierma-Zeinstra, S., Brandt, K.D., Croft, P., Doherty, M., Dougados, M., Hochberg, M., Hunter, D.J., Kwoh, K., Lohmander, L.S., and Tugwell, P. (2008) 'OARSI recommendations for the management of hip and knee osteoarthritis,

Part II: OARSI evidence-based, expert consensus guidelines', *Osteoarthritis and Cartilage*, 16: 137–62.

Zwakhalen, S.M., Hamers, J.P., bu-Saad, H.H., and Berger, M.P. (2006) 'Pain in elderly people with severe dementia: A systematic review of behavioural pain assessment tools', *BMC Geriatrics*, 6: 3.

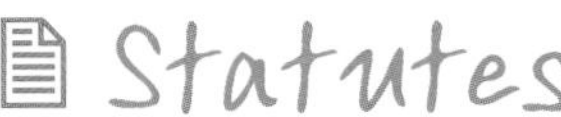

Mental Capacity Act 2005

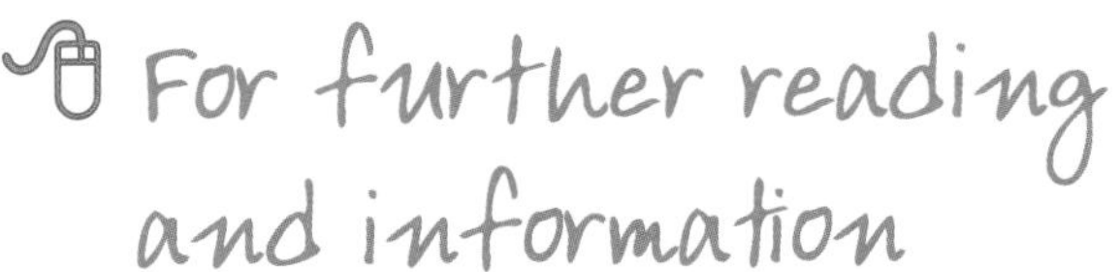

Department of Health (2001) *Medicines and Older People: Implementing Medicines-related Aspects of the NSF for Older People*, available online at http://www.dh.gov.uk/en/Publicationsandstatistics/Publications/PublicationsPolicyAndGuidance/DH_4008020 [accessed 26 October 2009]

Kumar, A. and Allcock, N. (2008) *Pain in Older People: Reflections and Experiences from an Older Person's Perspective*, available online at http://www.britishpainsociety.org/book_pain_in_older_age_ID7826.pdf [accessed 26 October 2009]

http://www.britishpainsociety.org/

http://www.pain-talk.co.uk/

Online Resource Centre

You can learn more about pain and its pharmacological management in older adults at the Online Resource Centre that accompanies this book: **http://www.oxfordtextbooks.co.uk/orc/hindle/**

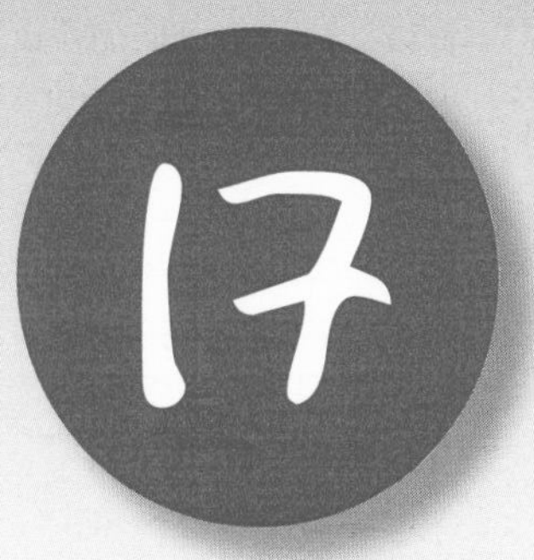

Sleep in older people

Lesley Hayes

Learning outcomes

By the end of the chapter, you will be able to:

- identify the 'normal' process of the sleep cycle and key changes that occur with age;
- recognize the key influences on sleep and associated effects;
- understand how disrupted sleep may be manifested; and
- identify the role of the healthcare provider in enhancing sleep.

Introduction

This chapter focuses on the subject of sleep, its impact on the lives of some older people, and how good-quality sleep can be promoted through facilitation and collaboration. Although the importance of sleep can be underestimated, it has consistently been found that disrupted or poor-quality sleep can affect people's lives in many ways. Although patterns of sleep are often said to change as people get older, they may also live in environments or with routines that can actively hinder sleep.

Sleep is a process that includes a number of different stages and is essential to healthy functioning. The need for sleep, however, differs between individuals and cultures, and so depends on many physiological and social/cultural influences. Some individuals, for example, require minimal sleep (as little as four hours per night); some cultures have siestas, whilst some individuals are awake at night due to their current or past employment. In some ways, therefore, there is no 'normal' sleep pattern; rather, there is the sleep pattern that is appropriate for the individual, and it is this that should be facilitated in health care.

Good-quality sleep can be defined as sleep that is of appropriate length, nature, and occurs at an appropriate time for the individual. This is relatively non-problematic where individuals have health and sufficient independence in their lifestyle for self-care, but this individualization can create significant challenges where they have health conditions, or are living in locations that do not adequately support their natural routine. It is important, however, that individuals' needs are considered. So, healthcare processes, organization, and approaches need to take account of this variance in individual needs.

Sleep can be affected by a wide range of factors, which can be internal—such as chronic illness (that is, illness that is ongoing and not short-term)—and external—such as a change of routine or residence, as in a period of hospitalization, or the move into residential care (Asplund, 1996; Ersser et al., 1999; Park et al., 2002; Montgomery and Dennis, 2003; Ancoli-Israel and Cooke, 2005; Richards et al., 2005; Lee et al., 2007). Support that facilitates independent living may include assistance with going to bed, but this may result in changed routines if services cannot accommodate individual's specific needs. Older people commonly experience hospitalization, or supported living, and so may be more influenced by these internal and external factors than younger adults.

Such factors may contribute to the consistently higher levels of dissatisfaction with sleep that are reported by older people compared to the general population (Montgomery and

Dennis, 2003; Liao et al., 2008). Dissatisfaction with sleep is reported by up to 20 per cent (Liao et al., 2008) and chronic insomnia has been reported by a significant proportion of older people—sometimes, up to a third (Ohayon et al., 2001; Liao, 2002). Addressing these concerns should therefore be an integral part of nursing care.

Normal sleep patterns

'Sleep architecture' is the term used to describe the structure of sleep. A normal sleep pattern (as illustrated in Figure 17.1) comprises a sleep cycle that is repeated four to six times during a 7–9-hour period of sleep (Bullock and Henze, 1999; National Sleep Foundation, 2006). Sleep normally follows a 24-hour periodic sequence and generally occurs at night, whatever the individual's specific sleep pattern (Bullock and Henze, 1999; Cole and Richards, 2007).

Figure 17.1 illustrates the different stages of normal sleep. As Bullock and Henze (1999), and Porth and Matfin (2009) outline, each part of the sleep cycle has different characteristics. Rapid eye movement (REM) sleep comprises sleep during which there is rapid eye movement and muscular twitching. Non-rapid eye movement (NREM) sleep has four substages (Stages 1–4); progression through these stages results in deeper sleep.

As a person falls into sleep, they move through Stage 1 and enter the NREM sequence, during which sleep becomes deeper (going from Stage 2 to Stage 4), followed by sleep becoming lighter (reversing process going back to Stage 2). At that point, they experience a period of REM sleep, after which they return to Stage 2. This sequence (deeper sleep through NREM stages, reversing back to lighter sleep, followed by REM sleep) is called the 'sleep cycle' and is repeated several times during a 'night's' sleep, with the depth of sleep reducing as each cycle is repeated, and waking then occurring by moving through Stage 1 to wakefulness at the end of the period of sleep.

Changes to patterns of sleep in older people

In older people, changes to this cycle often occur, including reduced strength of the circadian rhythm (that is, the biological cycle that parallels the cycle of night and day, and which generally leads to being awake during the day and asleep at night). It also inhibits the depth of sleep (Stages 3 and 4), meaning that sleep is effectively lighter (Ancoli-Israel and Cooke, 2005; Cajochen et al., 2006; National Sleep Foundation, 2006). There can also be a time shift, so that sleep begins earlier in the evening (Wolkove et al., 2007).

Experiencing consistently poor sleep is also often reported (Ancoli-Israel and Cooke, 2005; Irwin et al., 2006). This disruption can be associated with daytime sleeping or napping, disrupted cycles of sleep/wakefulness, or insomnia, which itself can take several forms (Bullock and Henze, 1999; Irwin et al., 2006; Bergeron et al., 2007), including:

- difficulty getting to sleep;
- difficulty staying asleep for a sufficient period of time;
- repeated waking through the night; and
- inability to return to sleep after waking.

All of these disruptions are more likely to be experienced by older people compared to those who are younger (Ersser et al., 1999; Irwin et al., 2006; Liao et al., 2008).

Disrupted sleep is therefore commonly experienced amongst older people and may have an associated, but not inevitable, impact on their lives when compared to those without sleep

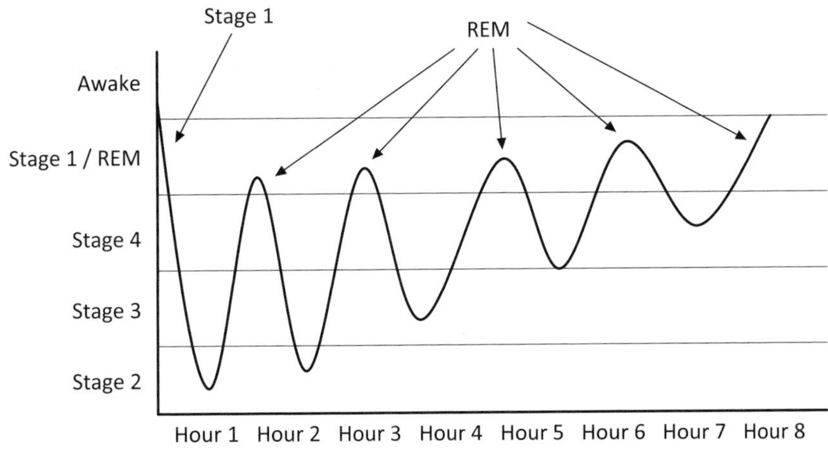

Figure 17.1 The sleep cycle stages
Source: Based on Bullock and Henze (1999).

disruption (Lichstein et al., 2001; Ellis et al., 2002; Alessi et al., 2005; Cole and Richards, 2007). It has been found that objective assessment of sleep does not always link clearly to a person's overall perception of their sleep quality (Edinger et al., 2000; Carlson and Garland, 2005).

Sleep can be affected by many things, and Figure 17.2 illustrates the wide range of internal and external factors that can affect sleep, along with the aspects of a person's life that can be affected when sleep is disrupted.

Underlying conditions are an example of factors that can affect the type of sleep disturbance experienced. Physical disability has been found to lead to waking with a feeling of not being rested, whilst symptoms associated with depression are more associated with waking at night (Maggi et al., 1998).

External factors include such things as the environment in which the older person is attempting to sleep. For example, sleep disturbance in hospital and nursing homes is common, and is often caused by noise (Ersser et al., 1999).

However, despite the magnitude of potential influences upon sleep and the effect that sleep disturbances can have upon daily living, its promotion can be undervalued in health care (Ancoli-Israel, 1997; Foley et al., 2004; Carlson and Garland, 2005; National Sleep Foundation, 2006; Liao et al., 2008).

Evidence base, and relation to best practice and care

Promoting changes that are ineffective is inappropriate, so awareness of the evidence base is essential (NICE, 2007).

Fundamental values and principles of care outlined by the Department of Health (undated; NHS Modernization Agency, 2003), Nursing and Midwifery Council (NMC), and the Royal College of Nursing (RCN) should be embedded within healthcare provision; addressing sleep disturbances in older people should therefore be based on these. These values include listening (embracing the whole person—that is, taking a holistic approach), caring, and being respectful towards others, as outlined in *The Code* (NMC, 2008), *Guidance for the Care of Older People* (NMC, 2009), and by the RCN (2004). In its public health guidance (health promotion guidance), the National Institute for Health and Clinical Excellence (2007) reiterates the importance of such values. They are firmly embedded

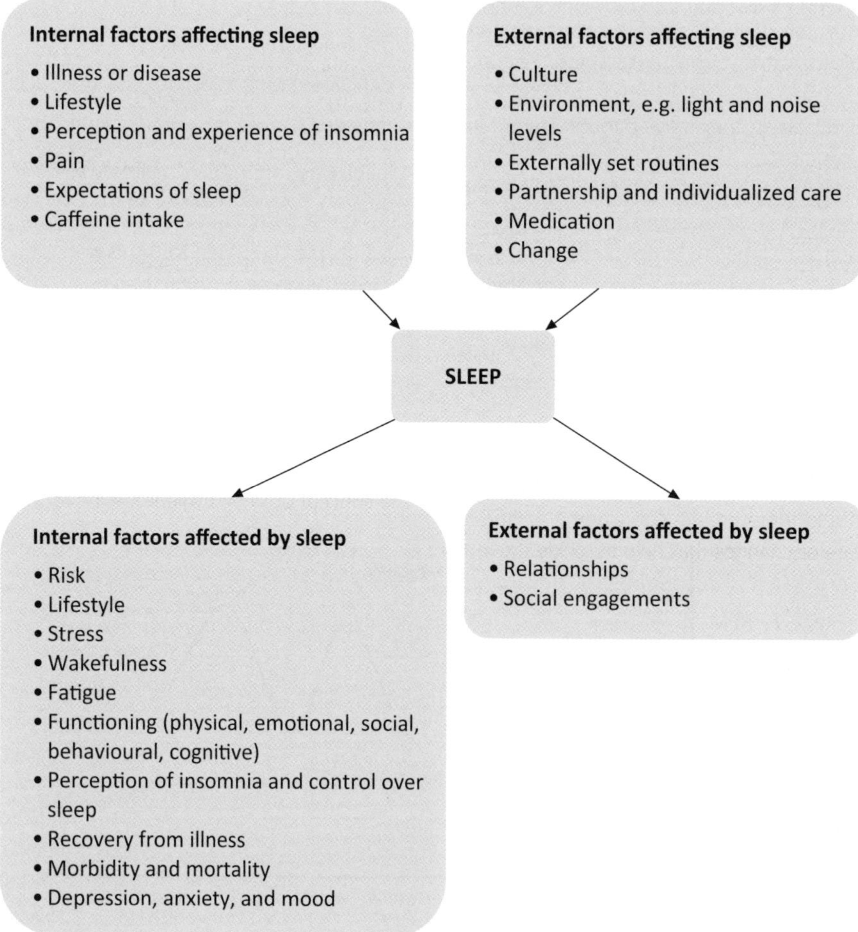

Figure 17.2 Factors that can affect and can be affected by sleep

within health promotion and are essential to enhancing sleep for older people. It is important therefore to recognize how these principles should inform the way in which older people are supported.

Supporting healthier choices requires activity that engages with and works in partnership with individuals, facilitates informed choice, and is empowering (DH, 2006). Working with older adults requires a collaborative approach to achieve these and to assist the provision of person-centred care (DH, 2001b). This should form part of holistic nursing care and appropriately embrace multiple approaches in order to meet individuals' needs. Indeed, Alessi et al. (2005) illustrated the benefits of multifaceted approaches to sleep disruption amongst older people living in nursing homes. Consequently, health promotion that emphasizes partnership has an important role in preventing and addressing sleep disruption.

Failure to work in partnership results in neglect of patients' or clients' specific needs and effectively disempowers them. This will result in health care that is less effective than it could otherwise be—particularly given the subjective component to the experience of sleep. Indeed, the subjective experience may be more significant than objective assessment. For example, older adults with insomnia—whether primary (for which there is no identifiable cause) or secondary (for which contributing factors can be identified)—can be affected differently in their ability to function, although there may be no significant differences in their actual sleep (Lichstein et al., 2001). This could arguably be due to the interaction of individual need, perceptions, actual sleep disturbance, and individual expectations, and reiterates the importance of determining and taking account of the individual's self-reported experiences. Doing so will facilitate partnership and concordance (that is, agreement between patient and healthcare provider of the patient's health priorities and ways in which these will be addressed).

Whilst many changes can be made by individuals, it is also important to recognize that beneficial change is not always within the control of the older person. Changes that facilitate sleep, and which can be made by organizations and healthcare providers, including nurses, should be identified and tackled. Nurses should therefore address external factors, as well as facilitate care or changes that help to tackle the internal factors that contribute to sleep disturbance. Being proactive in health care is essential, because few older people actively seek support (Irwin et al., 2006).

Current research

Research highlights two key approaches to addressing sleep disturbance: medication and non-medication.

Using medication to promote sleep

Hypnotic drugs are commonly prescribed to facilitate sleep. This medication, which focuses on internal causes or symptoms, is a common way of treating sleep disruption, but is problematic. It can work in the short term, but may result only in temporary improvements, with sleep disturbance recurring once medication is stopped (Irwin et al., 2006). There are also additional risks associated with the use of medication. Many older people take a number of medications, so adding to these increases the risk of negative effects—particularly with polypharmacy (that is, the concurrent administration of four or more medicines), which is experienced by almost 40 per cent of those over the age of 75 (DH, 2001a; BMA/RPSGB, 2009). This is an important issue, because both polypharmacy and taking hypnotic drugs are associated with an increased risk of falls (DH, 2001a). The British Medical Association (BMA) and Royal Pharmaceutical Society of Great Britain (RPSGB) (2009) therefore recommend that hypnotic drugs are not prescribed for older people due to the risk of adverse effects.

Taking medication to facilitate sleep has also been found to be associated with sleep difficulties (Maggi et al., 1998). So other strategies for addressing these, as well as the factors that also contribute to sleep disruption, should be explored (McCrae and Lichstein, 2002).

Non-medication approaches to promote sleep

Non-medication approaches address factors that are internal and external to the individual, and so include a variety of approaches to change. A range of approaches can therefore be recommended and used in preference to medication—particularly because they have none of the risks associated with medications (Montgomery and Dennis, 2003; Alessi et al., 2005).

Non-medication approaches to sleep promotion fall into four general categories:

- behavioural;
- cognitive;
- environmental; and
- underlying health-related.

The concept of sleep hygiene will be found to be integrative.

Behavioural and cognitive approaches

Behavioural and cognitive techniques focus on assisting individuals to make positive changes in behaviour and perceptions, respectively. Pallesen et al. (1998) provided audio and visual training, with information on behavioural and cognitive techniques, and found that the former helped to reduce the impact of insomnia with benefits that included reducing number of wakenings, increasing duration of sleep, and importantly increasing the feelings of being rested and reducing the use of hypnotics. Changing negative perceptions of sleep has also been shown to be beneficial in addressing sleep difficulties (Morin et al., 1993; Irwin et al., 2006), whilst cognitive behavioural therapy (CBT)—a therapy that facilitates changing perceptions and behaviour to make positive life changes—can help to maintain sleep and improve sleep efficiency (Montgomery and Dennis, 2003; Irwin et al., 2006).

A meta-analysis of research on sleep has found that focusing on changing behaviour helps with difficulties such as sleep quality, insufficient sleep, and number of wakenings in those over the age of 55 with primary insomnia (Irwin et al., 2006). Relaxation, behavioural, and CBT techniques all had similar effects. Teaching techniques such as meditation to reduce stress also produces a number of benefits, including reduction of sleep disturbances, reduced stress, and reported improvements in sleep quality and psychological status—that is, less irritability and depression—in patients with cancer (Carlson and Garland, 2005). Such approaches may therefore also be beneficial for others.

Interestingly, Morin et al. (1993) compared older adults who had chronic (long-standing) difficulties in sleeping with those who reported that they slept well. They found differences in attitudes to sleep and perceptions of control over sleep: those with insomnia had more negative attitudes and a lower sense of control over sleep. Determining attitudes therefore may also help to identify those experiencing difficulty with sleep; working to change these perceptions could arguably enhance an individual's experience of sleep and their subsequent management of it. Varied behavioural interventions have been shown to enhance sleep, including both the perception of sleep quality and patterns of sleep (Alessi et al., 2005; Irwin et al., 2006), and a range of interventions can be aimed at addressing such perceptions (Montgomery and Dennis, 2003).

Facilitating social integration and daily activities

Campos et al. (2005) found that social routines were important. In a study of individuals over 50 years old, they found that those post-stroke tended to have a lower quality of sleep compared with those who had not had a stroke. They also slept longer and awoke later. Social routines were found to influence participants' sleep routines, but those having had a stroke tended not to re-establish these as part of their recovery. Although small numbers were involved in this study, it provides a strong argument for facilitating social and other daytime activity that motivates individuals or groups to develop and maintain a positive routine.

Richards et al. (2005) found that daytime activity tended to support good-quality sleep by helping to establish, or re-establish, the sleep–wake cycle. They found that although daytime napping was reduced by only 45 minutes, participants fell asleep more rapidly, had better sleep efficiency, and slept longer.

Environmental approaches

Changed environmental routines, as occurs in hospitalization, can have a major impact on sleep, not only disrupting it, but also resulting in sleep deprivation and daytime napping (Southwell and Wistow, 1995; Lee et al., 2007). Feeling disempowered, being in a ward environment, and the associated lack of activities all had an impact. Lai and Good (2005) found that soothing music could assist sleep and enhance the perception of sleep—both of which are aspects important to the sleep experience.

Where sleep is disrupted, factors that could directly affect an individual's comfort should also be considered. Price et al. (2003), for example, found that mattress overlays could improve sleep by reducing pain levels in those with chronic pain, with the added benefit of pain relief being reduced for some.

➲ Addressing underlying health issues that affect sleep quality

Older people with multiple medical conditions report greater disruption and dissatisfaction with sleep (Ancoli-Israel and Cooke, 2005). Some conditions are increasingly common with ageing: restless legs and impaired breathing, such as sleep apnoea, can disrupt sleep, yet the person may be unaware of them (Lichstein et al., 2001; Ancoli-Israel and Cooke, 2005). Experiencing illnesses such as depression, anxiety, dementia, or having chronic pain, or waking to pass urine can also have these effects and influence sleep quality (Ersser et al., 1999; Lichstein et al., 2001; Montgomery and Dennis, 2003; Ancoli-Israel and Cooke, 2005; Cole and Richards, 2007). Any such underlying health issues that may impact on the quality of sleep need to be assessed and addressed to resolve the health issue or ameliorate its affect.

Improving general health

Changing general health can also help older people to sleep better (Ohayon et al., 2001). Physical exercise, including resistance training and brisk walking, has been found to be effective for older people when individualized for them (Montgomery and Dennis, 2002).

Sleep hygiene

The concept of 'sleep hygiene' is an important integrative concept that refers to the activities undertaken when preparing for sleep. It encompasses behavioural, cognitive, and environmental activity that can support or hinder sleep. Good sleep hygiene will therefore encompass activities that positively and proactively facilitate sleep for individuals, and are tailored to their needs.

It emphasizes the creation of an environment that is conducive to sleep through changes that are relevant to the individual. These may include broad lifestyle changes that aim to orientate the individual to the wake–sleep cycle, or behaviours that directly help the person to get to and stay asleep. Activities may change over time as needs change. Working with the individual may highlight changes that cannot be made directly by the individual. Noise levels in hospital are one example; these should be addressed by the organization.

Promoting good sleep hygiene with the individual emphasizes the benefits of making changes that facilitate sleep and can therefore enhance an individual's quality of sleep. Such facilitation is important; it empowers the individual by enabling change at the individual level through provision of information and broader health promotion.

Those reporting sleep disruption were more likely to have poor sleep hygiene/sleep habits—for example, taking medication, taking caffeine after 2 p.m., having irregular sleep patterns, being involved in cognitive activity before sleeping, and having a noisy bedroom (Ellis et al., 2002). Consequently, these should all be addressed. However, although they can all contribute to poor quality sleep (Ellis et al., 2002), their impact is not always clear-cut. Behaviour, such as napping during the day, was not greater for those reporting having normal sleep and those with sleep difficulties, so understanding the individual experience and care planning to address individual need is essential. Focusing on sleep hygiene is one way of achieving this.

Interventions that can depend on referral to other professionals should also be considered where improving sleep hygiene is problematic or insufficient to address an individual's needs.

Bootzin et al. (1991), cited in Montgomery and Dennis (2002), provides a simple framework for re-establishing sleep that follows the circadian rhythm. It is recommended that individuals should go to bed to sleep only when tired. If sleep does not occur, then they should get out of bed and go to bed again only when they again feel tired. They should get up at the same time each morning and avoid napping during the day.

In summary, the research above indicates that the following are important to facilitating good quality sleep:

- facilitating activity that helps to reduce stress and which may include relaxation or listening to relaxing music;
- enhancing positive perceptions of sleep;
- addressing worries that are affecting sleep, which may be about sleep or other concerns that inhibit sleep;
- facilitating development of an environment that better supports sleep—that is, an environment that is comfortable physically, psychologically, and socially, so that sleep takes place in an appropriate location, with an appropriate temperature, light, and noise level;
- addressing factors such as pain;
- avoiding stimulants such as caffeine later in the day;
- addressing any underlying medical conditions that tend to disrupt sleep and encouraging better general health/fitness; and
- facilitating development of an appropriate daily routine, which embraces social and physical activity, and reduces napping, and which may also include routines around preparing for bed.

The above points need to be viewed within a wider context with health promotion that is individualized and empowers the individual to make choices, both generally and specifically in relation to sleep. This will include enhancing knowledge and skills, so that the individual knows what choices there are and has the confidence to make decisions to meet their needs.

Reflection point

When admitted to hospital, the environment can be a busy and dynamic place in which lots of healthcare activity occurs. It is an experience that can rapidly disrupt an individual's routine, the effects of which can be exacerbated by the reasons for, and management of, the reasons for admission:

I felt that I still wanted to sleep. However, I had to wash my face. I was slow. I went to the toilet and did the grooming slowly. Then my blood pressure and other things had to be measured, then it was breakfast. I had to wake up.

(Lee et al., 2007: 341).

Reflect on the experience of this patient.

- What were his needs?
- Did the healthcare provision take account of these needs?
- What could have been done to facilitate this patient's needs better?

Assessment

Helping individuals to address their sleep disruption needs an organized and focused approach, and assessment facilitates this. Assessment is essential to care planning, and should be a collaborative exploration of the influencing factors, effects, and management of sleep within which individuals' sleep histories and sleep hygiene are obtained (Dougherty and Lister, 2008; Barrett et al., 2009). A sleep diary could be kept for a period to aid this assessment (Stimmel and Aiso, 2004;

Ancoli-Israel and Cooke, 2005). The Pittsburgh Sleep Quality Index may also be useful (Smyth, 2008). Obtaining the older person's perspective is essential: it identifies their views of what is causing wakening and their self-perception of their sleep experience. This will support key healthcare principles that facilitate empowerment (DH, 2000b).

The assessment process is a partnership that underpins and encourages delivery of individualized and effective patient care, which takes account of individuals' personal skills and needs, provides information to enable care planning and a review of success, and which embraces self-management. It should therefore be holistic, embracing '*physical, psychological, emotional, spiritual, social and cultural dimensions*' (Dougherty and Lister, 2008: 16).

Reference to a nursing model to inform your assessment—for example, the activities of living, which explicitly includes sleep (Holland et al., 2008; Barrett et al., 2009)—will assist this process. They are guiding frameworks that remind healthcare providers to consider the broad-ranging interacting factors that influence patient experience, as illustrated above in Figure 17.2.

Subsequent care planning, which forms part of the nursing process, should be based upon this collaborative assessment, and will therefore emphasize priorities and targets that are jointly agreed, relevant, and tenable for the individual. Such collaboration aims to enhance motivation, and enable better identification and achievement of targets. This will maintain and enhance patient esteem, and their ability to self-manage successfully. Evaluation (review) of the success of the care planned and subsequent health delivery is also essential. Needs and priorities of the individual may change; ongoing review enables assessment of success and challenges, and modification of the plan to meet any ongoing needs.

It is essential that patient assessment takes account of underlying physical, emotional, or psychological factors that may be contributing to sleep disruption, or exacerbating its effects. Observation (with consent) may be appropriate in helping to determine if these could be affecting sleep quality and tools do exist to guide this (Onen et al., 2008; Smyth, 2008).

Any underlying medical condition that disrupts sleep needs to be addressed. Where assessment identifies any such contributory medical condition, then additional referral and/or treatment may be appropriate. For example, urinary incontinence, including nocturnal micturition, which is common in older people (Ersser et al., 1999; DH, 2000a), can have many causes and disrupt sleep. Assessing for infection by screening urine and determining if the person has any symptoms such pain on urinating and the frequency or recent onset of or increase in wakening to urinate is therefore important. If night waking for urination is frequent, then referral for a continence assessment may be appropriate. Information, guidance, and support for completing pelvic floor exercises and addressing patterns of fluid intake may eradicate or reduce night waking and significantly enhance the quality of an individual's sleep. There are guidelines on assessment and treatment pathways: for example, DH (2000a) and Thüroff et al. (2005). Local policies are also likely to be in situ. These policies and guidelines will guide referral for assessment where initial assessment and treatment for a urine infection fails to resolve the issues.

See Chapter 14 for more on continence.

Locus of intervention

There are different levels of influence or action at which any given intervention could be aimed, although the particular focus will differ according to where the older person lives and their use of services. As can be seen in Figure 17.2 above, however, the individual should be the focus. Staff working with the individual can address sleep behaviour and knowledge through health promotion activity. Organizations, such as hospitals, residential, and nursing homes, can also make changes that facilitate good-quality sleep. Key actions are summarized below.

Actions that individuals can take to enhance their sleep

The individual can:

- undertake activity to reduce stress, which may include changing their routine to eradicate stress, undertaking relaxation to minimize the impact of stressors, or working to change their attitude towards sleep;
- develop appropriate and regular routines, and sleep hygiene measures, as highlighted above—for example, avoid daytime napping;
- change the environment so that it better supports sleep—for example, ensuring that it is noise-free, not too warm, and dark; and
- avoid stimulants, such as caffeine, later in the day.

Staff and organizational actions to promote sleep

Staff and organizations can encourage the development of environments that appropriately promote sleep for individuals. This requires development of flexible organizational practices and support within the organization for this, including:

- identifying individuals' needs regarding sleep, which may include observing for signs of sleep disturbance;

- raising awareness of activity or illness that can promote or inhibit sleep and how positive change can be made by the individual—including sharing information with colleagues and promoting change at an organizational level;
- empowering older people, in order to facilitate appropriate individual routines, and assisting individuals to follow their individual routines—including making use of day rooms, communal dining, and social activity where possible; and
- developing health-promoting activities to enhance sleep hygiene—for example, teaching relaxation techniques or finding ways of reducing noise levels.

Case study

Three days ago, Maddy moved into the residential home at which you are based. She was widowed eight months ago and has just been discharged from hospital after a fall in which she broke her hip. Her aim, following rehabilitation, is to return home to live independently as before. At the moment, she keeps herself to herself and complains about the constant light from the factory next door at night. She spends much of the day in her room and naps.

- **What would you do to help Maddy to address her sleeping pattern?**
- **Of what might the daytime napping be the result?**
- **How can Maddy re-establish her usual pattern of sleep?**

Empowerment is important!

Reflection point

Consider a time when you, or someone you know, has had difficulty sleeping. Identify what contributed to this.

- Was there one trigger, or were several factors influential?
- Were they psychological, social, physical, or environmental?
- How was the sleep difficulty addressed and did it work?

Now consider how the experience that you have identified reflects the issues illustrated in the research.

You will probably find that sleep was affected by a number of factors and addressed by making a number of changes. This highlights the need for a person-centred approach to overcoming sleep difficulties, and the importance of working in partnership with individuals to determine what changes they want to make and to assist them in making them.

NURSING PRACTICE INSIGHT: GET TO KNOW YOUR PATIENTS

When you work predominantly with older people, you will find that while many will readily explore health-related issues with you, others will need support and encouragement to do so. Getting to know the individual helps the nurse to understand why some factors cause problems for the patient, whilst others do not.

Working positively and in a person-centered way means that individual needs are jointly identified and discussed. Actions identified in this way are more likely to be followed because they are important to the individual and their relevance is evident.

Conclusion

Although there is a 'normal' pattern to the sleep cycle, individual needs vary. Research has found that sleep problems increase with age, and that these difficulties have wide-ranging causes and effects. There are a number of options for addressing these and which can be implemented to facilitate change. Non-medicine options should be considered given the risks associated with medication. Making changes to enhance sleep can occur at the individual and organizational level. Working in partnership with the individual, however, is essential if appropriate and relevant techniques are to be identified for them.

Questions and self-assessment

Now that you have worked through this chapter, answer the following questions.

- What are the key influences affecting sleep?
- How does disruption of sleep affect people's lives?
- What can done to help to address the issues?
- Think about assessing older people in your healthcare setting—for example, on admission or entry onto the team caseload—and consider the following.
  - How often do you discuss sleep with older people?
  - How can discussion be introduced or enhanced?
  - How can respect be retained when assessing for any sleep disturbances?
- Imagine that you are asked to lead on promoting good-quality sleep in an older person whom you support within

your healthcare environment. Their sleep is disrupted due to anxiety, and it is making them feel lethargic during the day and increasingly unwell.

- What additional information do you need to obtain in order to promote health successfully with this person?
- How can you facilitate an individualized response within your healthcare environment?
- Does the organization need to change its practice in order to enhance your ability to promote sleep? If so, what would be the key changes that you would like to see and what benefits would they bring for this person?

Self-assessment

- Having read the chapter, how will you change your practice?
- Identify up to three areas relating to sleep in which you need to develop your knowledge and understanding further.
- Identify how you are going to develop this knowledge and understanding, and set deadlines for achieving this.

References

Alessi, C., Martin, J., Webber, A., Kim, C., Harker, J., and Josephson, K. (2005) 'Randomized, controlled trial of a nonpharmacological intervention to improve abnormal sleep/wake patterns in nursing home residents', *Journal of the American Geriatrics Society,* 53: 803–10.

Ancoli-Israel, S. (1997) 'Sleep problems in older adults: Putting myths to bed', *Geriatrics*, 52(1): 20–7.

Ancoli-Israel, S. and Cooke, J. (2005) 'Prevalence and comorbidity of insomnia and effect on functioning in elderly populations', *Journal of the American Geriatrics Society*, 53: S264–S271.

Asplund, R. (1996) 'Daytime sleepiness and napping amongst the elderly in relation to somatic health and medical treatment', *Journal of Internal Medicine*, 239: 261–7.

Barrett, D., Wilson, B., and Woollands, A. (2009) *Care Planning a Guide for Nurses*, Harlow: Pearson Education.

Bergeron, C., Creculius, C., Murphy, R., Maguire, S., Osterwell, D., Simonson, W., Spivack, S., Stwalley, B., and Zee, P. (2007) 'Improving sleep management in the elderly', *Annals of Long-term Care*, available online at http://www.annalsoflongtermcare.com/article/8283.

Bootzin, R.R., Epstein, D., and Wood, J.M. (1991) 'Stimulus Control Instructions', in P. Hauri (ed.) *Case Studies in Insomnia*, New York, NY: Plenum Medical, pp.19–23, cited in P. Montgomery and J. Dennis (2002) 'Physical exercise for sleep problems in adults aged 60+', *Cochrane Database of Systematic Reviews*, 4, Art. No. CD003404, DOI: 10.1002/14651858.CD003404, available online at http://www2.cochrane.org/reviews/en/ab003404.html.

British Medical Association/Royal Pharmaceutical Society of Great Britain (2009) *British National Formulary 57*, available online at http://www.bnf.org/bnf.

Bullock, B. and Henze, R. (1999) *Focus on Pathophysiology*, Philadelphia, PA: Lippincott.

Cajochen, C., Münch, M., Knoblauch, V., Blatter, K., and Wirz-Justice, A. (2006) 'Age-related changes in the circadian and homeostatic regulation of human sleep', *Chronobiology International*, 23(1/2): 461–74.

Campos, T., Genes, F., Franc, F., Dantas, R., Araujo, J., and Menezes, A. (2005) 'The sleep–wake cycle in the late stage of cerebral vascular accident recovery', *Biological Rhythm Research*, 36(1/2): 109–13.

Carlson, L. and Garland, S. (2005) 'Impact of mindfulness-based stress reduction (MBSR) on sleep, mood, stress and fatigue symptoms in cancer outpatients', *International Journal of Behavioral Medicine*, 12(4): 278–85.

Cole, C. and Richards, K. (2007) 'Sleep disruption in older adults', *American Journal of Nursing*, 107(5): 40–9.

Department of Health (2000a) *Good Practice in Continence Services*, London: DH, available online at http://www.dh.gov.uk/en/Publicationsandstatistics/Publications/PublicationsPolicyAndGuidance/DH_4005851.

Department of Health (2000b) *The NHS Plan: A Plan for Investment, A Plan for Reform*, London: DH, available online at http://www.dh.gov.uk/prod_consum_dh/groups/dh_digitalassets/@dh/@en/documents/digitalasset/dh_4055783.pdf.

Department of Health (2001a) *Medicines and Older People: Implementing Medicines-related Aspects of the National Service Framework for Older People*, London: DH.

Department of Health (2001b) *National Service Framework for Older People*, London: DH.

Department of Health (2006) *Essence of Care Benchmarks for Promoting Health*, London: DH, available online at http://www.dh.gov.uk/en/Publicationsandstatistics/Publications/PublicationsPolicyAndGuidance/DH_075613.

Department of Health (undated) *Patient and Public Empowerment*, available online at http://www.dh.gov.uk/en/Managingyourorganisation/PatientAndPublicinvolvement/index.htm.

Dougherty, L. and Lister, S. (2008) *The Royal Marsden Hospital Manual of Clinical Nursing Procedures*, 7th edn., Chichester: Wiley-Blackwell.

Edinger, J., Sullivan, R., Bastian, L., March, G., Dailey, D., Hope, V., and Young, M. (2000) 'Insomnia and the eye of the beholder: Are there clinical markers of objective sleep disturbances among adults with and without insomnia complaints?', *Journal of Consulting and Clinical Psychology*, 68(4): 586–93.

Ellis, J., Hampson, S., and Cropley, M. (2002) 'Sleep hygiene or compensatory sleep practices: An examination of behaviours affecting sleep in older adults', *Psychology, Health and Medicine*, 7(2):157–62.

Ersser, S., Wiles, A., Taylor, H., Wade, S., Walsh, R., and Bentley, T. (1999) 'The sleep of older people in hospital and nursing homes', *Journal of Clinical Nursing*, 8: 360–8.

Foley, D., Ancoli-Israel, S., Britz, P., and Walsh, J. (2004) 'Sleep disturbances and chronic disease in older adults: Results of the 2003 National Sleep Foundation Sleep in America Survey', *Journal of Psychosomatic Research*, 56(5): 497–502.

Holland, K., Jenkins, J., Solomon, J., and Whittam, S. (2008) *Applying the Roper–Logan–Tierney Model in Practice*, London: Churchill Livingstone.

Irwin, M., Cole, J., and Nicassio, P. (2006) 'Comparative meta-analysis of behavioral interventions for insomnia and their efficacy in middle-aged adults and in older adults 55+ years of age', *Health Psychology*, 25(1): 3–14.

Lai, H. and Good, M. (2005) 'Music improves sleep quality in older adults', *Journal of Advanced Nursing*, 53(1): 134–46.

Lee, C., Low, L., and Twinn, S. (2007) 'Older men's experiences of sleep in the hospital', *Journal of Clinical Nursing*, 16: 36–343.

Liao, W. (2002) 'Effects of passive body heating on body temperature and sleep regulation in the elderly: A systematic review', *International Journal of Nursing Studies*, 39: 803–10.

Liao, W., Chiu, M., and Landis, C. (2008) 'A warm footbath before bedtime and sleep in older Taiwanese with sleep disturbance', *Research in Nursing & Health*, 31(5): 514–28.

Lichstein, K., Durrence, H., Bayen, U., and Riedel, B. (2001) 'Primary versus secondary insomnia in older adults: Subjective sleep and daytime functioning', *Psychology and Aging*, 16(2): 264–71.

Lichstein, K., Wilson, N., and Johnson, C. (2000) 'Psychological treatment of secondary insomnia', *Psychology and Aging*, 15(2): 232–40.

Maggi, S., Langlois, J., Minicuci, N., Grigoletto, F., Pavan, M., Foley, D., and Enzi, G. (1998) 'Sleep complaints in community-dwelling older persons: Prevalence, associated factors, and reported causes', *Journal of the American Geriatrics Society*, 46(2): 161–8.

McCrae, C.S. and Lichstein, K.L. (2002) 'Managing insomnia in long-term care', *Annals of Long Term Care*, 10(4): 38–43.

Montgomery, P. and Dennis, J. (2002) 'Physical exercise for sleep problems in adults aged 60+', *Cochrane Database of Systematic Reviews*, 4, Art. No. CD003404, DOI: 10.1002/14651858.CD003404, available online at http://www2.cochrane.org/reviews/en/ab003404.html.

Montgomery, P. and Dennis, J. (2003) 'Cognitive behavioural interventions for sleep problems in adults aged 60+', *Cochrane Database of Systematic Reviews*, 1, Art. No. CD003161, DOI: 10.1002/14651858.CD003161, available online at http://www2.cochrane.org/reviews/en/ab003161.html.

Morin, C., Stone, J., Trinkle, D., Mercer, J., and Remsberg, S (1993) 'Dysfunctional beliefs and attitudes about sleep among older adults with and without insomnia complaints', *Psychology and Aging*, 8(3): 3–467.

National Health Service Modernization Agency (2003) *Essence of Care Patient-focused Benchmarks for Clinical Governance Guidance and Benchmarks April 2003*, London: NHS.

National Institute for Health and Clinical Excellence (2007) *Behaviour Change at Population, Community and Individual Levels*, London: NICE, available online at http://guidance.nice.org.uk/PH6.

National Sleep Foundation (2006) *Sleep–Wake Cycle: Its Physiology and Impact on Health*, available online at http://www.sleepfoundation.org/primary-links/how-sleep-works.

Nursing and Midwifery Council (2008) *The Code: Standards of Conduct, Performance and Ethics for Nurses and Midwives*, available online at http://www.nmc-uk.org/aArticle.aspx?ArticleID=3056.

Nursing and Midwifery Council (2009) *Guidance for the Care of Older People*, London: NMC.

Ohayon, M., Zulley, J., Guilleminault, C., Smirne, S., and Priest, R. (2001) 'How age and daytime activities are related to insomnia in the general population: consequences for older people', *Journal of the American Geriatrics Society*, 49(4): 360–6.

Onen, S., Dubray, C., Decullier, E., Moreau, T., Chapuis, F., and Onen, F. (2008) 'Observation-based nocturnal sleep inventory: Screening tool for sleep apnea in elderly people', *Journal of the American Geriatrics Society*, 56(10): 1920–5.

Pallesen, S., Nordhus, I., and Kvale, G. (1998) 'Non-pharmacological interventions for insomnia in older adults: A meta-analysis of treatment efficacy', *Psychotherapy*, 35(4): 472–82.

Park, Y., Matsumoto, K., Seo, Y., Kang, M., and Nagashima, H. (2002) 'Effects of age and gender on sleep habits and sleep trouble for aged people', *Biological Rhythm Research*, 33(1): 39–51.

Porth, C. and Matfin, G. (2009) *Pathophysiology Concepts of Altered Health States*, Philadelphia, PA: Wolters Kluwer Health/Lippincott Williams and Wilkins.

Price, P., Rees-Mathews, S., Tebble, N., and Camilleri, J. (2003) 'The use of a new overlay mattress in patients with chronic pain: impact on sleep and self-reported pain', *Clinical Rehabilitation*, 17: 488–92.

Richards, K., Beck, C., O'Sullivan, P., and Shue, V. (2005) 'Effect of individualized social activity on sleep in nursing home residents with dementia', *Journal of the American Geriatrics Society*, 53: 1510–17.

Royal College of Nursing (2004) *Caring in Partnership: Older People and Nursing Staff Working towards the Future*, London: RCN, available online at http://www.rcn.org.uk/__data/assets/pdf_file/0003/27453/caring_partnership.pdf.

Smyth, C. (2008) 'Evaluating sleep quality in older adults', *American Journal of Nursing*, 108(5): 42–50.

Southwell, M. and Wistow, G. (1995) 'Sleep in hospitals at night: Are patients' needs being met?', *Journal of Advanced Nursing*, 21(6): 1101–9.

Stimmel, G. and Aiso, J. (2004) 'Managing insomnia in the elderly', *Psychiatric Times,* 21(3): 107–10.

Thüroff, J., Abrams, P., Andersson, K.E., Artibani, W., Chartier-Kastler, E., Hampel, C., and van Kerrebroeck, P.H. (2005) *Guidelines on Urinary Incontinence*, Arnhem, The Netherlands: European Association of Urology.

Wolkove, N., Elkholy, O., Baltzan, M., and Palayew, M. (2007) 'Sleep and aging: Part 1—Sleep disorders commonly found in older people', *Canadian Medical Association Journal*, 177(4): 376–7.

For further reading and information

National Institute for Health and Clinical Excellence (2007) *Quick Reference Guide: Behaviour Change*, available online at http://www.nice.org.uk/nicemedia/pdf/PH006quickrefguide.pdf

Royal College of Nursing (2009) *Dignity*, available online at http://www.rcn.org.uk/newsevents/campaigns/dignity

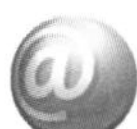

Online Resource Centre

You can learn more about sleep in older people at the Online Resource Centre that accompanies this book: **http://www.oxfordtextbooks.co.uk/orc/hindle/**

End-of-life care

Lisa Beeston

Learning outcomes

By the end of the chapter, you will be able to:

- identify what end-of-life care involves;
- describe how we might improve the experience of care at the end of life for older people and those close to them;
- recognize that end-of-life care can be difficult (particularly emotionally) not only for the person involved and their loved ones, but also for nursing staff concerned with their care.

Introduction

In 2004, the World Health Organization (WHO) pointed out that most deaths in European countries occur in people aged over 65. As life expectancy increases, numbers of people living into very old age are rising and more people are dying from serious chronic diseases rather than acute illness.

The *National Service Framework for Older People* (DH, 2001a) contained key recommendations on the subject of quality care and service provision. It also included recommendations about palliative care services, care in the community, and residential and nursing homes. Palliative and end-of-life care needs have often been overlooked in old age—particularly because death and dying are seen as part of the ageing process, and therefore 'predictable'. However, failure to provide good-quality palliative and end-of-life care for older people who are dying has been cited as one of the most serious consequences of age discrimination in terms of impact on quality of life (Philip, 2002). Publications such as the National Institute for Clinical Excellence (NICE) document *Improving Supportive Care and Palliative Care for Adults with Cancer* (2004), and the National End-of-Life Programme's *End-of-Life Care Strategy* (2008) and the *National Dementia Strategy* (2009), have focused attention on the need to promote high-quality care for all adults at the end of life.

What is meant by 'end of life?'

End-of-life care is a concept that brings into consideration issues such as:

- living well at the end of life;
- care in the last days of life;
- care after death; and
- support for carers after death.

It also considers issues such as what patients, clients, or carers might consider to be a 'a good death'. Individuals might have different ideas about this, but for many, it would involve:

- **Being treated as an individual, with dignity and respect**
- **Being without pain or other distressing symptoms**
- **Being in familiar surroundings**
- **Being in the company of close family and / or friends**

(National End-of-Life Programme, 2008).

Costello (2006), in a study of nurses' experiences of 'good and bad' deaths in hospital, concluded that 'effective communication' with patients and families about diagnosis and prognosis is needed, and that palliative care should begin at diagnosis and become integral to ongoing care.

The National Council for Palliative Care (2006) has pointed out that it is crucial to understand what meaning can be attached to the term 'end-of-life care' and how the term can be defined. The NCPC highlights a set of prognostic indicators that may help in making decisions about when 'end-of-life care' begins, which can be summarized as considering:

- whether or not you would be surprised if the patient were to die in the next 6–12 months;
- patient choice or need—for example, patients with advanced disease may make a choice for comfort care only and not for aggressive treatment;
- clinical indicators, such as general predictors of end-stage illness and ensuring comprehensive assessment, which will recognize the point at which dying is diagnosed.

It is suggested (NCPC, 2006) that end-of-life care is focused around this time and that, for most people, it will be likely that this will not begin earlier than one year before death; for most, it will come later than that.

End-of-life and palliative care

End-of-life care is also a term that encompasses the concept of palliative care although is not synonymous with it. It is important to note that 'palliative care' begins from diagnosis to beyond death. Palliative care has been defined by the WHO (2002) as an approach that improves the quality of life of patients and their families, facing the problems associated with life-threatening illness, through the prevention and relief of suffering by means of early identification and impeccable assessment, and treatment of pain and other problems, physical, psychosocial, and spiritual.

Provision of and access to end-of-life care

The provision of end-of-life care is complex, and will often require a combination of health and social care services, in hospital, in the community, in care homes, or in hospices. It is crucial to remember that significant care is also provided by family, friends, and relatives, and that 'informal carers' will need support at such times.

It is essential to remember that end-of-life care is relevant for anyone with any life-limiting condition and in any setting. For example, more than 500,000 people aged 65 or older live in care homes in this country and many will end their lives in these care settings (SCIE, 2005). Indeed, older people are reported to have trouble accessing good-quality palliative care and end-of-life care services (Seymour et al., 2001). Co-morbidity in older patients can complicate matters in that if a patient with advanced cancer also has dementia, then they are unlikely to be admitted to a specialist palliative care unit, with their mental health issues acting as a barrier to accessing other services (Lloyd Williams et al., 2005). This diagnostic overshadowing is something that the Disability Rights Commission (DRC) has highlighted in its recent report (2006). Indeed, the report pointed out that for people with learning disabilities and/or mental health problems reaching the end-of-life, hospice and other palliative care was not generally geared to their needs, and that physical symptoms could be inappropriately attributed to mental health issues or 'old age'. This emphasizes the need for appropriate holistic assessment, and for each symptom and need to be adequately assessed.

The evidence base for best practice and care

Evidence-based practice has been defined as the conscientious, explicit, and judicious use of current best evidence in making decisions about the care of individual patients (Sackett et al., 1996), and also should take into account individual clinical expertise and patient or client values, choices, and expectations.

Health care needs to be based not only on evidence-based practice, but also on the value of fair access to care, a person-centred approach, and whole-systems working (Lothian and Philip, 2001). To this end, one of the key issues that we need to address in healthcare practice, and literature surrounding this, is to extend the reviewing of literature to include evidence of the processes involved in implementing 'best evidence' (Harden, 2006) and also to consider what actually constitutes best evidence. We need to bear in mind the perspectives and experiences of the people (patients/users and carers) who are in need, or receipt, of such care. These sorts of issues are inextricably bound up with how we care, the values with which we operate, and the impact that this has—although these sorts of issues are the very ones that might be missing from effectiveness reviews, since the measurement of such aspects of care can be more nebulous. Evidence as to why structural factors (that is, how our services are devised and set up), organizational issues (that is, how organizations operate), and values-based decisions (that is, things that we do on the basis of our values and beliefs) limit or hamper its implementation is harder to come by—but equally as important if we are to improve end-of-life care for older people and their families (Popay, 2006). This leads on to the important issue of user and carer involvement in service provision—that is, how those who receive care perceive the service that they get.

Service user and carer review

The knowledge and experience held by the patient has for too long been an untapped resource [...] that could greatly benefit the quality of patients' care and ultimately their quality of life.

(DH, 2001b)

Patients and carers have a unique and essential contribution to offer healthcare planning, and organization and delivery, based on their insights and knowledge that can only be gained from the direct experience of using services (Rhodes and Nocon, 1998). Understanding these experiences is, therefore, a must for patient involvement at practice level and in planning services. There is a need to create a culture of involvement, listening, and feedback, in which the patients' and carers' experience is the catalyst for improving services (DH, 2003). User and carer involvement is perhaps particularly pertinent in caring for older people, as part of the struggle to overcome adverse attitudes towards the elderly (Katz et al., 2000). It is also particularly pertinent at the end of life, since adoption of a family-centred approach—with a focus on physical and psychosocial well-being, and a focus on palliative care—could reduce the experience of dissatisfaction for many service users (Rogers et al., 2000).

Support for carers and families with their loved ones at the end-of-life stage is essential nursing care—especially if the spouse, relative, or carer is also older and frail. Their needs should always be addressed, whether that involves practical arrangements such as providing drinks, or psychological concerns relating to bereavement. Rather than providing specialized skills in counselling, support for people who are dying and their carers normally only requires the nurse to be '*demonstrate a willingness to stay near, listen and try to understand*' (Johnson, 2006).

See Chapter 5 for more on the family and carers.

NURSING PRACTICE INSIGHT: THE LITTLE THINGS MAKE A BIG DIFFERENCE

As well as being aware of research and evidence, and incorporating this into our practice, it is also important to consider the small acts of human kindness, and the importance of valuing someone as a person first and foremost when we care for those facing the end of their lives.

The following anecdotal evidence prompted the author to reflect upon end-of-life care in a broader sense, in terms of how, as health care practitioners, we operate in our day-to-day practice:

I was at a conference where a carer recounted her experience of respite care for her husband who was suffering with dementia. He was a gifted musician who was still able to play complex pieces of music on the piano, despite not being oriented to time, place, or person. This activity, along with listening to classical music, provided relief from agitation, and calmed and distracted him, so his wife bought him a digital radio. However, every time she visited him, it was tuned in to Radio 1 and was loudly playing the type of music that he detested, and he therefore seemed to be increasingly agitated. One can only assume that this music was a favourite with members of staff[...]

We need to consider the behaviour of the staff: implicit in their act was the belief that it was 'OK' to retune the radio and that the environment in which this person was being nursed was 'their domain' rather than the patient's domain.

With this scenario in mind, you may wish to explore some of the work by Wolfensberger (1998), Sinclair (2007), and Kitwood (1997), who highlight the issues faced by devalued people and groups of people.

It may seem a little odd that a 'Nursing Practice Insight' should be to read more, but what we put into our heads has an important outcome in our behaviour. This is something that is well explored in educational literature (Wee and Hughes, 2007). For example, Fish and Coles (1998) use the iceberg as a metaphor for practice: if you can imagine that the part of the iceberg above water represents 'what we do' in our practice, such as tasks and skills, then the part below the waterline is not as easily viewed, and relates to our values, beliefs, attitudes, assumptions, feelings, expectations, and knowledge. This is the part that is harder to measure, because it is not directly observable—but it is central in influencing our actions and behaviours when we are caring for others.

Conceptualizing end-of-life care for our own practice

Work by Kellehear (2008) explores the seemingly contradictory positions of health promotion, and palliative and end-of-life care. He states, for example, that we have commonly equated palliative care with terminal care—being cared for in the last few days, weeks, or months of life—and this has made the issue of health promotion counter-intuitive for some practitioners. Palliative and end-of-life care both refer to the holistic management of symptoms and care for people with any life-threatening condition. This also involves keeping individuals as well as possible and ensuring that they can live as well as they are able until the end of life. This might involve rethinking how we conceptualize palliative and end-of-life care. For example, Kellehear (1999) outlines the importance of allowing non-medicalized approaches to palliative care to evolve. This may, on first reading, be rather difficult to understand, but if we consider—as Corner and Dunlop (1997) point out—that the current way in which we view palliative and end-of-life care is inherently biomedical—that is, often focused on nursing or medical issues, as determined by physical symptoms—then one way of rethinking such care may involve recognition that some of the social aspects of dying are complex and lie outside clinical/medical constructions. For example, simply recognizing that physical symptoms may not be the root cause of someone's suffering or angst may be a starting point.

So how do we conceptualize end-of-life care for our own practice? End-of-life care for older people raises many complex issues, which can be discussed and analysed on several different levels. One way of thinking about how we, as individual practitioners, engage in such care and support people might be to consider applying the 'logical levels' model developed and outlined by Robert Dilts (1990) (see Table 18.1). The function of each level is to organize the information on the level below. Changing something on a lower level could, but would not necessarily, affect the upper levels, but changing something in the upper level would change things below. For example, if my spiritual beliefs are such that I believe in heaven, hell, and purgatory, then my behaviour may be focused around seeking reconciliation and forgiveness for certain aspects of my life. Likewise, if my identity is primarily as a mother and grandmother, then it might be very important to me that my family is with me at the end of my life.

Table 18.1 Logical levels

6. Spirituality/purpose (Who else/for whom?)	This can be thought of as being part of a' bigger picture': 'What is my purpose in life?'
5. Identity/mission (Who?)	Who are we as human beings, or as individuals, and how does this impact on what we want in our lives?
4. Beliefs/values (Why?)	Why do we do certain things? What do we value or believe in, and how does this influence us?
3. Capabilities/strategies (How?)	How do we do things? What are our capabilities, strategies, or action plans? Do we foster capabilities and strategies in others?
2. Behaviours (What?)	This can be seen in what we do. Consider the ways in which we behave towards people, and how behaving differently may enhance end-of-life care.
1. Environment (Where/when?)	This refers to external constraints and influences. Consider what we can add, or change, within the environment to improve end-of-life care.

Source: Adapted from Dilts (1990)

The model can provide a useful framework for ways of reflecting on our selves, others, organizations in which we work, and the society in which we live.

Reflection point

Some of these points are expanded upon below, but you might also wish to think of other situations in your own practice that fit within this framework, and reflect upon how you might improve end-of-life care for older people and their loved ones.

Environment

One of the key issues facing those at the end of life is that of the environment in which they wish to receive care. Research suggests that, when faced with a terminal illness, most people would prefer to be at home and die at home (Higginson and Sen Gupta, 2000; Higginson, 2003), although this preference may change as death becomes more imminent and access to more intensive support is needed or requested.

According to the National Audit Office (2008), mortality statistics show that 35 per cent of people die at home or in a care home, while between 46 per cent and 77 per cent of deaths occur in a hospital, allowing for regional variations. Place of death also varies by condition, with cancer patients more likely to die in a hospice or at their home (94 per cent of all hospice deaths are people with cancer, whereas deaths from dementia predominantly occur in care homes). Variation in place of death is complex and will obviously depend upon preferences, choices, resources, support, finances, and the complexity of symptom management issues. It is also related to the dominant paradigm of care, with the expectation that it is normal for formal care to be provided in, or linked to, institutions such as hospitals, care homes, and hospices. Sinclair (2007) points out that no valued person chooses to live their normal day-to-day life in institutional care, so it is not therefore surprising that, when given a choice, people will prefer to be cared for and die at home.

This is addressed to some extent in the Department of Health guidelines *Preferred Priorities for Care* (2007), and the *Gold Standards Framework* (National GSF Framework Team, 2010). These guidelines incorporate a document that people hold for themselves and take with them if they receive care in different places. It has space for the individual's thoughts about their care and the choices that they would like to make, including stating where, if possible, they would want to be when they die and with whom. Information about choices and who might be involved in their care can also be recorded, so that any care staff can read about what matters to the individual and what they wish to happen—thereby ensuring continuity of care. If anything changes, this can be written in the plan, so that it stays up to date. The *Preferred Priorities for Care* guidelines provide an opportunity for individuals and staff to work together to develop advanced care plans in accordance with the Mental Capacity Act 2005.

Details of documents relating to the end-of-life care programme can be found online at http://www.endoflifecareforadults.nhs.uk/.

NURSING PRACTICE INSIGHT: DISCUSSING END-OF-LIFE ISSUES WITH PATIENTS

End-of-life discussions will provide patients with the opportunity to talk about their goals and expectations.

However, it is important to remember that conversations about such issues can be sensitive, and can require a great amount of skill when raising issues and dealing with responses. Discussing wishes and future care with patients is complex.

For further discussion and advice, read *Advance Care Planning: A Guide for Health and Social Care Staff* (National End-of-Life Programme, 2008).

Dying at home

The National Council on Ageing (2002) has published a paper that makes recommendations regarding equality, adequacy, and appropriateness of palliative care services for older people, including issues about the place of death. Although a US organization, many of its recommendations are relevant whatever the country in which older people live. Many studies confirm that most people prefer to die at home (Higginson et al., 1998; Higginson and Sen-Gupta, 2000), yet in the UK only a quarter of cancer patients, for example, do so. This is a complex situation, since people's preferences may change over a period of time and depending upon their situation, with regard to the support that they need and the type of symptoms that they may be experiencing (Higginson and Sen-Gupta, 2000). The main reasons for admission to a hospital, hospice, or care home are a combination of carer breakdown, poor symptom control, and poor communication.

In a review of out-of-hours palliative care in the community, Thomas (2001) points to the fact that there is evidence to suggest that the provision of good care at home is more difficult to achieve for patients who are:

- socially/economically deprived;
- elderly;
- experiencing poor symptom control;
- unable to access 24-hour support; and
- suffering from a chronic illness with an ill-defined terminal stage.

The key issue here—and one of the core values of palliative or end-of-life care—is that people have some choice in their place of death. Anticipating what may interfere with this choice, or stop someone from achieving their wishes, is something that healthcare professionals can bear in mind and for which they can make plans with regard to care packages and support required.

Sinclair (2007) gives a more analytical and moving account of the importance of 'place':

The story *My Place* by Sally Morgan (1987) [...] confirmed to me how much more complex and vital the link between identity and place or home is compared to the 'sophisticated' modern view. As a child I had seen my great aunt and uncle dying in their home. Their dying at home seemed to crown their home and taught me in instinctive ways a deeper appreciation of the meaning of 'my place'. Now, as an adult, what I saw happening to people who were dying, especially in institutions, made me want to make certain for them a death in their own place, in their own way.

(Sinclair, 2007: 2).

However, whilst this may be true, we must be aware of assumptions. Holloway writes that:

[F]usion of private circumstance and professional care is regarded as 'best practice' but in reality this can result in home being turned into a place populated by strangers where family assume unfamiliar roles and technology replaces homeliness.

(Holloway, 2007: 17).

The key thing is discussion and establishing preferences with those who are involved or affected. In the case of older people who are confused and especially those at end-stage dementia, it is a much more complex process and thus imperative that the person affected have their wishes adhered to, which, in an ideal scenario, have been discussed and recorded prior to deterioration of cognitive status. It is thus the next of kin or family and carers that would be able to relay this information, and who should therefore be involved in communicating and ensuring that the patient's care preferences, and choice of place at end of life, are carried out where possible.

Behaviours

Our behaviours are influenced by our abilities, our beliefs and values, our identity, and our purpose in life, but in broad terms we can think about our caring behaviours in the following way.

- **What we do too much of and need to do less of**—For example, when we set our visiting times on wards, it might be that a dying person wishes to spend more time with their family, yet this is only allowed between the hours of 4 p.m. and 8 p.m.
- **What we do too little of and need to do more of**—For example, we may not include people in decisions about their care (even down to what, when, and where they would like to eat) and need to think about how we can be more flexible in this area.
- **What we do in a certain way that we might do differently**—For example, we may do things *for* people rather than *with* them. We may do drug rounds at certain times because it is common practice, rather than think about whether the person would be better managing their own medication regime in a way that suits them and which gives better symptom relief.

We need to consider whether we have ritualistic practices, or whether our behaviours are based in well-thought-through and evidence-based information, which includes patient preferences and makes best use of available resources (Sackett et al., 1996).

Capabilities and strategies

If we are to care well for those who are at the end of their lives, we need the capabilities and strategies to do this, and we also need to consider what capabilities and strategies those for whom we are caring need, in order to function and feel as well as they can. This is complex and involves a great deal of self-awareness on our part. Sometimes, we are inclined to avoid situations that we know will be difficult to deal with or in which we fear saying the wrong thing.

Caring for those who are dying and for their loved ones or those close to them is often difficult and distressing. Dealing with intense emotion, loss, grief, and bereavement on a daily basis can be very stressful for carers in the health and social care field (Renzenbrink, 2004). Handling difficult discussions is something at which we need to become more skilled and, sometimes, such conversations are avoided because of the uncomfortable feelings that they bring up for us.

Table 18.2 provides some examples of how we might phrase things when we might not know what to say. It also gives some idea of the sort of questions that might prompt therapeutic interactions.

Beliefs and values

The following offers a brief overview of the way in which our beliefs can impact our behaviours.

Student activity

Visit the Online Resource Centre that accompanies this book and review Scenario 1.

How do you think your own beliefs and values have been influenced by the culture in which you live in, the things that you see, hear, and read, and how your beliefs and values impact upon what you do?

For example, in Table 18.4 later in this chapter, the concept of ageism is briefly outlined. Consider how you personally view older people, consider how you think society views them, and consider if you think this has an influence on the care that they receive, bearing in mind that:

- what we believe influences how we behave; and
- how we behave influences how others behave towards us.

- **We can have beliefs about our own or others' limitations**—For example, we might believe that 'Mrs Smith' cannot cope with bad news, so we may avoid any discussion that may bring the topic up, rather than try to establish what she wants to know.
- **We can have beliefs about what is possible**—For example, we might believe that it is not possible for 'Mr Jones' to see his dog, because he is in a ward and dogs are not allowed into wards, so we do not try to find flexibility in the rules.
- **We can have beliefs about cause and effect**—For example, a patient may believe that morphine is a 'bad' drug, which causes addiction, so they will not take the painkillers that would be effective.
- **We can have beliefs about correlation**—For example, we can believe that, because a person is uncommunicative with us or does not wish to join in with certain activities, they are depressed—but it may be the case that they simply wish to be on their own and do not like the formal activities, which they see as contrived and lacking in personal meaning.

The other important thing to say about beliefs is to highlight the concept of 'motivated reasoning'—that is, the way in which we tend to scrutinize evidence that goes against our preferences and accept more uncritically evidence that supports what we believe. Reasoning is often guided by our desires (Sutherland, 2007). So for those of us who are supporting the dying or bereaved, it is useful to have given some thought to our own beliefs and values, and how these impact our reasoning. We also need to ensure that we are not imposing these in a conscious or unconscious way on those for whom we are caring (Cobb, 2001).

Identity or mission

Our beliefs cluster together to give us a sense of who we are and how our world is. You will probably have a sense of

Table 18.2 Diagnostic questions and examples of therapeutic interventions to conserve dignity

	Diagnostic questions	Therapeutic interventions
	Illness-related concerns	
	Symptom distress	
Physical distress	'How comfortable are you? Is there anything that we can do to make you feel more comfortable?'	Vigilance to symptom management; frequent assessment and application of comfort care.
Psychological distress	'How are you coping with what is happening to you?'	Assume a supportive stance; empathic listening; referral to counselling.
Medical uncertainty	'Is there anything further about your illness that you would like to know? Are you getting all of the information that you feel you need?'	Upon request, provide accurate, understandable information, and strategies to deal with possible future crises.
Death anxiety	'Are there things about the later stages of your illness that you would like to discuss?'	
Level of in dependence	'Has your illness made you more dependent on others?'	Have patients participate in decision-making, regarding both medical and personal issues.
Cognitive acuity	'Are you having any difficulty with your thinking?'	Treat delirium; when possible, avoiding sedating medication(s).
Functional capacity	'How much are you able to do for yourself?'	Use orthotics, physiotherapy, and occupational therapy.
	Dignity-conserving repertoire	
	Dignity-conserving perspectives	
Continuity of self	'Are there any things about you that this disease does not affect?'	See the patient as worthy of honour, respect, and esteem; soliciting stories, life review or narrative; sharing of photographs or crafts.
Maintenance of pride	'What about yourself or your life are you most proud of?'	
Role preservation	'What things did you do before you were sick that were most important to you?'	
Hopefulness	'What is still possible?'	Encouraging and enabling the patient to participate in meaningful or purposeful activities.
Generativity/legacy	'How do you want to be remembered?'	Life project (e.g. making audio/video, writing letters or journal), dignity psychotherapy.
Autonomy/control	'How in control do you feel?'	Involve in treatment and care decisions.
Acceptance	'How at peace are you with what is happening to you?'	Support the patient in their outlook; encourage doing things that enhance their sense of well-being (e.g. meditation, light exercise, listening to music, prayer).
Resilience or fighting spirit	'What part of you is strongest right now?'	
	Dignity-conserving practices	
Living in the moment	'Are there things that take your mind away from illness and offer you comfort?'	Allow the patient to participate in normal routines, or to take comfort in momentary distractions (e.g. listening to music, daily outings).
Maintaining normalcy	'Are there things that you still enjoy doing on a regular basis?'	
Finding spiritual comfort	'Is there a spiritual or religious community that you are connected with, or would like to be connected with?'	Make referrals to chaplain or spiritual leader; enable the patient to participate in their particular spiritual and/or culturally based practices.

Table 18.2 *(Continued)* Diagnostic questions and examples of therapeutic interventions to conserve dignity

	Diagnostic questions	Therapeutic interventions
	Social dignity inventory	
Privacy boundaries	'What about your privacy or your body is important to you?'	Ask permission to examine patient; proper draping to safeguard and respect modesty.
Social support	'Who are the people that are most important to you? Who is your closest confidante?'	Liberal policies about visitation, rooming in; enlisting involvement of a wide support network.
Care tenor	'Is there anything in the way in which you are treated that is undermining your sense of dignity?'	Treat the patient as worthy of honour, esteem, and respect; adopt a stance conveying this.
Burden to others	'Do you worry about being a burden to others? If so, to whom and in what ways?'	Encourage explicit discussion about these concerns, with those whom they fear they are burdening.
Aftermath concerns	'What are your biggest concerns for the people whom you will leave behind?'	Encourage the settling of affairs, preparation of an advanced directive, making a will, funeral planning.

Source: Chochinov (2006).

identity for yourself as a nurse, and this will influence your behaviour.

Student activity

Visit the Online Resource Centre that accompanies this book and review Scenario 2.

Consider how you view the role of the nurse.

- Are some of the aspects of care outlined in the scenario central to what caring for someone is about?
- If this is part of your identity and belief, are you more likely to behave in this way?

From a patient's point of view, or a relative or carer's point of view, when facing death, people may be prompted into rethinking their beliefs about the way in which they view their world (Cobb, 2001). Their identity may, for example, be challenged.

Reflection point

Imagine how you would feel if you were to define yourself by the role that your employment gives to you, but this was taken away because you could no longer work due to illness.

Spirituality or purpose

Spirituality, or purpose, is perhaps about the really big question: 'Why?' It is about the search for meaning in our lives. This is not only about someone's religious beliefs, but also about their general beliefs and values—that is, their sense of purpose in life. Lloyd (1997) gives a definition of 'spirituality' as a dimension that brings together attitudes, beliefs, feelings, and practices, reaching beyond the wholly rational and material.

It is important to recognize that there might be differences between spiritual and religious beliefs for our patients, as the following definitions clarify.

- **Religion** can be seen to refer to an organized system of beliefs, practices, rituals, and symbols designed to facilitate closeness to the sacred or transcendent (that is, 'God', a 'higher power', or an 'ultimate truth/reality').
- **Spirituality** can be seen to refer to the personal quest for understanding answers to ultimate questions about life, about meaning and about relationship with the sacred or transcendent, which may (or may not) lead to, or arise from, the development of religious rituals and the formation of community (Koenig et al., 2001).

Spiritual and /or religious beliefs and practices can play a considerable role in the lives of those who are seriously ill and dying, and for those close to them. As well as providing a foundation or underpinning for the decisions that people make, spiritual and religious traditions often provide a conceptual framework for understanding the human experience of death and dying, and for making meaning of illness and suffering (Daaleman and VandeCreek, 2000).

The importance of spiritual and religious beliefs in coping with illness, suffering, and dying is outlined by various studies, as well as individual personal accounts. Patients can derive comfort from their religious or spiritual beliefs as they face the end of life, and some find reassurance through a belief in continued existence after physical death, even if that existence is perhaps living on in the memory of those who still live.

Moss asserts that:

> **[W]e can no more give a sense of meaning and purpose to someone else than we can eat or breathe for them. But to share that journey with them can help them feel valued, which is the first step to regaining a purpose and meaning.**
>
> (Moss, 2002: 44).

So in the context of care at the end of life, perhaps our role is partly this. We need to ensure that symptoms are well managed, we need to make holistic assessments, we need to provide the best care that we can, and we need to recognize that people have differing spiritual and religious beliefs, which are important to them as they face the end of their lives. Spiritual issues need to be acknowledged in care as part of what makes people tick; Part of the reason why they might be overlooked may be that, as nurses, we are not always aware of how to incorporate such issues into our own practice and what questions to ask.

NURSING PRACTICE INSIGHT: USING SPIRITUAL ASPECTS OF CARE IN YOUR PRACTICE

The acronym in Table 18.3 may provide you with some points for consideration when thinking about how to incorporate spiritual aspects of care into your practice and how to start a conversation with someone that brings these issues up for discussion.

Issues of loss

When we think about loss, we automatically assume that is related to bereavement and death. One of the issues that nurses need to bear in mind when caring for older people is that loss can be complex and multiple. Loss is a broad concept, which encompasses more than issues relating to death. For example, if you consider the case of an older person being admitted into care, they will face the loss of their home, many of their possessions, the familiarity of their surroundings, neighbours, perhaps pets, the view from their window, a lifetime of memories associated with things such as pictures on their walls, the sense of being 'grounded' somewhere and belonging to a community, and loss of some degree of independence, spontaneity, and choice in day-to-day life matters, and control over ordinary activities that we take for granted. These losses may be compounded by losses associated with ill health.

Thompson (2002) highlights the relative lack of attention given to older people's experiences of loss, arguing that ageism, as a form of discrimination, pushes older people's

Table 18.3 FICA: A spiritual assessment tool

F	Faith	*'What do you believe in that gives meaning to your life?'* *'Do you consider yourself to be a religious or spiritual person?'* Both 'religious' and 'spiritual' are used as terms, because individuals may relate to one and may even take offence at the other. Some people who will say they are 'not religious' will admit to being 'spiritual', which should prompt a discussion of what this means to them. However, an answer such as, 'Yes, I'm Catholic', tells you something, but you will need to explore what this means.
I	Importance/ influence	*'How important is your faith (or religion or spirituality) to you?'* Just hearing that the person is spiritual or a member of a particular religion tells you little. How important is this? How is it important? There is a big difference between a Catholic who has not been to Mass since childhood and one who goes to Mass daily.
C	Community	*'Are you a part of a religious or spiritual community?'* Particularly for those who participate in an organized religion, community is often a central part of their spiritual and social experience. It is not uncommon that just when this community becomes most important, when death approaches, the individual can be cut off from that community because of illness and healthcare needs.
A	Address or Application	*'How would you like me to address these issues in your health care?'* *'How might these things apply to your current situation?'* *'How can we assist you in your spiritual care?'* Patients and families often feel better simply because they have been given permission to share their beliefs. That you have inquired is usually seen as a sign of respect. However, there may be very specific things that you can do to be of assistance. Asking if patients have any special concerns or fears and then addressing them may be of help and/or provide reassurance that these things will be thought of in the plan of care.

Note: A more detailed version can be found online at http://www.mywhatever.com/cifwriter/library/70/4966.html

Source: Adapted from Pulchalski (1999).

needs and perspectives into the margins, and that their experiences of loss are trivialized, made invisible, or seen as 'less than' the losses of those who are younger. She argues that ageism operates on personal, cultural, and structural levels, as outlined in Table 18.4.

Illness trajectories and symptoms

In end-of-life care, good symptom management is important and relief from distressing symptoms is crucial—but to go into detail here about symptom relief for each major illness would be beyond the scope of this chapter. Instead a brief outline of 'illness trajectories' is provided below to highlight the typical courses that illnesses can take and to draw your attention to the fact that people will have different experiences of illness before death. Watson et al. (2009) offer a more detailed account of the assessment and management of different symptoms.

See Chapter 10 for more on the key health conditions that affect older people.

Many older people experience some chronic illness (Lyn and Adamson, 2003), but different illnesses and conditions will impact differently upon individuals. Older people are more commonly affected by multiple medical problems of varying severity (WHO, 2004). When planning our healthcare services, and the support and intervention required, it is useful to consider how trajectories of chronic illness impact upon service needs across time. One way of organizing such care for older people who are likely to die as a result of their condition is to consider a trajectory of decline over time. Figure 18.1—adapted from Lyn and Adamson (2003) and highlighted by the WHO (2004)—illustrates this, and each trajectory corresponds to a different rhythm and set of priorities in care. It can, however, be difficult to predict the course of many chronic illnesses affecting older people, and it is important to remember that care should be based on patient and family need, not only perceived prognosis. Many chronically ill older people will have an indistinct medical prognosis and diagnosing when death is imminent can be difficult.

The three typical illness trajectories for people with progressive chronic disease described by Lyn and Adamson (2003) have been considered as frameworks that may help clinicians and carers to plan and deliver appropriate care.

- **Short period of evident decline**—This trajectory is typical of cancer. Most patients with cancer remain well and able to function for a significant period of time, but if the condition is not curable, once the illness becomes overwhelming, the patient usually declines rapidly in the final weeks and days preceding death.
- **Long-term limitations with intermittent exacerbations and sudden dying**—This trajectory is typical of organ system failure. Patients within this category may live with their condition for a relatively long time and only experience minor limitations in everyday life. On occasion, there may be some physiological stress, which overwhelms the body's normal homeostasis and leads to a worsening of symptoms. Patients can survive some of these episodes, but may then die from a complication or exacerbation in a way that appears rather sudden.
- **Prolonged dwindling**—This trajectory is typical of dementia or disabling stroke. The median length of survival from diagnosis to death in dementia is eight years (WHO, 2004), and during this time there can be a progressive deterioration in ability and awareness.

We need to challenge how we conceptualize health and illness. Chronically ill older people can experience multiple conditions (Lyn and Adamson, 2003) and the 'conventional' model of care (see Figure 18.2) does not apply well to such groups of people because it presumes a sharp transition in which the person suddenly becomes terminally ill, when in fact there may be a gradual decline. Patients may need both curative treatment for one particular symptom, as well as palliative treatment aimed at treating or controlling other symptoms during their illness, and it will depend on what this trajectory is, what their symptoms are, and how these can best be managed.

Table 18.4 Ageism on a personal, cultural, or structural level

Ageism on a personal level	This is about the level of personal prejudice with which we operate. It is about our assumptions regarding older people, the generalizations that we make, and the attitudes and beliefs that we have.
Ageism on a cultural level	This is about the level of shared attitudes, assumptions, and meanings. It is about the way in which stereotypes are disseminated through the media. Increasingly, sexist and racist jokes are seen to be unacceptable in a society in which wealth, youth, and beauty are highly valued.
Ageism at a structural level	This is about how ageist attitudes are embedded within the structures of society.

Source: Adapted from Thompson (2002).

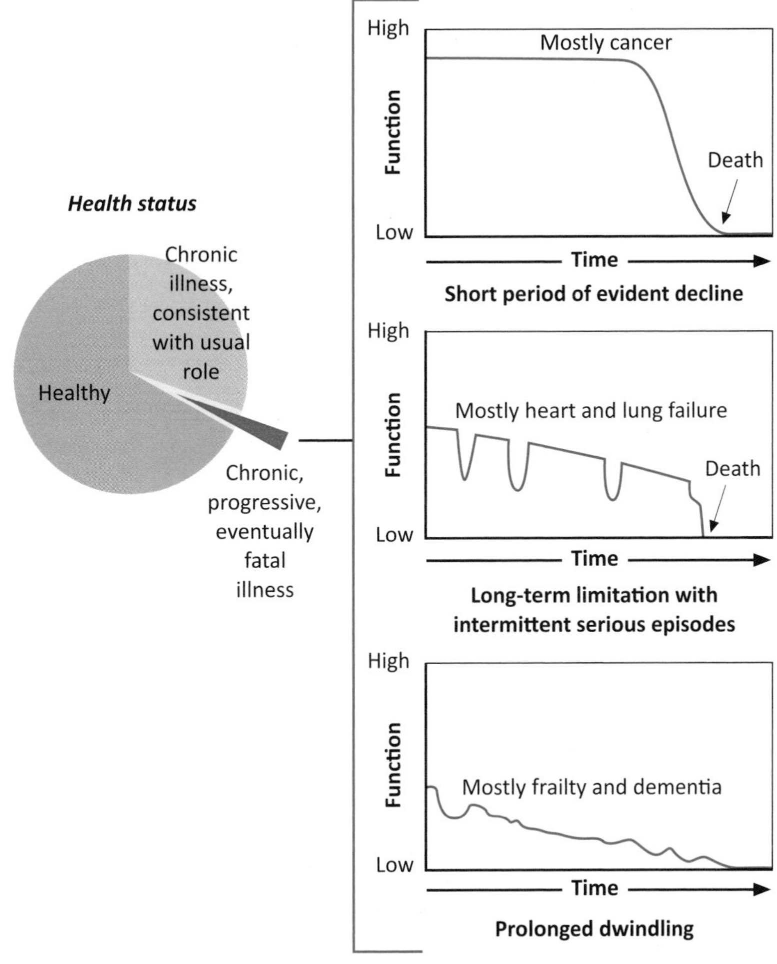

Figure 18.1 Chronic, progressive, and eventually fatal illness in the elderly typically follows three trajectories
Source: Used with permission from Lyn and Adamson (2003).

Liverpool Care Pathway

The Liverpool Care Pathway (LCP) is employed by healthcare staff to support people during the last 48 or 72 hours of life. This is an evidence-based integrated care pathway tool that provides guidance on the different aspects of care required, including the physical, psychological, and spiritual comfort of patients and their relatives. It was originally developed for use in hospitals, but can now be used in a variety of care settings.

The key elements include:

- a multidisciplinary team approach;
- initial assessment of the patient's condition and comfort;
- communication with the family and significant others;
- identification of religious and spiritual needs;
- an agreed plan of care;
- anticipatory prescribing;
- symptom control—pain, agitation, nausea and vomiting, respiratory secretions, breathlessness;
- agreeing and ceasing unnecessary interventions;
- ongoing assessment, recording, and amendment to plan if required;
- care after death—that is, informing the general practitioner (GP); and
- providing appropriate information to the family.

Care after death

Good end-of-life care does not stop at the point of a person's death. As healthcare practitioners, we need to be familiar with good practice for care of the deceased person's body, and we need to be responsive to their wishes and viewpoints with regard to any cultural or spiritual and religious beliefs. We also need to care for and support those who have been bereaved.

As a nurse, there may be a desire to 'do something' immediately following a death—but take time to consider how

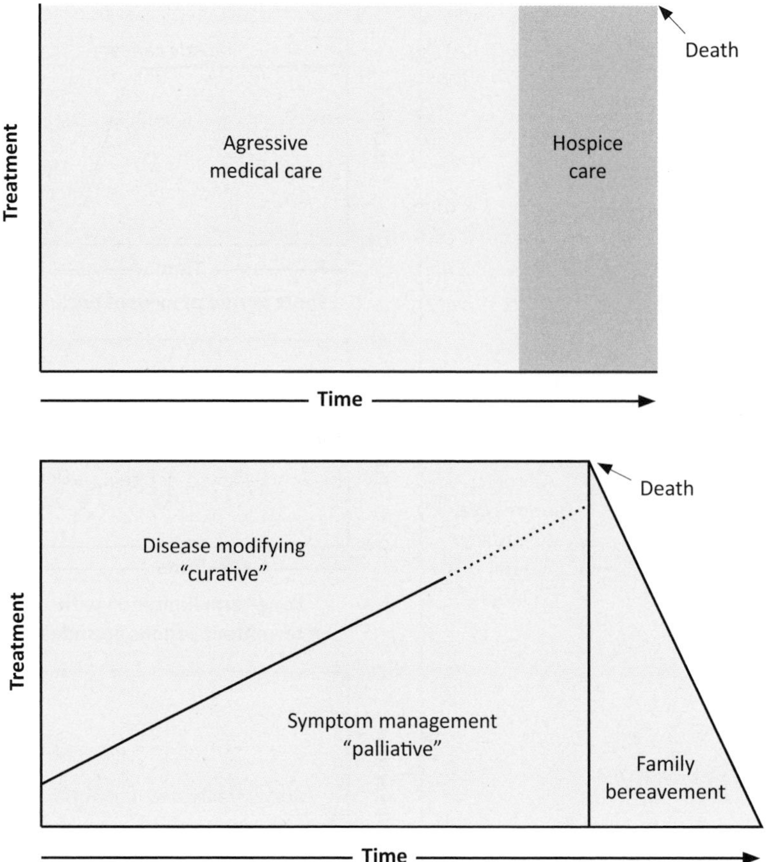

Figure 18.2 The 'conventional' model of care versus the 'trajectory' model
Source: Used with permission from Lyn and Adamson (2003).

those who are bereaved might feel. After a death, nothing has to be done immediately. Some people may want to stay in the room with the body, others prefer to leave. One thing that is practical is that you might want to have someone make sure the body is lying flat before the joints become stiff and cannot be moved. This rigor mortis begins sometime during the first hours after death. Be aware that this may be someone who has been designated by the family, or in line with religious practices. Also, it is important to notify the person who is going to be responsible for death verification or certification. The complexities of this are outlined in the *End-of-Life Care Strategy* (National End-of-Life Programme, 2008).

Staff will need to be aware of the legal issues surrounding certification of death. For example, if a death occurs at home, the out-of-hours GP may be unable to certify a death if the death does not comply with existing legal requirements. To certify a death, a medical practitioner must have attended the deceased during their last illness (which is rarely the case for GP out-of-hours providers). However, even when a death has been certified, unless the doctor has seen the deceased in the 14 days preceding death or viewed the body after death, the registrar is statutorily required to report the death to the coroner. Where a death cannot be certified, it must be referred to the coroner. If the patient is in the community, it will, in many cases, be possible for the patient's own GP to certify the death on the following day, but this may mean that the body of the deceased remains at the place of residence for several hours. Staff will need to explain this to the family as necessary.

NURSING PRACTICE INSIGHT: HELPING RELATIVES AND CARERS

Local policies will vary, but it is important that you make yourself aware of what these are and how you may access them.

Sometimes, carers or relatives might want to be involved with the care and preparation of the deceased—either out of religious beliefs or out of love for that person who has died. This needs to be established before anything is done to the dead person that may offend.

The period following a death is usually a time of intense emotional turmoil for those close to the person. People's reactions to a death will vary and there is no 'expected way to behave'.

During this period of loss and emotional turmoil, there will also be a need for relatives or carers to sort out the deceased person's affairs. This can be a difficult time, and people might not know what they need to do in the days and weeks following the death. A checklist of things to consider following a death is available online at http://www.direct.gov.uk/en/prod_dg/groups/dg_digitalassets/@dg/@en/documents/digitalasset/dg_170740.pdf.

It is useful as a nurse to be aware of what these things are—even if they do not require immediate action or discussion. It may also be useful for you to read *When a Patient Dies: Advice on Developing Bereavement Services in the NHS* (DH, 2006).

Conclusion

In conclusion, around 500,000 people die each year in England, of whom almost two-thirds are over 75 years of age (National End-of-Life Programme, 2008). The *End-of-Life Care Strategy* highlights some of the issues that we, as health care workers, need to consider for our practice. It is important to remember that we should aim to provide high-quality care for all adults approaching the end of life, irrespective of age, gender, ethnicity, religious belief, disability, sexual orientation, and diagnosis.

As nurses, it is perhaps true to say that much of our care focuses on the 'where', 'when', 'what', and 'how' (that is, environment, behaviours, capabilities, and strategies) of care. We also need to consider how the 'why', 'who', and 'for whom' (that is, the beliefs, values, spirituality, identity, and purpose) fits in with the care that we provide. End-of-life care is complex. It raises concerns for us all about death and the meaning of life; it raises moral, legal, and ethical issues about the best way in which to care for those who are dying and support those who have been bereaved or face loss. This chapter has touched on some of these issues and provided an overview, along with some suggested further reading and information.

Everyone will die, and perhaps a starting point for those of us involved with caring is to consider our own mortality and what we might value for our own care—and then consider if this comes close to what we are providing for those who have been deemed 'patients' in our care.

Questions and self-assessment

Now that you have worked through the chapter, answer the following questions.

- What does the term 'end-of-life care' mean?
- How might services for end-of-life care be organized and delivered to ensure that care meets the needs of individuals and those close to them?
- How might individualized care support provide emotional support to the person reaching the end of life and those who care for them?

Self-assessment

- Having read the chapter, how will you change your practice?
- Identify up to three areas relating to end-of-life care in which you need to develop your knowledge and understanding further.
- Identify how you are going to develop this knowledge and understanding, and set deadlines for achieving this.

References

Chochinov, H.M. (2006) 'Dying, dignity and new horizons in palliative end-of-life care', *A Cancer Journal for Clinicians*, 56: 84–103.

Cobb, M. (2001) *The Dying Soul: Spiritual Care at the End of Life*, Buckingham: Open University Press.

Corner, J. and Dunlop, R. (1997) 'New Approaches to Care', in D. Clark, J. Hockley, and S. Ahmedazai (eds.) *New Themes in Palliative Care*, Buckingham: Open University Press, pp. 288–302.

Costello, J. (2006) 'Dying well: Nurses' experience of 'good and bad' deaths in hospital', *Journal of Advanced Nursing*, 54(5): 594–601.

Daaleman, T.P. and VandeCreek, L. (2000) 'Placing religion and spirituality in end-of-life care', *Journal of the American Medical Association*, 284: 2514.

Department of Health (2001a) *National Service Framework for Older People*, available online at http://www.dh.gov.uk/en/publicationsandstatistics/publications/publicationspolicyandguidance/DH_4003066.

Department of Health (2001b) *The Expert Patient: A New Approach to Chronic Disease Management for the 21st Century*, London: DH

Department of Health (2003) *Strengthening Accountability: Involving Patients and the Public*, London: DH.

Department of Health (2005) *When a Patient Dies: Advice on Developing Bereavement Services in the NHS*, available online at http://www.dh.gov.uk/en/Publicationsandstatistics/Publications/PublicationsPolicyAndGuidance/DH_4122191.

Department of Health (2008) *End-of-Life Care Strategy: Promoting High-quality Care for All Adults at the End of Life*, available online at http://www.dh.gov.uk/publications.

Department of Health (2009) *Living Well with Dementia: A National Dementia Strategy*, available online at http://www.dh.gov.uk/prod_consum_dh/groups/dh_digitalassets/@dh/@en/documents/digitalasset/dh_094051.pdf.

Dilts, R. (1990) *Changing Belief Systems with NLP*, Capitola, CA: Meta Publications.

Disability Rights Commission (2006) *Equal Treatment: Closing the Gap—A Formal Investigation into Physical Health Inequalities Experienced by People with Learning Disabilities and/or Mental Health Problems*, available online at http://www.learningdisabilitiesuk.org.uk/docs/DRCrpt.pdf.

Fish, D. and Coles, C. (1998) *Developing Professional Judgement in Health Care: Learning Through the Critical Appreciation of Practice*, Oxford: Butterworth–Heinemann.

Harden, A. (2006) 'Extending the Boundaries of Systematic Reviews to Integrate Different Types of Study: Examples of Methods Developed within Reviews on Young People's Health', in J. Popay (ed.) *Moving Beyond Effectiveness in Evidence Synthesis: Methodological Issues in the Synthesis of Diverse Sources of Evidence*, London: NICE.

Health Advisory Service (2000) *Not Because They Are Old: An Independent Inquiry into the Care of Older People on Acute Wards in General Hospital*, London: HAS.

Higginson, I. (2003) *Priorities and Preferences for End-of-Life Care in England, Wales and Scotland*, London: NCPC.

Higginson, I. and Sen Gupta, G. (2000) 'Place of care in advanced cancer: A qualitative systematic literature review of patient preferences', *Journal of Palliative Medicine*, 3(3): 287–300.

Higginson, I., Astin, P., and Dolan, S. (1998) 'Where do cancer patients die? Ten year trends in the place of death of cancer patients in England', *Palliative Medicine*, 12(5): 353–63.

Holloway, M. (2007) *Negotiating Death in Contemporary Health and Social Care*, Bristol: Policy Press.

Johnson, M. (2006) 'Dying, Bereavement and Loss', in S.J. Redfern and F.M. Ross (eds.) *Nursing Older People*, London: Churchill Livingstone.

Katz, A.M., Conant, L., Inui, T.S., Baron, D., and Bor, D. (2000) 'A council of elders: Creating a multi-voiced dialogue in a community of care', *Social Science and Medicine*, 50(6): 851–60.

Kellehear, A. (1999) *Health Promoting Palliative Care*, Melbourne: Oxford University Press.

Kellehear, A. (2008) 'Health Promotion and Palliative Care', in G. Mitchell (ed.) *Palliative Care: A Patient-centred Approach*, Oxford: Radcliffe Publishing.

Kitwood, T. (1997) *Dementia Reconsidered: The Person Comes First*, Buckingham: Open University Press.

Koenig, H.K., McCullough, M.E., and Larson, D.B. (2001) *Handbook of Religion and Health*, Oxford: Oxford University Press.

Lloyd, M. (1997) 'Dying and bereavement, spirituality and social work in a market economy of welfare', *British Journal of Social Work*, 27(2): 175–90.

Lloyd Williams, M., Payne, S., and Dennis, M. (2005) 'Specialist palliative care in dementia: Patients with dementia are unable to access appropriate palliative care', *British Medical Journal*, 330: 671–2.

Lothian, K. and Philip, I. (2001) 'Maintaining the dignity and autonomy of older people in the healthcare setting', *British Medical Journal*, 322: 668–70.

Lyn, J. and Adamson, D. (2003) *Living Well at the End of Life: Adapting Health Care to Serious Chronic Illness in Old Age*, Rand Health White Paper, available online at http://www.rand.org/pubs/white_papers/WP137/.

Morgan, S. (1987) *My Place*, Freemantle: Freemantle Arts Centre Press.

Moss, B. (2002) 'Spirituality: A Personal Perspective', in N. Thompson (ed.) *Loss and Grief: A Guide for Human Services Practitioners*, Basingstoke: Palgrave.

National Audit Office (2008) *End-of-Life Care*, Report by the Comptroller and Auditor General, London: HMSO, available online at http://www.nao.org.uk/publications/0708/end_of_life_care.aspx.

National Council for Palliative Care (2006) *End-of-Life Care Strategy*, available online at http://www.ncpc.org.uk/download/publications/NCPC_EoLC_Submission.pdf.

National Council on Ageing (2002) *End-of-Life Issues*, Policy Position Paper, available online at http://www.ncoa.org/.

National End of Life Programme (2007) *Preferred Priorities for Care*, available online at http://www.endoflifecareforadults.nhs.uk/publications/ppcform.

National End of Life Programme (2008) *Advance Care Planning Guide*, available online at http://www.endoflifecareforadults.nhs.uk/publications/pubacpguide.

National GSF Framework Team (2010) *Gold Standards Framework*, available online at http://www.goldstandardsframework.nhs.uk/.

National Institute for Health and Clinical Excellence (2004) *Improving Supportive Care and Palliative Care for Adults with Cancer: The Manual*, London: NICE, available online at http://www.nice.org.uk/nicemedia/pdf/csgspmanual.pdf.

Philip, I. (2002) 'Introduction', in J. Hockley and D. Clark (eds) *Palliative Care for Older People in Care Homes*, Buckingham: Open University Press.

Popay, J. (2006) *Moving Beyond Effectiveness in Evidence Synthesis: Methodological Issues in the Synthesis of Diverse Sources of Evidence*, London: NICE.

Pulchalski, C. (1999) *Palliative Care Perspectives*, available online at http://www.mywhatever.com/cifwriter/library/70/4966.html.

Renzenbrink, I. (2004) 'Relentless Self-care in Living with Dying', in P. Silverman and J. Berzoff (eds.) *A Handbook for Health Practitioners in End-of-Life Care*, New York: Columbia University Press.

Rhodes, P. and Nocon, A. (1998) 'User involvement and the NHS reforms', *Health Expectations*, 1(2): 73–81.

Rogers, A., Karlsen, S., and Addington-Hall, J. (2000) '"All the services were excellent: It is when the human element comes in that things go wrong"—Dissatisfaction with hospital care in the last year of life', *Journal of Advanced Nursing*, 31(4): 768–74.

Sackett, D., Rosenberg, W., Muir Gray, J., Haynes, R., and Richardson, W. (1996) 'Evidence-based medicine: What it is and what it isn't', *British Medical Journal*, 312: 71–2.

Seymour, J., Clark, D., and Phillip, I. (2001) 'Editorial: Palliative care and geriatric medicine—Shared concerns, shared challenges', *Palliative Medicine*, 15: 269–70.

Sinclair, P. (2007) *Rethinking Palliative Care: A Social Role Valorization Approach*, Bristol: Policy Press.

Social Care Institute for Excellence (2005) *SCIE Research Briefing 10: Terminal Care in Care Homes*, available online at http://www.scie.org.uk/publications/briefings/briefing10/index.asp.

Sutherland, S. (2007) *Irrationality*, London: Pinter and Martin.

Thomas, K. (2001*) Out-of-hours Palliative Care in the Community*, London: Macmillan Cancer Relief.

Thompson, S. (2002) 'Older People', in N. Thompson (ed.) *Loss and Grief: A Guide for Human Services Practitioners*, Basingstoke: Palgrave.

Watson, M., Lucas, C., Hoy, A., and Wells, J. (2009) *Oxford Handbook of Palliative Care*, 2nd edn, Oxford: Oxford University Press.

Wee, B. and Hughes, N. (2007) *Education in Palliative Care: Building on a Culture of Learning*, Oxford: Oxford University Press.

Wolfensberger, W. (1998) *A Brief Introduction to Social Role Valorization: A Higher Order Concept for Addressing the Plight of Societally Devalued People, and for Structuring Human Services*, 3rd edn, New York: Syracuse University.

World Health Organization (2002) *Definition of Palliative Care*, available online at https://apps.who.int/dsa/justpub/cpl.htm.

World Health Organization (2004) *Better Palliative Care for Older People*, Copenhagen: WHO, available online at http://www.euro.who.int/.

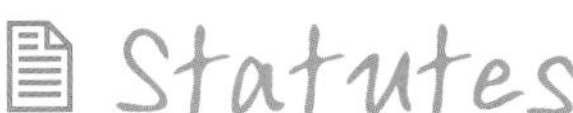

Statutes

Mental Capacity Act 2005

For further reading and information

Books

Earle, S., Komaromy, C., and Bartholomew, C. (2009) *Death and Dying: A Reader*, London: Sage

Payne, S., Seymour, J., and Ingleton, C. (2008) *Palliative Care Nursing: Principle and Evidence for Practice*, 2nd edn, Oxford: Oxford University Press

Vries, K. de (2003) 'Palliative Care for People with Dementia', in T. Adams and J. Manthorpe (eds) *Dementia Care*, London: Edward Arnold, pp. 114–35

Watson, M., Lucas, C., Hoy, A., and Wells, J. (2009) *Oxford Handbook of Palliative Care*, 2nd edn, Oxford: Oxford University Press

Websites

The following websites may provide you with valuable information and evidence-based guidelines for practice and support.

http://www.caresearch.com.au/
An initiative of the Australian Government Department of Health and Ageing, funded through the National Palliative Care Program.

http://www.cicelysaundersfoundation.org/
Cicely Saunders International focuses on carrying out quality research to improve the care and treatment of all patients with progressive illness, and to make high-quality palliative care available to everyone who needs it.

http://www.crusebereavementcare.org.uk/
Cruse Bereavement Care exists to promote the well-being of bereaved people, and to enable anyone bereaved by death to understand their grief and cope with their loss. Services are free to bereaved people. The organization provides support, and offers information, advice, education, and training services.

http://www.dh.gov.uk/en/socialcare/deliveringadultsocialcare/olderpeople/nationaldementiastrategy/index.htm
Department of Health (2009) *National Dementia Strategy*, London: DH

http://www.endoflifecareforadults.nhs.uk/
This website is aimed at health and social care staff, and provides information on a variety of aspects relating to end-of-life care. This includes more than 100 case studies that highlight good practise; new cases are constantly being added. They are taken from different care settings—for example, care homes, hospitals, primary care, and hospices—and stages of the care pathway. They also cover engaging with users and carers, commissioning, strategic direction, and knowledge and skills. In addition, there is a section containing latest news, useful websites, links, and resources.

http://www.euro.who.int/__data/assets/pdf_file/0009/98235/E82933.pdf
World Health Organization (2004) *Better Palliative Care for Older People*, Copenhagen: WHO

http://www.goldstandardsframework.nhs.uk/
The aim of the Gold Standards Framework (GSF) is to develop a practise-based system to improve the organization and quality of care for patients in the last stages of life in the

community, so that more live and die well in their preferred place of choice.

http://www.growthhouse.org/

This website is a gateway to resources for life-threatening illness and end-of-life care. Its primary mission is to improve the quality of compassionate care for people who are dying, through public education and global professional collaboration. It offers a comprehensive collection of reviewed resources for end-of-life care.

http://www.helpthehospices.org.uk/

A charity supporting hospice care throughout the UK. The charity provides information and support to carers and patients.

http://www.hospicecare.com/

A site that promotes communication, facilitating and providing education, and by becoming an information resource for patients, professionals, healthcare providers, and policy-makers around the world.

http://www.hospicepatients.org/clinicalpracticeguidelines1994.html

Agency for Health Care Policy and Research (1994) *Clinical Guideline Number 9*, Rockville, MD: AHCPR—a clinical practice guideline that originates from the USA, but provides a valuable source of clinical information about pain management

http://www.ncpc.org.uk/

The National Council for Hospice and Specialist Palliative Care Services provides information about palliative care, current news, and links to other sites.

http://www.medicine.ox.ac.uk/bandolier/booth/painpag/index2.html

Bandolier hosts the Oxford Pain Internet site and provides valuable evidence-based information about palliative and supportive care, and pain management.

http://www.kingsfund.org.uk/library/

The King's Fund Information and Library Service holds material about improving the quality of life for people facing the impact of end of life. This includes NHS policy documents and guidance, as well as information about developments in services. This online reading room collates details of books, reports, and journal articles, plus links to relevant organizations and other information resources.

http://www.macmillan.org.uk/

Macmillan Cancer Support provides practical, medical, emotional, and financial support for people affected by cancer, and campaigns for better cancer care.

http://www.mariecurie.org.uk/

Marie Curie Cancer Care provides free, high-quality nursing to give terminally ill people the choice of dying at home supported by their families.

http://www.mcpcil.org.uk/liverpool-care-pathway/

The Liverpool Care Pathway (LCP) for the dying patient has been developed to transfer the hospice model of care into other care settings.

http://www.cochrane.org/

There are approximately 50 Cochrane 'review groups', each preparing systematic reviews for a specific area of health care. The Cochrane Pain, Palliative and Supportive Care Group (PaPaS) focuses on reviews for the prevention and treatment of pain, the treatment of symptoms at the end of life, and supporting patients, carers, and their families through the disease process.

http://www.ncpc.org.uk/

The National Council for Palliative Care is the umbrella organization for those involved in providing, commissioning, and using hospice and palliative care services in England, Wales, and Northern Ireland. It promotes the extension and improvement of palliative care services, regardless of diagnosis, in various health and social care settings.

http://www.palliativedrugs.com/

This site provides information for health professionals concerning the use of drugs in palliative care.

http://www.palliative-medicine.org/

The Association for Palliative Medicine of Great Britain and Ireland offers information on palliative care issues and educational opportunities.

http://www.scie.org.uk/publications/briefings/briefing10/index.asp

Social Care Institute for Excellence (2005) *SCIE Research Briefing 10: Terminal Care in Care Homes*, London: SCIE

http://www.suerydercare.org/

Sue Ryder Care supports people with a wide range of neurological diseases and life-limiting illnesses.

http://www.who.int/cancer/palliative/en/

The World Health Organization cancer pages offer links to WHO publications and recommended guidelines for practice in cancer and palliative care.

Online Resource Centre

You can learn more about end-of-life care at the Online Resource Centre that accompanies this book:

http://www.oxfordtextbooks.co.uk/orc/hindle/

Index

Note: page references to figures, tables, diagrams and photographs are given in italics.

A

Abbey pain scale *224*
abdominal examination 187–8
abuse, definition 14
  see also elder abuse
accident and emergency (A&E) admission 72
acoustics 24
'active ageing' 123–4
acute care 111
acute otitis media 26
acute pain 216–17, 221
adherence to medication 85–7, *86*, 90–1
adjuvant analgesics 225, *226*
Adult In-patient Survey 2008 19, *20*
advanced decisions/directives (ADs) 49–50
advocates 16
  mental capacity 50
  self-advocacy 155
Age Concern (now Age UK) 173–4, 181
age discrimination 9–10, 44, 253–4, *254*
age-related macular degeneration (AMD) 34
Age UK 3, 12, 44, 49
ageism 9–10, 44, 253–4, *254*
alcohol abuse 150–1
alcohol hand rubs 206, 207
alphabet, manual *37–8*
alphabet model 126–7
Alzheimer's disease 142, 160
anal sphincter disorders 193–4, 195
analgesic ladder *226*
angina pectoris 131
antidepressants
  tricyclic, side effects *76*
  use of, for pain relief 216, 225, 226
anxiety disorders 148–9
aprons 208–9
arthritis 136–7
assessments
  of capacity 50
  of carers 59, 60–2, *61*
  as concept central to person-centred care 17
  dementia 142–3, 160
  for incontinence 188, 191–3, *192–3*, 196, *197–8*, 198
  of loneliness 56
  nutritional intake 175–6
  of pain 220–3, *222*, *223*, *224*
  relating to sleep 239–40
  risk assessments for falls 70–4, *71–4*
  single assessment process (SAP) 87, 103–5, *104–5*
assisted suicide 51–2
atrial fibrillation 134
attitudes 4, 10, 13
augmentative and alternative communication (AAC) methods 156, 158

B

balance disorders 27
behaviours
  approaches to improving sleep 237–8
  medication-taking 13, 85–7, *86*, 90–1, 227
  of nurse relating to end-of-life care 249–52
  risk indicators of suicide 147
  therapies for bladder training 189
beliefs 10
  impact on behaviours 250
  on pain-relieving drugs 225
  religious 10, 252–3
bipolar affective disorder 149
bisexuality 56
bladder 186–9
Bland case 51
bone mineral density (BMD) 77
Bournewood Case 16, 44
bowels 193–8, *193*, *197*, *198*
British Medical Association (BMA) 50, 52

C

capacity *see* mental capacity
cardiovascular conditions 131–5
care delivery
  care plans 101, *102*
  in relation to dignity 18–19
  systematic approach to 114–15, *114*
care homes
  as end-of-life environment 248–9
  in relation to long-term care 105–7
  in relation to nutrition 181
Care Quality Commission (CQC) 19, 106, 202–3
carers and caring 5
  action plan for *62*
  carers' assessments 59, 60–2, *61*
  concept of caring 17–18
  conditions requiring care 58
  definitions 57
  and ethnicity 63
  as experts 60
  factors impacting on 60–1
  job description *58*
  monitoring and evaluating *20*
  older people as carers 59
  policy and legislation 59–60
  skills and qualities 112
  support for 61–3, 63–4, 247, 256–7
  value and importance of 58
  working with carers 143
Carers (Equal Opportunities) Act 2004 59, 60
Carers UK 57, 58, 63
Caring with Confidence programme 61–2
Caroline Walker Trust 181
cataracts 34
catheters 190
cerebral palsy 160, 163
cerumen impaction 26
Champions for Older People Programme 3, 12–13, 111
choice
  as concept central to person-centred care 17
  in relation to food 176–7, *177*
chronic heart failure 133–4
chronic illness
  psychosocial aspects of 124–6
  trajectories for 254, *255*
chronic obstructive pulmonary disease 135–6
chronic pain 218–20, *219*
Clostridium difficile 201–2
co-morbidity 110, 246

Code: standards of conduct, performance and ethics for nurses and midwives, The 43, 48, 53, 106, 236
cognitive behavioural therapy (CBT) 147, 149, 150, 237–8
cognitive impairment
  and assessment of pain 221–2
  impact on nutrition 180–1
colon *193*
colonic investigations 195
common law 46–8
communication
  as concept central to person-centred care 16
  as part of champions' action plan 13
  in relation to hospital care 112, 117
  in relation to people with dementia 143–4
  in relation to people with hearing loss 29–31
  in relation to people with learning disabilities 156–8, *157*
  in relation to people with sight loss 36–7, *37*, *38*
community-acquired pneumonia 136
community care services 5, 97–8
  intermediate care 105
  long-term care 105–7
  nursing in home environment 101–3
  personalized care plans 101, *102*
  self-care 98–101, *99*
  single assessment process (SAP) 103–5, *104–5*
community learning disability teams (CLDTs) 164
compensation 45
concordance with medication 13, 85–7, 90–1, 227
confidentiality 48
consent
  informed 48–9
  and mental capacity 47–8
  in relation to people with learning difficulties 158
constipation 193–5
continence *see* elimination and continence
'continuing NHS care' 46
contract 45
coronary artery atheroma *131*
Court of Protection 50
Crossroads Care 61, 63
Crown Prosecution Service (CPS) 52
culturally competent care 10

D

dehydration, potential causes of *169*
delirium (acute confusional state) 145–6
dementia 6, 142
  causes and assessments of 142–3, *142*, 160
  and depression 148
  family carers 143
  and people with learning disabilities 160, *161–2*
  provision of nursing care 143–5
  in relation to incontinence 195
  in relation to nutrition 180–1
  see also mental health
Department of Health (DH)
  definitions 11, 14, 57, 105
depression 146–8
  see also bipolar affective disorder
Deprivation of Liberty Safeguards (DoLS) 16
dexterity assessment 188
diabetes 126–8
  diabetic retinopathy 34–5
diarrhoea 194, 196
dietary factors
  in relation to constipation 195
  in relation to falls 75
  see also nutrition and fluids
Dietary Reference Values (DRVs) 170–1
digital rectal examination 187, 194
Dignitas clinics 51–2
dignity 4, 11–12
  and communication 112–13
  dignity model *13*
  as Essence of Care benchmark 17, *18*
  initiatives to improve and promote 12–13, *13*, 111
  monitoring and evaluating 19–20
  preservation of, during end-of-life care *251–2*
  in relation to people with sight loss 39–40
  supporting dignified care 18–19
Director of Public Prosecutions (DPP) 51–2
Disability Rights Commission (DRC) 154, 163, 246
discharge planning 118–19
'do not resuscitate' (DNR) 50
Doloplus-2 pain assessment tool 221, *223*
Dosette boxes 13, 86–7
Down's syndrome 154, 160, *161–2*
Dudley Postural Stability Programme *79*
dying *see* end-of-life care
dysphagia 163, 179

E

ear wax impaction 26
ears
  anatomy and physiology 24–6, *25*
  common ear conditions 26–7, *28*
  see also hearing loss
'Eat Well Plate' 171, *172*, *173*
education
  nurse 13, 85, 91, 164
  patient 84, 91, 133, 158
elder abuse
  definition 14
  legislation 15–16, 44–5
  raising concerns of suspected 16
  types of 14–15
electrical stimulation treatment 189
electroconvulsive therapy (ECT) 147
elimination and continence 6, 13, 185
  faecal incontinence 193–8
  urinary incontinence 185–93
emotional abuse 14
empathy, as concept central to person-centred care 17
empowerment
  as concept central to person-centred care 17
  in relation to sleep 241
end-of-life care 7, 245
  after death 255–7
  conceptualizing 247–8, *248*
  conservation of dignity at end-of-life *251–2*
  defining 'end-of-life' 245–6
  and environment 248–9
  evidence base for best practice 246
  illness trajectories and symptoms 254, *255*, *256*
  information resources for 259–60
  issues of loss 253–4, *254*
  Liverpool Care Pathway (LCP) 255
  nursing behaviours and beliefs 249–52
  and palliative care 246
  provision of and access to 246
  responsibility of nurse *117*
  service user and carer review 247
  spirituality 252–3, *253*
End-of-Life Care Strategy 60, 245, 256, 257
end-of-life legislation 50–2
endocrine conditions 126–8
enduring power of attorney (EPA) 49
environment 18
  and end-of-life care 248–9
  for people with dementia 144
  in relation to continence 188
  in relation to nutrition *177*, 181–2
  in relation to sight loss 38
  in relation to sleep 238
  see also home environment
Essence of Care (EoC) 16–18, *17*, *18*, 181
estimated average requirement (EAR) 170, *170*
ethics 5, 45–6
ethnicity 63–4
European Court of Human Rights (ECtHR) 44, 52

euthanasia 51–2
evaluation of dignity in care 19–20, *20*
exercise
for constipation 195
for pelvic floor muscles 188, 196
in relation to falls 75, 78–9
in relation to obesity 173
Expert Patient Programme 61–2, 100
eye clinic patient support workers 40
eyes
anatomy of 33, *33*
see also sight loss

F
faecal incontinence 6, 193
assessments 196, *197–8*, 198
causes of 193–4
investigations into cause 194–5
normal faecal elimination 193
nursing care 196
and skin care 191
treatment of 195–6
falls 5, 69
causes of 70, *71*, *72*, *76*
consequences of 77–8
definition 69
facts about 69–70
falls care pathway *73*
fear of falling 78
hip fractures 70
National Service Framework for Older People, on 70
nursing practice following 78
occupational therapist perspective 80
osteoporosis 76–7, *77*
prevention 39, 75–6, 78–80, *79*
risk assessments 70–4, *71–4*
see also mobility
families 5, 57, 58, 143
FAST (for diagnosis of strokes) 130
financial abuse 14–15
'Five Moments for Hand Hygiene' 206, 208
fluid balance charts 187, *192–3*
fluids *see* nutrition and fluids
Focus on Older People 55–6, 57
food *see* nutrition and fluids
food diary 194, *198*
foot care 75
functional incontinence 186–7

G
gate control theory *217*
gay people 56
generalized anxiety disorder (GAD) 148
Geriatric Depression Scale (GDS) 146, *147*
gerontological nursing, definition 118
glaucoma 34
gloves 208–9
Gold Standards Framework 248–9, 259–60
Guidance for the Care of Older People 3, 43, 103, 111, *113*, 236

H
haemorrhagic stroke 129
hand hygiene 206–8, *207*
health care sectors, interface with social care sectors 119
healthcare-associated infections (HCAIs) 202–3, 209–10
Healthcare Commission 12
hearing aids 30–1, *31*
hearing loss 4–5, 23–4
acoustics 24
communication aids 30–1
definitions 24
effective communication 29–30
and mental health 29
perspective of people with 31–2
problems experienced with 27, 28–9
social and psychological impact of 28, *29*
types of *28*
what it 'sounds' like 29
see also ears
heart conditions 131–5
Help the Aged 3, 44, 69
High-quality Care for All: NHS next-stage review final report 11
hip fractures 70
holism, as concept central to person-centred care 17
home environment
dying in 249
nursing in 101–3
in relation to falls 75–6, 78–80
tele-care and tele-health 76, 101
hospital care 5, 109–10
acute care 111
admission into hospital 112–13
consequences of living longer 110
delivery of 113–15
discharge planning 118–19
importance of communication 112, 117
improvements to 111
infection risk in hospital setting 203, 205
media representation 111
number of people in hospital *110*
organization of 112–13
patient comfort rounds 115, *116*
preserving independence 118
in relation to nutrition 117–18, *177*, 181–2
return to traditional nursing practices 115
skilled workforce 118
skills and responsibilities of nurse 115, *116–17*, 117
and social care sectors 119
as support for carers 62–3
hospitals, as support for carers 62–3
House of Lords 51, 52
Human Rights Act 1998 44, 51, 52
Hungry to be Heard 173–4
hygiene and infection control 6, 201–2
chain of infection 203–5
healthcare-associated infections (HCAIs) 202–3
infection control 205–9, *207*
precautions 209–10
risk factors 203
sleep hygiene 238–9
Hygiene Code 202–3
hypoglycaemia 127–8

I
incontinence *see* elimination and continence
independence, for people with sight loss 39–40
infection control *see* hygiene and infection control
infections
entry, exit and transmission 204–5
organisms, as cause of 203–4
precautions against 209–10
source of 204
susceptible host factors 205
information, provision of, for people with sight loss 36
intermediate care 105
involvement, as concept central to person-centred care 16
ischaemic heart disease 131–3
ischaemic stroke 129–31
isolation
nursing 209–10
social 56–7

J
Johnson, Alan, MP 113

L
labels 10
lasting power of attorney (LPA) 49–50
law *see* legislation
laxatives *195*
leadership 18
learning disabilities 6, 154–5
causes of 159
cerebral palsy 160, 163
challenges in services 163–4

learning disabilities (*Cont.*)
communication strategies for people with 156–8, *157*
consent 158
and dementia 160, *161–2*
Down's syndrome 154, 160, *161–2*
effect on health and ageing 159–60
health initiatives in relation to 163
life experiences of people with 158–9
pain management 163
rights and principles 155–6
specialist services 164–5
terminology 155
leg ulcers 134–5
legislation 5, 43
advanced decisions/directives (ADs) 49
ageism and age discrimination 44
assisted suicide 51–2
common law 46–8
confidentiality 48
consent 47–8, 48–9, 158
continuing NHS care 46
contract, tort and compensation 45
Court of Protection 50
definitions 45
and end-of-life issues 50–2
ethical rights 45–6, 155–6
mental capacity 45, 47–8
power of attorney 49–50
relating to caring 59–60
in relation to abuse 15–16, 44–5
in relation to carers 59–60
social care provision 46
statutes and statutory instruments 54
withdrawal of treatment 51
lesbian people 56
liaison nurses 40, 164
lighting, environmental 38
Liverpool Care Pathway (LCP) 255
living wills 49–50
local authorities 61
loneliness 56–7
long-term care 58, 105–7
long-term conditions 5–6
personalized care plans 101
and self-care *99*, 100
stepped care model *102*
loss 253–4
low-vision support services 40

M

Making Safeguarding Everybody's Business 141
malnutrition 173–4, *174*
Malnutrition Universal Screening Tool (MUST) 175
Maslow's hierarchy of needs 125, *126*
media representation 111
medication
for constipation 195, *195*
for incontinence 189, *190*
for pain 225–7, *226*, *228*
in relation to falls *71*, 76, *76*
use of, to promote sleep 237
medication management 5, 83–4
definition and need for 84–5
drug interactions 84–5
medication errors 87–9, *90*
medication review 84, 87, *88*, *89*
medication-taking behaviour 13, 85–7, *86*, 90–1, 227
nursing practice 85, 91
in relation to pain 223–30, *226*, *228*, *229–30*
Mediterranean diet 171–2
Mencap 154
mental capacity
assessment of 50
legislation 45, 47–8, 49
Mental Capacity Act 2005 16, 45, 47–50, 106
mental health 6, 13, 141–2
in relation to hearing loss 29
in relation to incontinence 188
see also specific mental conditions, e.g. dementia
'mercy killing' 51–2
mixed sex hospital accommodation 113
mixed urinary incontinence 187
mobility 5, 69, 134, 188
see also falls
monitoring dignity in care 19–20, *20*
Montreal Declaration on Learning Disabilities 155–6
multidisciplinary teams (MDTs) 113, 118–19, 220
multifactorial falls risk assessment 70–2
musculoskeletal conditions 136–7
myocardial infarction 131–2

N

National Audit Office 110, 142, 248
National Carers Strategy 55, 57
National Council for Palliative Care 246
National Dementia Strategy 60, 142, 143, 245
National End-of-Life Programme 245, 249, 256, 257
National Health Service *see* NHS
National Institute for Health and Clinical Excellence *see* NICE
National Patient Safety Agency (NPSA) 72–3, 87, 181–2, 206
National Service Framework for Older People, in relation to:
assessments 103
care, on basis of needs 53
community care services 98
continence services 185
depression 146
dignity 4, 11
end-of-life care 245
falls 70, *71*
hospital care 109–14, 118
intermediate care 105
learning disabilities 163
medication management 84, 85, 87
social care provision 46
neglect 15
negligence 47
neurological conditions 128–31
and incontinence 194, 195–6
neurological model of care *102*
neuropathic pain 218, *219*
neurotransmitters 215
NHS
employee liability in negligence 47
and healthcare-associated infections 202–3
impact on older people services 109
and long-term care 106–7
patient choice and empowerment 4, 100
Patient Survey Programme 111
revitalizing food services 181
statutory obligations for care 46
vision and values 11, 98
NICE, in relation to:
end-of-life care 245
evidence base 236
falls 70–2, 73, 80
incontinence 188, 189, 193
mental health 143, 147, 149
nutrition and fluids 173, 175, 178
No Secrets 14, 15
nociceptive pain 218, *219*
non-steroidal anti-inflammatories (NSAIDs) 225
'not for resuscitation' (NFR) 50
Nursing and Midwifery Council (NMC), on:
assisted suicide 52
consent 158
covert administration of medication 50
dignity and respect 155
medication management 83, 85, 90
medication-taking behaviour 91
nursing skills 112, 156, 187
preregistration nursing programmes 4
see also Code: standards of conduct, performance and ethics for nurses and midwives; *Guidance for the Care of Older People*
nursing care
for anxiety disorders 149
for bipolar affective disorder 149

for delirium 145–6
for dementia 143–5
for depression 147
for incontinence 196
of isolated patients 209
for people with drink problems 151
relating to medication management 85
for schizophrenia 150
nursing practice insights into:
administration of medicines 90
caring for carers 57–8, 63–4
dignity and respect 19–20, 155, 241
elder abuse 16
end-of-life care 247, 249, 253, 256–7
falls 75, 78
hearing loss 24, 30
heart conditions 132, 133–4
home assessments 103
hospital care 110
hypoglycaemia 127
incontinence 188, 196
inhaler use 136
learning disabilities 159, 163
legislation and rights issues 47, 48, 49, 50
medication-taking behaviour 91
mental health 143, 147, 149, 150, 151
nutrition and fluids 171, 180
pain 218, 220, 221
sight loss 37
strokes 130
nursing skills and responsibilities 112, 115, *116–17*, 117, 118, 164
nutrition and fluids 6, 168
assessment 175–6
dehydration, causes of *169*
difficulties in eating 179–81
'Eat Well Plate' 171, *172*, *173*
fluid 171, *173*
in hospital 117–18, *177*, 181–2
impact of age-related changes 168–9, *169*
improving intake strategies 178–9, *179*
malnutrition 173–4, *174*
Mediterranean diet 171–2
nutritional status 170
obesity 173
organizational initiatives to improve 181–2
in relation to cognitive impairment and dementia 180–1
requirements and guidelines 170–2, *170*
screening 174–5
selection, choice and consumption 176–7, *177*
texture of food and drinks 179

O

obesity 173
obsessive compulsive disorders 148–9
occupational therapist, perspective of 80
Office for National Statistics (ONS) 3, 55–6, 57, 63
opioids 225, *226*
osteoarthritis 136–7
osteoporosis 76–7, *77*
otosclerosis 26
Our Health, Our Care, Our Say: a new direction for community services 59, 97, 163
overactive bladder 186, 189–90
overflow incontinence 187

P

pads 190, 196
pain management 6–7, 13, 213
acute pain 216–17, 221
assessments 220–3, *222*, *223*, *224*
gate control theory *217*
and medication management 223–30, *228*, *229–30*
neurotransmitters and pain signals 215, *216*
pain pathway *214*
for people with learning disabilities 163
persistent pain 218–20, *219*
physiology and ageing 213–16
stages of 214
palliative care *see* end-of-life care
paracetamol 225–6
Parkinson's disease 128–9
participation, as concept central to person-centred care 16
partnership, as concept central to person-centred care 16–17
patient-centred medication review 84, 87
pelvic floor muscles 188–9, 196
penile sheaths 190
perforated ear drum 26
permanent vegetative state 51
persistent pain 218–20, *219*
person-centred care 4, 16–17, *17*
person-centred planning 164
personalized care plans 101, *102*
phobias 148
physical abuse 14
physical activity
in preventing falls 78–9, *79*
in relation to obesity 173
physical care, for people with dementia 144–5
physical examination, of people with incontinence 194
physiological effects of ageing *125*
pneumonia, community-acquired 136
policy 11, 59–60
polypharmacy 163, 225–7
postural management *79*, 163
preregistration nursing curricula 4
presbyacusis 27
Pretty case 52
prevention measures
for dementia 145
for falls 75–6, 78–80, *79*
for healthcare-associated infections 209–10
for osteoporosis 77
primary care *see* community care services
primary care trusts (PCTs) 61
Princess Royal Trust for Carers, The 61, 63
privacy, as EoC benchmark 17, *18*
Protection of Vulnerable Adults (PoVA) 15, 118
protective clothing 208–9
psychological abuse 14
psychological support
for people with sight loss 36
for stroke sufferers 131
psychosocial impact of illness 28, 124–6
Purdy case 51–2

R

rectal examination, digital 187, 194
rectum 193–6, *193*
religion 10, 252–3, *253*
reservoir (source of infection) 204
respiratory conditions 135–6
rheumatoid arthritis 137
risk assessments for falls 70–4, *71–4*
routine, importance in promoting sleep 238, 240
Royal College of Nursing (RCN)
on dignity 12
example of nursing care plan *104–5*
on incontinence 195
on resuscitation 50
on sleep 236
Royal National Institute for the Blind (RNIB)
on communication and psychological support 36
manual alphabet *37–8*
statistics 33, 34
Royal National Institute for the Deaf (RNID) 24, 27

S

safety at home, in relation to falls 75–6
schizophrenia 149–50
self-care 98–101, *99*
service delivery models 113–14
sexual abuse 15
sexuality 10, 56
sight loss 4–5, 23, 33, *33*
common causes of 33–5
eyesight, looking after 75
supporting people with 35–40, *37–8*
what it feels like 40
single assessment process (SAP) 87, 103–5, *104–5*

single householders 5, 55–6
sip feeds 178–9, *179*
skin care and incontinence 191
sleep and rest 7, 234–5
  actions to promote sleep 240–1
  addressing underlying health issues 238–9
  assessments 239–40
  changes to sleep patterns 235–6
  empowerment 241
  evidence base and best practice 236–7
  factors affected by and affecting sleep *236*
  normal sleep patterns 235, *235*
  research into promoting sleep 237–8
social care
  policy 11, 59–60
  provision 46
  sectors, interface with health care sectors 119
social isolation 56–7
social role inventory 125–6
somatoform disorders 149
specialist services for people with learning disabilities 164–5
spectacles, care of 75
spirituality 10, 252–3, *253*
stereotypes 10
stools 194, *198*
stress incontinence 186, 188–9
strokes 35, 59–60, 129–31
suicide 147–8
  assisted 51–2
surgery
  for anal sphincter and lower rectum disorders 195
  for incontinence 189
systematic approach to care delivery 114–15, *114*

T

tele-care and tele-health 76, 101
texture of food and drinks 179
tinnitus 27
toileting *see* elimination and continence
tort 45
Transforming Community Services 98, 107
transient ischaemic attack (TIA) 35, 59–60, 129–31
treatment, withdrawal of 51
trust, as concept central to person-centred care 16

U

UK Council of Deafness (UKCoD) 27
UN Convention on the Rights of Disabled People 155–6
urethral bulking agents 189
urgency incontinence 186, 189–90
urinary incontinence
  assessments 191–3, *192–3*
  causes and types 186–7
  investigations into cause 187–8
  normal elimination and the ageing process 185–6
  and skin care 191
urinary tract *186*
urine testing 187

V

vaginal cones 189
vaginal examination 188
values 4, 10, 13
  of NHS 11
  of nurse 250
Valuing People 155–6
Vetting and Barring Scheme 15
visual disturbance 35
vulnerable adult, definition 14
  see also elder abuse

W

withdrawal of treatment 51
workforce, skilled 118
World Health Organization (WHO)
  on 'active ageing' 123–4
  on ages at which death and illness occur 245, 254
  analgesic ladder *226*
  hand hygiene 206, 208
  on palliative care 246